HISTORIES OF HEALTH IN SOUTHEAST ASIA

HISTORIES OF HEALTH
IN SOUTHEAST ASIA

Perspectives on the Long Twentieth Century

Edited by Tim Harper and Sunil S. Amrith

Indiana University Press

Bloomington & Indianapolis

This book is a publication of

Indiana University Press
Office of Scholarly Publishing
Herman B Wells Library 350
1320 East 10th Street
Bloomington, Indiana 47405 USA

iupress.indiana.edu

Telephone orders   800-842-6796
Fax orders   812-855-7931

♾ The paper used in this publication meets the minimum requirements of the American National Standard for Information Sciences—Permanence of Paper for Printed Library Materials, ANSI Z39.48-1992.

Manufactured in the United States of America

Library of Congress Cataloging-in-Publication Data

Histories of health in Southeast Asia : perspectives on the long twentieth century / edited by Tim Harper and Sunil S. Amrith.
    p. ; cm. — (Philanthropic and nonprofit studies)
    Includes bibliographical references and index.
    ISBN 978-0-253-01486-3 (cl : alk. paper) — ISBN 978-0-253-01491-7 (pb : alk. paper) — ISBN 978-0-253-01495-5 (eb)
    I. Harper, T. N. (Timothy Norman)- editor. II. Amrith, Sunil S.- editor. III. Series: Philanthropic and nonprofit studies.
    [DNLM: 1. History of Medicine—Asia, Southeastern.
  2. History, 20th Century—Asia, Southeastern. WZ 70 JA25]
    RA541.S68
    362.10959′0904—dc23
                                                            2014022237

1 2 3 4 5   19 18 17 16 15 14

Contents

Acknowledgments

THE EDITORS WOULD like to thank the China Medical Board for its generous support of this volume, which is published in connection with the CMB's hundredth anniversary. This volume owes its existence, in particular, to the vision and initiative of Dr. Lincoln Chen, who has encouraged us in this endeavor from the start. At the China Medical Board, we would also like to thank Jennifer Ryan, whose support has been vital to us throughout the process of preparing the volume for publication, and CMB board member Harvey Fineberg. Mary Wilson, who is a contributor to this volume, also participated in these early planning sessions. We are grateful to the editors of the companion volume on the history of health in China—Mary Bullock and Bridie Andrews—for many helpful conversations.

The project from which this volume arises has been based at the Joint Centre for History and Economics, which hosted the initial workshop from which the volume developed, and the Centre has supported the development of this book in countless ways since then. The editors are especially grateful to the Centre's director, Emma Rothschild, and to Inga Huld Markan, for their untiring support of our work. We would also like to thank Amy Price for her work designing and maintaining the project's website.

The discussions at the 2011 Cambridge workshop that launched this book project were greatly enriched by the participation of Seema Alavi, Komatra Chuengsatiansup, Bambang Purwanto, and Amartya Sen. A second workshop, held in Yogyakarta in July 2012, brought together most of the contributors to this volume in a discussion of draft chapters. We are deeply grateful to Professor Bambang Purwanto and to the Universitas Gajah Mada; they were most generous hosts, and they provided an atmosphere for productive conversations.

The development of the volume for publication was aided by Kirsty Walker's superb editorial work on the chapters. We are grateful, too, to Sandy Aitken for her work on the index, and to Mary-Rose Cheadle for her role in liaising with the authors and arranging copyright permissions.

Alongside the publication of this volume, a key outcome of the CMB-supported project on Transnational Histories of Health in Southeast Asia was a two-week summer school held in Cambridge in July 2013, bringing together six outstanding young scholars from Southeast Asia—Jeffrey Acaba, Vivek Neelakantan, Heong Hong Por, Ravando, Sreytouch Vong, and Patricia Wong. One of them, Vivek Neelakantan, has contributed to this volume; we are confident that the others will make their mark in the field as their projects develop. The editors learned a great deal from their work. In connection with the summer school, we are particularly grateful to Lily Chang for her energy and initiative in organizing it. Her efforts were crucial to its success. We would also like to thank Professor Loh Wei Leng (another of our contributors) for her inspiring role in making the summer school a success.

Last but not least, we would like to thank Indiana University Press for the speed and efficiency with which they have brought this book to press. The volume as a whole benefited from the detailed critical comments of the anonymous reader for the Press.

HISTORIES OF HEALTH
IN SOUTHEAST ASIA

Introduction

Sunil S. Amrith and Tim Harper

In 1914, THE life expectancy of an average Indonesian man was under thirty-five years. On the rubber plantations of Perak, in Malaysia, the death rate among Tamil migrant workers was over 85 per 1,000. The health of Southeast Asia's people, the distribution of its population, and the region's ecology had all been transformed by decades of tumultuous change. The map of Southeast Asia had been redrawn by imperial conquest and competition; the balance of its population has been altered by some of the largest migrations in modern history; its forest frontier was breached by new forms of commodity production. Its cities and towns were in intellectual ferment as Southeast Asia entered its "age in motion." The outbreak of World War I intensified the contradictory forces that would shape the health and well-being of Southeast Asia's peoples in the twentieth century. The war catalyzed political conflicts that would last for decades: through them, the lives of millions of Southeast Asians would be affected by warfare and epidemics, mass displacement, and natural disasters.[1]

Yet it also marked a threshold in the development of modern medicine and public health in the region—in connection with parallel developments in South Asia and East Asia. The China Medical Board was founded in 1914, the first in a series of initiatives to bring American-style public health education to Asia. Over the next three decades, the Rockefeller Foundation would take its experiments in public health to the Philippines and Indonesia, Sri Lanka, and Thailand. Dutch, French, and British colonial states embarked on the gradual expansion of their medical facilities, as did the independent kingdom of Siam—hospital treatment, medicalized childbirth, pharmaceutical advertising, and rural health centers entered the life experience of a larger—although still limited—number of people. Southeast Asian health workers and doctors emerged as key players in international debates, however unequal the terms of the discussion. And indigenous medical practitioners across the region adapted to new circumstances with ingenuity and eclecticism.

Health patterns in Southeast Asia have changed in profound respects over the past century. In 2014, Southeast Asia is a microcosm of global health. The health of its peoples has improved in dramatic ways, thanks to a combination of medical intervention, rapid economic development, political activism, and long-term demographic change. Nevertheless, widespread inequalities remain both within individual countries and across the region: inequalities in life expectancy, inequalities in access to healthcare, inequalities in treatment outcomes. Southeast Asia's ecological diversity and its rapid growth have combined to make it a hotbed of new and emerging infectious diseases, even as it suffers from an epidemic rise in non-communicable chronic disease. Natural disasters have always been a particular threat to health in Southeast Asia: there are strong indications that both their intensity and their effects have worsened in recent years, and stand to become more severe with accelerating climate change.

The chapters in this volume reflect on a century of change from a range of disciplinary perspectives: its contributors include social historians and cultural anthropologists, a political scientist, and an epidemiologist. The history of medicine in Southeast Asia is a vibrant and growing field of research, and contributors to this volume have been among its most active participants. Since the 1990s, important monographs have appeared on individual countries within the region, along with a handful of collective volumes on the region as a whole.[2] The field has been institutionalized through the work of institutions such as the group on the History of Medicine in Southeast Asia (HOMSEA), which has hosted a series of important conferences and overseen the recent publication of an important collection of essays.[3]

Recent historical scholarship has focused on medical encounters in the colonial period, informed by the tools of cultural history and critical theory. A number of the contributors to this volume—Au, Komatra, Walker, and Loh Kah Seng in particular—develop these perspectives, and they reinforce the finding that medicine was a field of negotiation between colonial and indigenous epistemologies; they show that colonial hegemony over healing was never complete, and that the peoples of the region negotiated between biomedicine and an eclectic range of indigenous practices drawn from across Asia. Taken as a whole, however, this volume is not a history of medicine in Southeast Asia. Rather, it examines the social, cultural, demographic, and political dimensions of health in the widest possible sense. As such, the chapters herein engage with many other fields of scholarship that have a distinguished pedigree in Southeast Asian studies, including demography, epidemiology, and public policy. The chapters intercut deeply local perspectives with a comparative and connected view of the region as a whole: some are single-country studies, others are transnational in approach. Taken together, they provide new insights on both the underlying structures and the urgent crises shaping health and welfare in Southeast Asia.

Southeast Asia in the Longue Durée

The approach advertised is "transnational." The term can be overused such as to lose its meaning or become merely a gesture to the global context. But in a vital sense, as a crossroads of migrations, cultures, ideas, and social practices, the experience of Southeast Asia has always been transnational. Few inhabitants of the region think of themselves as "Southeast Asian." Few scholars in the region write on a Southeast Asian scale. For most, the framework in which people conduct their lives is more local; the larger politics that matters is national. "Southeast Asia" is itself a Cold War construct, first used in a concrete political sense with the formation of the South East Asia Command by the Allies in 1943, as a theater of war.[4] Often smaller regions are more of a factor than the idea of Southeast Asia: such as the Malay World, or "sea of Melayu," and the "Sulu Zone." Many of these geographies can only be understood when connected to entities beyond the region, such as the Bay of Bengal, the wider Indian Ocean, South China, or looking inland to the uplands of "Zomia." Disease, of course, despite the best efforts of state epidemiologists, is no respecter of geographical boundaries. The health institutions that have played a major role in the region—not least the China Medical Board itself—have had a broader geographical remit. Although an early generation of scholars placed an emphasis in finding unities within the diversity of the Southeast Asia experience, more recently scholars have questioned the usefulness of this, even arguing that scholars should dispense with the term altogether.[5]

We have not gone so far. We acknowledge that Southeast Asia—not least through ASEAN's experience and continuing demands on the circulation of professionals through policies such as the ASEAN Economic Community—has been important to the health experience of the region and will remain so in the future. From the outset of the project, we encouraged our authors to write on a Southeast Asian scale. But we have also recognized the importance of nuanced local case studies. And we have also sought to stress internal and external interconnections. Southeast Asia—the Southeast Asian experience—is perhaps best understood as a set of regions that segue into one another, a set of horizons. We, following the example of Denys Lombard, have sought to identify "networks and synchronisms" across and beyond the region.[6]

Several themes stand out over the longer duration. One is the dynamism of the worlds of traditional health. These have always been syncretic, eclectic, sophisticated, and, above all, highly transnational. There was a cosmopolitan market in traditional medicines from the earliest times, and a significant long-distance circulation of specialist healers. The impact of colonial rule, from as early as the sixteenth century, did great violence to local therapeutic systems. This has been traced in the confrontation between animistic priestesses and the

Spanish authorities in the Philippines from the 1520s through to the seventeenth century. The repercussions of this were long term and diverse. The nature of traditional medicine began to change; for example, in the Philippines and elsewhere, religious hierarchies became more patriarchal as the healing functions of women were undermined.[7] In one sense, this was one of the first crises of health in an early globalizing age. But, overall, the picture has been of the persistent adaptability of traditional therapeutic systems into the modern period. In part, this was because colonial authorities were not uniformly hostile to it. As Atsuko Naono's chapter shows, at certain periods colonial officials could invest in it through a desire to unify health provision, and fall back on it in times of crisis. But, more importantly, it was the center of creative initiatives, of the kind outlined by Nopphanat Anuphongphat and Komatra Chuengsatiansup in their chapter on Thailand.

The short feature by Sokhieng Au, distilled from her outstanding book on traditional medicine in Cambodia, shows how so-called traditional medicine has been constructed as a field, complementary to Western systems. In Cambodia, the creation of a National Center for Traditional Medicine was funded by the Nippon Foundation in cooperation with the Cambodian Ministry of Health, in an initiative that was in line with the 2008 World Health Organization Beijing Declaration on Traditional Medicine. Traditional medicine remains a multinational enterprise; indeed one could argue that the sector—in the form of Aw Boon Haw's patented "Tiger Balm" remedy from the 1920s—pioneered overseas Chinese enterprises' adoption of Western business methods, notably advertising. Tiger Balm also shows how the consumption of Chinese medicine, or any kind of local medicinal product, transcended any one specific ethnic group.[8]

A second theme is that this is a world of constant movement, and the experience of migrants has been at the forefront of health history and health-care interventions in the modern period. Colonial medicine was pioneered by the need to control the health of mobile groups, particularly its own soldiers, not least in stemming the spread of sexually transmitted diseases.[9] As Warwick Anderson's study of American medicine in the Philippines shows, military logic precipitated many early public health measures in an urban context, and military men formed the core of a new civil force of sanitary inspectors.[10] Rural health measures, slow to emerge across Southeast Asia, followed the establishment of European plantations, and privileged their workforces at the expense of other rural people. Equally, the health of migrant peoples was also important to Asian initiatives. Health issues loomed large in the political life of the Chinese diaspora. Many of its leading figures in the early twentieth century—Sun Yat-sen, Wu Lien-teh, Lim Boon Keng—were medical men. Health, as the companion volume in this series shows, was central to philanthropic activity. It was also central to the political mobilization of the Chinese overseas, for example the fund-raising campaigns for China medical relief led by Tan Kah Kee, acquired, by the 1920s, an unprecedented mass dimension. In a similar way, by the 1930s, medical "missions" to Indians overseas in Malaya and elsewhere were central to Indian nationalists' engagement with the world outside the subcontinent.

This collection begins 1914, at a moment when the European conquest of the region was complete, and in a period of consolidation—of what the Burma civil servant J. S. Furnivall termed "the fashioning of Leviathan." It was an area of censuses, taxation, irrigation, and cadastral surveys. With it came the slow and partial extension of colonial education and welfare policy, of which the Ethical Policy in the Netherlands East Indies after 1901 was the most ambitious expression. The one territory outside formal Western control, Thailand, was undergoing not dissimilar processes of modernization and institutional reform. The improvement of local health was central to colonial visions of modernization. It has long been argued by historians that colonial health care provision was driven less by humanitarian concerns than the need to discipline Asian populations; to bolster the legitimacy of the colonial presence, where it was conspicuously lacking; that "ethical" interventions were motivated by the need to create more productive and efficient labor forces.[11] Debates on the health of Asian laborers were at the time, and remain for historians, at the heart of discussions on the moral culpability of Western imperialism in the region.[12] Yet this should not obscure the diversity of health initiatives and agendas in the colonial period, whether seen in medical research institutes, missionary work, philanthropic bodies such as the Rockefeller Foundation, or, as the chapter by Sunil Amrith discusses, in new international organizations. All of these were dependent on Southeast Asian involvement and initiative. The health of the body politic was, as Rachel Leow's chapter shows, central to the visions for national progress embraced by a new generation of Southeast Asian political leaders.

Health, War, and Crisis

A recurrent theme in these chapters is the relationship between health and crisis. The scale of disruptive change in modern Southeast Asia has provoked recurrent crises of subsistence, reproduction, and social cohesion. In Southeast Asia, as elsewhere in the world, a rise in the destructive power of warfare has been responsible for some of the most profound shocks to population health: the most dramatic spikes in mortality and morbidity have taken place during or immediately after periods of armed conflict. The vast increase in the speed and scale of transport and communications from the nineteenth century had profound effects on Southeast Asia's cultural and intellectual history—but also hastened the spread of epidemic disease. Episodes of crisis loom large in Southeast Asians' experience of illness; they have left their imprint on social memory. The chapters here are attentive to the texture of experience: Kirsty Walker's use of oral testimony; Eric Tagliacozzo's excavation of medical memoirs rich with detail; Greg Bankoff's attention to the role of religious ideas, including Buddhist meditation, in local responses to catastrophe.

Eric Tagliacozzo's chapter foreshadows many of the themes of the volume by focusing on the nexus between pilgrimage, globalization, and epidemic disease in the second half of the nineteenth century. The Hajj, one of the oldest regular movements of people over long distances, was transformed in the nineteenth century by the global revolution in transportation and communications. Larger numbers of Southeast Asian Muslims than ever before made the pilgrimage to Mecca, a large number of them from the Indonesian archipelago under Dutch colonial rule. Tagliacozzo shows that cholera was a constant threat accompanying the pilgrimage as it grew in scale. The threat of contagion provoked various efforts at inter-imperial and international cooperation to survey and regulate Hajj shipping; the quarantine station at Kamaran Island emerged as the front line in attempts to sanitize the Hajj. Epidemiological surveillance, improved water supplies, and medical intervention combined to reduce the threat of epidemics by the turn of the twentieth century. Yet these interventions also paved the way for greater imperial control over the mobility of Muslim subjects, motivated by political as much as by epidemiological concerns.

World War I revealed, more brutally, the propensity of technology to provoke crises in health. The war of 1914–18 played a more significant role in modern Southeast Asian history than most historians have recognized—the influenza pandemic of 1918 revealed the full extent of social, economic, and ecological disruption that the war had brought.[13] Kirsty Walker's moving chapter on the social history of the influenza epidemic shows the extent of devastation that it brought. Recent estimates of mortality suggest that in the Dutch East Indies alone, 1.5 million people died, together with around 35,000 in Malaya, and 85,000 in the Philippines. Walker shows that the pandemic's impact has been underestimated, and its social and cultural reverberations misunderstood. The influenza epidemic highlighted the fragile hold of colonial medicine—biomedicine offered few solutions to influenza; modern medical facilities were overstrained, and very often associated not with cure but with death. Walker shows that Southeast Asian victims of the pandemic turned to the whole range of healing practices—biomedical, indigenous, Ayurvedic, and Chinese—rooted in the region's history.

In its impact on mortality, morbidity, and the development of health systems in Southeast Asia, World War II was even more pivotal. The Japanese invasion of Southeast Asia from December 1941 precipitated a massive social crisis, the displacement of population—often into various forms of forced labor—which brought in its wake a resurgence of outbreaks of typhoid and cholera. The breakdown of regional systems for the distribution of rice and other foodstuffs left a long legacy of chronic malnutrition.[14] In many places, local mechanisms of disease control collapsed. But once the convulsions of the initial fighting had eased, this was also a time Southeast Asian medical practitioners came to the fore, freed from the professional hierarchies that dominated colonial health services. As the supply of imported medicines dried up, medical research was undertaken into locally sourced alternatives. A memoir of a doctor in Malaya's industrial Kinta Valley not untypically recounts how antimalarial measures were continued with rubber oil, vaccinations with resharpened needles, and how—after reading of the example of Victor G. Heiser of the Rockefeller Foundation in the Philippines—he began to educate his staff in preventative medicine.[15]

Throughout the second half of the twentieth century warfare remained a cause of premature death and widespread morbidity. The bleak succession of Cold War–era conflicts and "dirty wars" in Southeast Asia since 1945 had a devastating impact. Sexually transmitted diseases, disability, and mental trauma loom large among the health consequences of war. The environmental impact of jungle warfare, epitomized by the use of chemical defoliants during the Malayan Emergency and then by U.S. forces in Vietnam and Laos, had long-term effects both on population health and on local ecology and biodiversity. In Malaya, the counterinsurgency program of resettlement of the rural Chinese into "New Villages" had deleterious health effects on the upwards of 570,000 people "resettled" and 650,000 "regrouped." But it also necessitated the provision of aftercare, not only by the colonial state, but by Chinese political parties, Christian missions, and other bodies. This focus on the rural Chinese generated further political pressures for the more general extension of rural health care to the Malays, seen as mostly "loyal" to the Malayan government. The opening up of the interior of the Malay peninsula drawing the campaign aided this; for example, the spraying of malarial areas with DDT was an offshoot of resettlement. But this could equally lead to very uneven provision. In 1956, 40 percent of the rural people protected from malaria lived on the strategically central rubber estates, and the "malaria barrier" was the greatest impediment to rural development elsewhere.[16] It is striking how states of emergency are a backdrop to some of the most important events in health history in the mid-twentieth century. The command structures of counterinsurgency underpinned the development approach of postcolonial Malaya under its "father of development," Abdul Razak Hussein. A similar rhetoric of crisis and emergency was a feature of Singapore's great experiment in rehousing virtually all of its citizens.[17]

The most frequent, recurring crises in modern Southeast Asia, however, have been natural disasters. Greg Bankoff's chapter shows that Southeast Asia has been particularly and acutely vulnerable to natural disasters, experiencing a "disproportionate number of hazards per unit of surface area." Bankoff suggests that Southeast Asia has become more vulnerable to disasters over time, accounting for a rising proportion of deaths worldwide from natural disasters. Storms and floods have been responsible for the largest number of crises, followed by volcanic eruptions, and climatic events influenced by the El Niño Southern Oscillation. Scientists predict that the impact of climate change on Southeast Asia will increase the number of extreme weather events, increasing the region's vulnerability to catastrophic disaster. One consequence of this vulnerability, Bankoff shows, is that Southeast Asia has been a key testing ground for the development of the field of disaster medicine since the 1980s. Although health has not traditionally been high on its list of concerns, the effectiveness of ASEAN's interventions to provide relief after the Indian Ocean tsunami of 2004, and cyclone Nargis in Myanmar in 2008, suggest that this regional institution might yet play a greater role in Southeast Asia's response to the threat of natural disasters.

Perhaps the most striking insight of Bankoff's chapter is that, in the experience of most Southeast Asians, disasters are not so much exceptional crises as so-called normal hazards of everyday life. He cites an estimate that no fewer than 80 percent of the region's inhabitants have experienced directly trauma related to natural hazards. In their responses to this threat, too, Bankoff argues that Southeast Asia's peoples have drawn on a wide range of moral and spiritual resources, of which the practice of disaster medicine and the psychiatric treatment of post-traumatic stress disorder are only two elements—that is to say, Southeast Asia's resilience in the face of natural hazards owes something to its long history of religious and cultural exchange.

Uneven Transitions

However large crisis looms in communities' experiences and memories, a demographic perspective tells a different kind of story: a story of gradually and then dramatically reduced mortality, increased longevity, and changing population structure. A key tension that runs through the book emerges from the juxtaposition of social and demographic history: from that tension, many of the contradictions underlying the history of health in modern Southeast Asia emerge. Southeast Asia's transitions are fractured by widespread inequalities. Although life expectancy has increased across the region, it remains widely variable: from eighty-one years in Singapore, to just fifty-six in Myanmar. Many of these inequalities are rooted in Southeast Asia's political, cultural, and environmental past.

Peter Boomgaard's chapter shows that, at the broadest level of analysis, Southeast Asia has undergone a demographic transition in the second half of the twentieth century. Although Southeast Asia has historically been a region of very low population growth, Boomgaard shows that the nineteenth century saw a modest increase of population in Southeast Asia (a rate of nearly 1 percent), brought about by a combination of a slight decrease in mortality possibly combined with a rise in fertility. This was followed—between 1930 and 1960—by a more rapid population growth (nearly 2 percent), notwithstanding the cataclysm of World War II. This was followed by a period of very rapid population growth between 1960 and 1990: mortality fell rapidly, and fertility remained at its previous high levels. Fertility then dropped—a trend that began in Singapore, Malaysia, and Thailand, and then spread throughout the region. Spurred by the antibiotic revolution and mass vaccination, by economic development, and by the social change precipitated by industrialization and urbanization, death rates fell rapidly in postcolonial Southeast Asia. Those same social pressures encouraged later marriage and birth control by the 1970s—after 1990, the effects of this drop in fertility produced a slowdown in population growth that was as dramatic as its increase in the 1960s and 1970s. Average life expectancy in Southeast Asia rose from 42.4 years in 1950–55 to 68.0 years in 2000–5, though beneath these figures are wide inequalities across and between countries.

Over these years of demographic transition, rapid urbanization has transformed Southeast Asian society. Nearly half of Southeast Asia's population (43 percent) lives in urban areas today, although this average masks great intercountry variation, from 100 percent in Singapore to just 15 percent in Laos.[18] As Atsuko Naono's chapter shows, this had led to a shifting relationship between urban and rural health. "Rural" Southeast Asia, Naono shows, has usually been defined externally, and the perception of rural areas has changed over time. In the colonial period, curative medical facilities were heavily concentrated in urban areas. As chapters by both Naono and Amrith show, in the 1920s and 1930s, greater attention was paid to rural health: the League of Nations and the Rockefeller Foundation embarked on a series of experiments in rural hygiene and sanitation, supported by numerous indigenous initiatives—initially reluctant colonial states, too, began to invest more in rural health.

Naono shows that this began to shift after independence. The expansion of health services to rural areas became a common priority for Southeast Asian states with very different ideological complexions. She concludes that in the contemporary era, rural Southeast Asia is perhaps better served in terms of health coverage than the urban periphery. Geographer Jonathan Rigg makes a similar observation: urban poverty in contemporary Southeast Asia is much less understood than rural poverty.[19] This suggests that much work remains to be done on the health, and the healing practices, of Southeast Asia's urban poor. The pioneering work of James Warren and others in the 1980s would merit extension—Loh Kah Seng takes up the challenge in his contribution to this volume, and in his recent book.[20] At the same time, Alberto Gomes's chapter draws our attention to groups who have borne the heaviest cost of the transformation of Southeast Asia's rural landscapes—its forest peoples. Gomes shows that the Menraq of Malaysia have been displaced by a process of land clearance for economic development, state-directed policies of integration and resettlement, and cultural exclusion.

He highlights the toll this has taken in terms of malnutrition, illness, and high mortality.

Among the most fundamental effects of Southeast Asia's demographic transition, as Theresa W. Devasahayam's chapter shows, is an aging population. Increased longevity combined with declining fertility means that an increasing proportion of Southeast Asia's population is over the age of sixty. Devasahayam shows that this demographic shift has significant political (and indeed ethical) implications, particularly where it comes to provision of health and social care. Traditionally, families have been responsible for provision of care to the elderly in Southeast Asia; Devasahayam argues that common fears about the decline of family responsibility in the region have been overstated. Families remain the crucial source of care for the elderly; but Devasahayam shows that these intergenerational transfers do not work in only one direction. There has been a rise in financial transfers between grandparents and grandchildren (often to pay for grandchildren's education); as migration increases, the proportion of children raised by their grandparents across Southeast Asia is on the increase, particularly in rural areas and in countries of emigration, such as the Philippines.[21] More specifically, in the field of health, Devasahayam cites evidence from Thailand that parents, and mothers in particular, have taken primary responsibility for the care of adult children suffering from HIV/AIDS. Nevertheless, Devasahayam concludes that population aging is likely to require a more concerted response from Southeast Asia's states, and a greater public role in care for the elderly.

Aging and urbanization are among the forces shaping the most fundamental epidemiological shift in Southeast Asia's recent history: the rising toll of non-communicable, chronic diseases. Historical research on chronic disease in Southeast Asia remains in its infancy, and this subject is undoubtedly a gap in the present volume's coverage. Recent figures suggest that chronic non-communicable diseases are responsible for 60 percent of deaths in Southeast Asia: heart disease, stroke, cancers, and chronic lung disease are on the rise. Risk factors include rapid urbanization and its effect on diet and lifestyle; a lack of public health provision and early detection among poorer communities; and unhealthy patterns of consumption, epitomized by high levels of tobacco use.[22] Loh Wei Leng's chapter provides a long view on the history of the tobacco industry in Southeast Asia. The obstacles in the way of reining in tobacco use have deep roots in the close nexus between states and producers, in the financial benefits of tobacco use in terms of tax revenues, and in the power of the tobacco industry and its lobbyists. Pointing to the alarming rise in smoking among teenagers and particularly young women, Loh shows that tobacco companies have been skilled at using new social media and cultivating new cultures of consumption—at great cost to public health.

Southeast Asia's multiple health transitions are clearly delineated, yet they remain uneven. As Mary Wilson's chapter points out, epidemic disease remains a vital—even a growing—threat to Southeast Asia's health, even as chronic diseases exert the greatest toll in terms of mortality. Wilson shows that Southeast Asia is a hotbed of emerging infectious diseases. The region's tropical ecology, its population density, and its population mobility (the last of these deeply rooted in the region's history) have all made Southeast Asia vulnerable to epidemics. Outlining the challenge of infectious disease control in the region, Wilson highlights the impact of the 2003 SARS epidemic in Southeast Asia, the recent rise in dengue infections, the ever-present threat of avian influenza, the enduring impact of malaria, and the rise of drug-resistant strains of common infectious diseases: including artemisinin-resistant *Plasmodium falciparum*. Among the health-related effects of climate change, many epidemiologists fear an increase in vector-borne and water-borne disease transmission in Southeast Asia.[23]

The Politics of Health

Ideas about health and illness, debates about health policy, interventions to improve population health—these have all been linked inextricably with the larger political transformations of modern Southeast Asian history. The third major theme of the volume, then, concerns the politics of health in Southeast Asia.

Loh Kah Seng's chapter provides a nuanced view of the relationship between health care—hospitals and asylums in particular—and colonial power. In the process, he establishes new directions for the historiographical debate on colonialism and health in Southeast Asia. Loh highlights the two countervailing positions in the debate—the notion that colonial health provision was marked by its absence and parsimony; and the contrary view, that they were "total institutions." Acknowledging the many ways in which leprosaria indeed functioned as a "tool of empire," as well as the limits in their reach and their resources, Loh moves toward a more complex view: he shows that leprosaria were contested sites of social experiment and social engineering, and that patients found a margin of freedom to shape their own experiences of confinement.

As Loh points out, "the postcolonial states of Southeast Asia retained the focus on hospitals and curative medicine that was a hallmark of Western colonial practice." Many of the book's chapters show the centrality of health interventions to the ambitions of Southeast Asia's independent states. Naono shows that rural health missions formed part of an enthusiasm for development—and an association of rural areas with backwardness—that most of Southeast Asia's states embraced in the postcolonial era. Vivek Neelakantan's short feature on the eradication of smallpox in Indonesia reinforces this point: the internationally coordinated campaigns for the eradication of the "Big Four" infectious diseases relied, to a large extent, on the political enthusiasm of Asian states, and the agency and initiative of local health workers.[24]

Rachel Leow's chapter situates the place of health in the context of intellectual history. Beginning with the observation that medical doctors were represented disproportionately among the ranks of Southeast Asia's nationalist leaders, Leow argues that medical metaphors and medical analogies have shaped political discourse in the region in striking ways. Although such political metaphors as social "cancers" and the "cleansing" of the body politic are by no means confined to Southeast Asia, Leow shows that they have assumed particular inflections in a context where the problem of racial and ethnic diversity has been integral to political debate. The second part of her chapter engages in an illuminating contrast between two very different medical doctors representing countervailing strands of modern Malaysian politics. Malaysia's longest-serving prime minister, Dr. Mahathir Mohamad, was a biomedical doctor whose political ideology owed much to a rigid scientific modernism, that included a strong belief in eugenics. Leow contrasts Mahathir's intellectual background with that of Burhannudin al-Helmy, a homeopath trained in Delhi, whose religiously infused Malay nationalism was more flexible and more open to difference than Mahathir's rigid, statist vision. She concludes, provocatively, that "religion, spirituality and so-called 'unscientific' resources are frequently an unremarked idiom of social organization, national regeneration and critical thought." Debates on health in modern Southeast Asia, that is to say, are related intimately to visions of social cohesion, and in particular to debates about incorporating and managing cultural and ethnic diversity within the social and political body.

Moving into the last quarter of the twentieth century, Teresa Encarnacion Tadem's chapter examines the rise of health activism in the Philippines since the 1970s. She argues that non-governmental organization committed to "health for the poor"—an ambiguous and often contested notion—had complex political affiliations and multiple origins: from the revolutionary left, committed to armed struggle, to the activist networks of the Catholic Church. The lack of access to health care by poor and rural populations became a cause to rally opposition to the Marcos regime, and to mount a broader critique of social and economic inequality. Yet Tadem shows that tensions began to divide the Philippines' health activists: one fault line was distinctive to the Philippines—the Catholic Church's implacable opposition to women's reproductive health measures. Across the region, however, health activists have confronted the dilemmas of their Filipino counterparts where it came to the question of whether to accept office, and how far to work with the state.

Although Tadem's chapter focuses entirely on the Philippines, it paves the way for a wider comparative and connected history of nongovernmental activism for health in Southeast Asia: this is a promising area for future work. In many other countries in the region, health-related activism is linked to wider struggles for human rights and against social and economic inequality. The Interfaith Youth Coalition on AIDS in Myanmar (IYCA-Myanmar) has played an important role not only in raising awareness about HIV/AIDS, but also as a voice for peace in the aftermath of the anti-Muslim violence that swept the country in 2012 and 2013.[25] There are numerous other groups in Thailand, Malaysia, Singapore, and Indonesia that have fulfilled a similar role, each in a different political context. Historians could trace multiple genealogies for civil society involvement in health across Southeast Asia—in the long tradition of medical provision and philanthropy by Southeast Asia's Chinese, in the growing and self-conscious intervention of civil society groups in the public sphere from the early twentieth century, and in traditions of political radicalism and localist alternatives to state provision of services.[26]

There is one further political and economic transition underway across Southeast Asia—and it is mentioned only briefly in this volume: the growing privatization of health care. Even prior to the colonial era, private actors and private philanthropy played a leading role in the provision of healing to different sections of Southeast Asian society: the fluid world of itinerant doctors trained in multiple indigenous traditions was, in its own way, highly commercialized. The immediate postcolonial period saw a turn toward state provision, particularly in the field of preventive health: as we have seen, improvements in population health were an aim of nation builders' ambitions and an index of their attainment. Since the 1980s, in consonance with global trends, the private sector has increasingly penetrated public hospitals; the often unregulated world of private clinics and hospitals has burgeoned into a huge industry.

One recent study—part of a special issue of *The Lancet* on health in contemporary Southeast Asia—concludes that "the region is . . . unique, however, with respect to the rapid growth of trade in health services, including migration of health personnel and medical tourism."[27] The region has witnessed a significant migration of health and medical personnel—doctors, nurses, technicians, care workers: the Philippines is the largest source country, and Singapore the greatest magnet.[28]

These movements—linked in complex ways to Southeast Asia's long history of cross-border migration—are both a force of regional integration, and a source of regional inequality. The politics of health in Southeast Asia is, more than ever, bound up with the politics of migration: their relationship will continue to provoke debate.

Despite the growing role of for-profit private provision, access to healthcare remains a central element in debates over citizenship and state responsibility in Southeast Asia—arguably more so than it is in neighboring regions. Whereas in India, there has been a striking absence of public discussion of health, this has not been true in Southeast Asia. In recent years, the region is a site for interventions that have been watched keenly by global policy makers—including Thailand's move towards universal coverage, and Vietnam's innovative health fund. It seems likely that public provision of health services will continue to form an important element of states' legitimacy in the region. The conclusion to Loh Kah Seng's chapter is worth citing, for it is applicable far beyond Singapore and Malaysia:

> As healthcare decisions are increasingly overlaid by questions about how and how much Southeast Asians should organize their adult lives—to work, save and pay for illness—the nexus between the international and local will be of even greater importance within the framework of the global economy of the twenty-first century.

Future Directions

The workshop at which the chapters in this volume were originally presented was part of a wider initiative, undertaken with the support of the China Medical Board, to develop the study of health history in Southeast Asia. In summer 2013, six postgraduate students from Southeast Asian universities attended a two-week summer school at the University of Cambridge to advance their research on different dimensions of the history of health in Southeast Asia. The depth and breadth of their projects—which ranged from the study of mental health in Malaysia in the 1960s to women's health education in the colonial Philippines—were a testament to how vibrant and promising a field of research the history of health is today, and how many directions remain open for further exploration.

As the contents of this volume—and, as importantly, its gaps—suggest, there are many areas that would repay further investigation: the history of mental health and mental illness; a greater attention to health policy and health inequalities in the postcolonial period. There is scope for a much closer relationship between the history of health and environmental history, which is a lively but distinct field of scholarship in Southeast Asian studies—this is an urgent need if we are to place in a longer historical context the health challenges presented by climate change. It is clear that the rise of non-communicable chronic disease is one of the most important developments in Southeast Asia's twentieth-century history, and historians have only just begun to consider this history. Finally, there are hints in the chapters in this volume of how much remains to be done to uncover new sorts of archives of health and illness in modern Southeast Asia: from patient records to oral histories, indigenous chronicles and memoirs, there are many voices that state-centric histories of medicine have done little to explore, and which await further work by historians.

Notes

1. Ralph Shlomowitz and Lance Brennan, "Mortality and Indian Labour in Malaya, 1877–1913," *Indian Economic and Social History Review* 29, no. 1 (1992): 57–75; Takashi Shiraishi, *An Age in Motion: Popular Radicalism in Java* (Ithaca, NY: Cornell University Press, 1990).

2. Warwick Anderson, *Colonial Pathologies: American Tropical Medicine, Race, and Hygiene in the Philippines* (Durham, NC: Duke University Press, 2006); Lenore Manderson, *Sickness and the State: Health and Illness in Colonial Malaya, 1870–1940* (Cambridge and Melbourne: Cambridge University Press, 2002); Norman Owen, ed., *Death and Disease in Southeast Asia* (Oxford: Oxford University Press, 1987); and Judith L. Richell, *Disease and Demography in Colonial Burma* (Singapore: National University of Singapore Press, 2006).

3. See History of Medicine in Southeast Asia website, www.fas.nus.edu.sg/hist/homsea /index.html, accessed August 1, 2013; and Laurence Monnais and Harold J. Cook, *Global Movements, Local Concerns: Medicine and Health in Southeast Asia* (Singapore: NUS Press, 2012).

4. Donald K. Emmerson, "'Southeast Asia': What's in a Name?" *Journal of Southeast Asian Studies* 15, no. 1 (1984): 1–21.

5. Willem van Schendel, "Southeast Asia: An Idea Whose Time Is Past?" *Bijdragen Tot de Taal-, Land- En Volkenkunde / Journal of the Humanities and Social Sciences of Southeast Asia* 168, no. 4 (2013): 497–510.

6. Denys Lombard, "Networks and Synchronisms in Southeast Asian History," *Journal of Southeast Asian Studies* 26, no. 1 (1995): 10–16.

7. Barbara Watson Andaya, *The Flaming Womb: Repositioning Women in Early Modern Southeast Asia* (Honolulu: University of Hawai'i Press, 2006), e.g., 95–96.

8. Sherman Cochran, *Chinese Medicine Men: Consumer Culture in China and Southeast Asia* (Cambridge, MA: Harvard University Press, 2006), 119–36.

9. For an overview, see Philippa Levine, *Prostitution, Race, and Politics : Policing Venereal Disease in the British Empire* (London: Routledge, 2003).

10. Warwick Anderson, *Colonial Pathologies*.

11. See, for example, Lenore Manderson, *Sickness and the State: Health and Illness in Colonial Malaya, 1870–1940* (Cambridge: Cambridge University Press, 1996).

12. Jan Breman, *Taming the Coolie Beast: Plantation Society and the Colonial Order in Southeast Asia* (Oxford: Oxford University Press, 1989); and J. H. Houben, "Colonial History Revisited," *Itinerario* 17, no. 1 (1993): 93–98.

13. See, for example, Kees van Dijk, *The Netherlands Indies and the Great War, 1914–1918* (Leiden: KITLV, 2007).

14. See, in particular, Paul H. Kratoska, *The Japanese Occupation of Malaya: A Social and Economic History* (Honolulu, University of Hawai'i Press, 1997).

15. T. J. Danaraj, *Memoirs of a Doctor* (Kuala Lumpur: T. J. Danaraj, 1990), 104–10.

16. T. N. Harper, *The End of Empire and the Making of Malaya* (Cambridge: Cambridge University Press, 1999), 230–31.

17. Gregory Clancey, *Toward a Spatial History of Emergency: Notes from Singapore*, ARI Working Paper Series 8 (Singapore: Asia Research Institute, 2003); Loh Kah Seng, *Squatters into Citizens: The 1961 Bukit Ho Swee Fire and the Making of Modern Singapore* (Singapore: NUS Press, 2013).

18. Jose Acuin, Rebecca Firestone, Thein Thein Htay, Geok Lin Khor, Hasbullah Thabrany, Vonthanak Saphonn, and Suwit Wibulpolprasert, "Southeast Asia: An Emerging Focus for Global Health," *Lancet* 377 (2011): 534–35.

19. Jonathan Rigg, "From Rural to Urban: A Geography of Boundary Crossing in Southeast Asia," *TRaNS: Trans-Regional and -National Studies of Southeast Asia* 1, no. 1 (2013): 5–26.

20. James F. Warren, *Rickshaw Coolie: A People's History of Singapore, 1880–1940*, 2nd. ed. (Singapore: NUS Press, 2003); Loh, *Squatters into Citizens.*

21. Rhacel S. Parrenas, *Children of Global Migration: Transnational Families and Gendered Woes* (Stanford, CA: Stanford University Press, 2005); Rigg, "From Rural to Urban."

22. Antonio Dans, Nawi Ng, Cherian Varghese, E Shyong Tai, Rebecca Firestone, and Ruth Bonita, "The Rise of Chronic Non-communicable Diseases in Southeast Asia: Time for Action," *Lancet* 337 (2011): 680–89.

23. Richard J. Coker, Benjamin M. Hunter, James W. Rudge, Marco Liverani, and Piya Hanvoravongchai, "Emerging Infectious Diseases in Southeast Asia: Regional Challenges to Control," *Lancet* 337 (2011): 599–609.

24. See also Sunil S. Amrith, *Decolonizing International Health: India and Southeast Asia, c. 1930–1965* (Basingstoke, UK: Palgrave MacMillan, 2006).

25. Physicians for Human Rights, *Patterns of Anti-Muslim Violence in Burma: A Call for Accountability and Prevention* (New York: Physicians for Human Rights, 2013), 14.

26. Cochran, *Chinese Medicine Men*; Su Lin Lewis, "Rotary International's 'Acid Test': Multi-ethnic Associational Life in 1930s Southeast Asia," *Journal of Global History* 7, no. 2 (2012), 302–24.

27. Virasakdi Chongsuvivatwong, Kai Hong Phua, Mui Teng Yap, Nicola S. Pocock, Jamal H. Hashim, Rethy Chhem, Siswanto Agus Wilopo, and Alan D. Lopez, "Health and Health-Care Systems in Southeast Asia: Diversity and Transitions," *Lancet* 337 (2011): 429–37.

28. Megha Amrith, "'They Think We Are Just Caregivers': The Ambivalence of Care among Filipino Medical Workers in Singapore," *The Asia Pacific Journal of Anthropology* 11, nos. 3/4 (2010): 410–27.

PART I
THE LONGUE DURÉE

1 Krom Luang Wongsa and the House of Snidvongs

Knowledge Transition and the Transformation of Medicine in Early Modern Siam

Nopphanat Anuphongphat and
Komatra Chuengsatiansup

By the end of the seventeenth century, Ayutthaya, the Siamese capital, along with Melaka and Hoi An, had already become regional centers of trade and commercial exchange.[1] Located on an expansive Chao Phraya River with its maze of interconnecting waterways, the entrepôt of Ayutthaya, known to the European as the "Venice of the East," spawned barges and ships from the high seas as well as sampans from local canals. During its glorious days in the reign of King Narai, the Court of Siam at Ayutthaya was frequented by Portuguese, Dutch, English, and French visitors. They were traders, missionaries, and diplomats who brought along not only new commodities, new religions, and new contracts, but more importantly new knowledge. It was the time for new learning as the new episteme had called into question not only the modus vivendi that the Siamese had long held sway, but also the modus operandi in the technical domains of architecture, engineering, astronomy, and medicine.[2]

The royal court at Ayutthaya was seemingly keen to embrace all things Western. With Constantine Phalkon, a Greek adventurer, as his counselor, King Narai received ambassadors; endorsed foreign trade; made treaties; appointed foreign consultants; enlisted Western technical assistance in design and construction of forts, palaces, and water supply systems; accompanied French envoys to witness a lunar eclipse; and provided missionary facilities to build churches and granted them freedom to preach Christianity.[3] In medicine, Western doctors were appointed as court physicians. Records reveal that the Royal Court of King Narai had requested Daniel Brochebourde, a French surgeon from Vereenigde Oostindische Compagnie (VOC) to serve as court doctor where his descendant also served thereafter.[4] A hospital was also founded in 1669 in Ayutthaya to provide medical care for local people.[5] Western medicine seemed to be well received, as two hundred to three hundred people waited each day for their medicine.[6]

Medical knowledge in Ayutthaya at the time, according to Simon de La Loubère, was nothing but primitive. La Loubère, a French diplomat and missionary, arrived at Ayutthaya in 1687 during the reign of King Narai and spent three months in Siam seemingly intruding on all aspects of Siamese life. Upon his return, he wrote a report of his magisterial survey of Siam, *A New Historical Relation of the Kingdom of Siam,* which first appeared in French in 1691 and in English two years later. His rendering of "an exact account of the things" he had seen and learnt in Siam described in detail the geography, history, production, cultivation, education, habits, houses, food, marriage, art, government, king, custom of the court, climate, law, and astronomy, all observed and learned during his extraordinary stay from September 27, 1687, to January 3, 1688. In medicine, La Loubère said of the Siamese,

> They trouble not themselves to have any principle of Medicine, but only a number of Receipts, which they have learnt from their Ancestors, and in which they never alter any thing. They have no regard to the particular symptoms of diseases: and yet they fail not to cure a great many; because the natural Temperance of the Siameses [*sic*] preserves them from a great many evils difficult to cure. But when at last it happens that the Distemper is stronger than the Remedies, they fail not to attribute the cause thereof to Enchantment.[7]

If the state of medical knowledge in Siam as described by La Loubère seemed archaic, Western medicine, which was still in its infancy at the time, was not far removed from its Siamese counterparts. There were records of medical treatments among French missionaries in which holy water and consecrated oils were used to anoint the sick in church services; these were counted on to have therapeutic efficacy.[8]

While adopting and making good use of Western medicine, the court of Ayutthaya was not an empty vessel. Elaborated bodies of medical knowledge did exist. Records of herbal remedies and medical regimens prescribed to King Narai were found in a medical treatise with names of attending physicians and dates of prescription.[9] The indicated dates suggested that the records were made between the third and fifth years of King Narai's reign, 1659–61, more than two decades prior to the arrival of La Loubère. The text, known as *King Narai's Medical Treatise,* was compiled, with subsequent additions of medical formulae from the successive reigns, to have a total of eighty-one formulae and was supposedly intended as a reference for house doctors.[10] Among the names of physicians, however, only five of the nine doctors listed were Siamese. The others included one Indian doctor, one Chinese doctor, and two Western physicians.[11] Medical formulae on the list also included recipes for ointments prescribed to the king by Western physicians. This significant medical text attested to the eclectic attitude of Siamese royal court towards medical practices at the time when differing ideas contended and conjoined.

Western influence at the Siamese court ended with the death of King Narai. With the fall of Ayutthaya in 1767, evidence of traditional Thai medical knowledge as well as its interaction with Western medicine was further scattered. It was not until the early Rattanakosin era that efforts to restore knowledge in various fields were seriously attempted. In the field of medicine, restoration of medical knowledge was immediately carried out during the First Reign. Medical texts and statues of hermits demonstrating meditation and exercise postures were placed and proffered to the public at Wat Phra Chetuphon (Wat Pho), near the Grand Palace.[12] A compilation of pharmacopoeia (Tamra Rong Phra Osot) was undertaken during the Second Reign. Medical texts were collected from around the kingdom by the order of the king.[13] In the Third Reign, stone tablets engraved with traditional medical knowledge and anatomical diagrams of massage were placed at the corridors of Wat Rajaorasaram and Wat Pho for public viewing. During this period of medical revitalization, however, *King Narai's Medical Treatise* mysteriously disappeared. It only reemerged some 250 years later, when Siam was attempting to come to terms with a new threat of colonial aggression in the nineteenth century.

Although most of valuable texts and official records were destroyed during the fall of Ayutthaya, *King Narai's Medical Treatise* survived the destruction. A copy of this significant treatise was kept by Krom Luang Wongsa, the chief physician at the royal court during the reign of King Rama III and IV. Krom Luang Wongsa was himself a renowned traditional doctor from a lineage of famous healers. During his time, however, traditional medicine was fiercely challenged by Western medical knowledge. Rather than resisting changes, Prince Krom Luang Wongsa learned Western medicine from missionary doctors. His mastery of modern medicine earned him a certificate from the New York Academy of Medicine and made him a corresponding fellow of the institute.

As the new science made its headway into Siam, Krom Luang Wongsa's family, the Snidvongs, strove to carry on its customary duty. Krom Luang Wongsa's son maintained the family tradition, became a doctor, and served as court physician. Like his father, he learned and had good command of both traditional and Western medicine. Krom Luang Wongsa's grandson, however, could no longer hold on to the family medical tradition. He forwent traditional medicine and was the first Siamese to earn a bachelor degree in modern medicine from a Western university. The story of Krom Luang Wongsa's family embodies the dynamic interplay of power, changing contexts, and contested medical knowledge in nineteenth-century Siam. It is through the family history of Krom Luang Wongsa that this chapter seeks to understand how medicine from different knowledge traditions contested each other and combined.

Royal Court Physician and the Challenge of the New Science

The arrival of Western colonialism in the nineteenth century reintroduced a Western system of knowledge to Siam, a system of knowledge far more scientific than that acquainted by the court of King Narai some two hundred years earlier. Siamese conventional wisdom that appeared to defy the logic of science was increasingly challenged. It did not take long for the Siamese elites to realize the inevitability of change and the necessity to learn new science. Among those directly affected by the winds of change were the royal court physicians. Based on a totally different worldview, the two systems of healing often came to direct conflict and it was traditional medicine that kept losing its ground to the new science. An illustrative incident was when Dr. Dan Beach Bradley, an American missionary doctor, visited Vajirayan Bhikkhu to give him a medical checkup. Vajirayan Bhikkhu (who later became King Mongkut, but was at that time ordained as a monk), suffered from a kind of "wind disease."

Upon his examination, Bradley proposed an etiological explanation of the disease and openly expressed his disagreement with folk theory. He attempted to convince Vajirayan Bhikkhu and a host of Siamese physicians that the "wind theory" proposed by Siamese doctors was indeed a hoax:

> I found the poor man very much diseased. He had had a complaint in the right ear that had led to paralysis of the nerve that controls the muscles of the face. . . . This disease, I learned, is called "wind." It was said that it first began at the feet and gradually ascended to its present seat. It had been treated by local applications and internal medicines of a heating kind. I spent considerable time to convince the patient and physicians that the idea of "wind" being cause of the disease was all humbug.
>
> The patient and his brother were quick to perceive the truth of my illustrations, and then labored to bring over the native physicians to the faith. The latter were not willing to give up their notion which was the main pillar of their theory. I then proceeded to show what was the probable cause of the complaint, and was happy to find that I gained the confidence of those who heard me. The patient seemed willing to dismiss the former physicians and put himself solely under my care.[14]

Krom Luang Wongsa must have felt such challenges, for he was also serving as the royal court physician at the time. The new science might as well have aroused the intellectual curiosity of the young doctor who would eventually rise to the position of chief physician in charge of the Department of Royal Physicians.

The Life and Times of Krom Luang Wongsa

Among the Siamese elites eager to learn the knowledge of the West, Krom Luang Wongsa Dhiraj Snid was a crucial figure. The forty-ninth son of King Rama II, he was born July 9, 1808, and given the title "Phra Ong Chao Nuam." His mother was from a family of adept physicians; both of her parents were famous in traditional medical practice. They both served as royal court physicians during the reign of King Rama II. Their medical knowledge has been inherited and transmitted over generations. Phra Ong Chao Nuam joined the service as physician at the royal court during the reign of King Rama III. His service earned him the title "Krom Muen Wongsa Dhiraj Snid." During the reign of King Rama IV, he was in charge of the Royal Warehouse and the Ministry of the Interior, chief counselor to the king and, with royal bestowal, acceded to the title of "Krom Luang Wongsa Snid." He was known to be well versed in liberal arts, science, military, education, diplomacy and international affairs.[15] In medicine, Krom Luang Wongsa Dhiraj Snid (hereafter Krom Luang Wongsa) was court physician in charge of Department of Royal Physicians during the reigns of King Rama III and IV, and his descendants also succeeded him in serving as court physicians.

As was the custom at the time, children of the royal court went through a period of study. After learning the Thai language at a very young age, young men started studying Pali as well as regal conduct and etiquette in their early teens. Between the ages of thirteen and twenty-one, they were ordained as Buddhist novices to learn monastic discipline. After leaving the novitiate they pursued further education under the tutelage of respected authorities. They also learned statecraft and royal legislative procedures by conferring in administrative affairs at the palace hall. After the age of twenty-one, they entered monkhood and spent their time learning Buddhism as well as mastering the secret art of thaumaturgy. The gentlemen were considered mature and ready to serve as courtiers only after the completion of their monastic lives.[16]

As a novice, Krom Luang Wongsa was fortunate to have Somdet Phra Maha Samana Chao Kromma Phra Paramanujita Jinorasa, the supreme patriarch, as his mentor. Instructed by a master well versed in Buddhism, statecraft, arts, and literature, Krom Luang Wongsa was subsequently known as a man of multiple talents.[17] Krom Luang Wongsa inherited the medical knowledge from his maternal family and he had been concocting medications for his father, King Rama II, since his teens.[18] At the age of thirty-four, King Rama III appointed him the chief of court physicians in charge of the Department of Royal Physicians.[19] It was an important position, for the department was responsible for life and death of all the royal families.[20] To ensure they could take on the responsibility, all court physicians needed to be meticulously appraised.[21] Jean-Baptiste Pallegoix, vicar apostolic of Eastern Siam (1805–62) who resided in Siam during the reign of King Rama III and IV recorded in his journal the story of the court physician:

There is a chief mandarin for all royal doctors. The latter are divided in several groups providing the service in turn. They must be on guard in the palace day and night to give care to patients of the court. They accompany the army, princes and mandarins on their journeys. All doctors receive salary from the King and their dignity passes to their children.[22]

Krom Luang Wongsa's medical prowess was well established. After a single year of serving as royal court physician, one of the most beloved daughters of King Rama III was placed under his care.[23] His exceptional skill was so impressive that it was praised in a famous poem, "The Illness of Krom Muen Upsorn Sudadhep."[24] One verse read,

The Chamberlain's medication was indeed fit for the task.
Shortly after taking, [the patient] was merrily in good mood.[25]

In 1850 King Rama III fell seriously ill. Krom Luang Wongsa was duly in charge of caring for the King. The ailment had become untreatable and the King died the following year. When King Rama IV ascended to the throne, Krom Luang Wongsa was once more entrusted to carry on his duty as the chief physician in charge of the Department of Royal Physicians.[26]

The Exposure and Espousal of Western Medicine

Krom Luang Wongsa was no stranger to Westerners; most foreigners in Bangkok at the time were well acquainted with him. An article in the *Illustrirte Zeitung,* a news magazine published in Germany, described Krom Luang Wongsa's friendly character as follows:

Krom Luang Wongsa Dhiraj Snidh, Prince of Siam, was a brother of the reigning King. . . .[27] He is wealthy and generous. He owns, for instance, several ocean steamers in a business he operates. Although outwardly he might appear difficult to approach, he is in fact truly good natured and hospitable, especially to his European friends. He always allows visitors to borrow his steamers. Recently, he received Mr. Commerzienrath Wolf, a visitor from Gladbach, and let him use the steamer free of charge. Besides, whenever he is free from his duty, he always permits foreigners audiences and provides assistance when they are in need.[28]

Sir John Bowring, the British Ambassador who came to negotiate a treaty with King Rama IV, upon learning that the King had appointed Krom Luang Wongsa to chair the treaty commission, wrote in his records,

The King nominated his brother, the Prince Krom Hluang Wongsa, to the Presidency of the Commission; and he could not have made wiser choice, for the prince has had much intercourse with foreigners, among whom, as with the Siamese, he is extremely popular. His influence was undoubtedly flung into the balance of an emancipating and a liberal policy; and I have reason to believe he had no sinister interest likely to prejudice or mislead.[29]

In fact, as a man well versed in diplomatic affairs, Krom Luang Wongsa was in many instances appointed chief officer in the negotiations to amend treaties with European powers during the reign of King Rama IV.

Krom Luang Wongsa's interest in Western medicine probably sprang from his interaction with his many missionary friends and his favorable attitude towards Western civilization. Townsend Harris, the American envoy who negotiated the treaty between Siam and the United States during King Mongkut's reign in 1856, noted, "From there we called on Krom Luang Wong [Sa] Tirat Sanit, the King's brother and Chief Physicians to the royal family. . . . He spoke about the Siamese being a jungle people, and not so advanced in civilization as the nations of the West."[30] This self-deprecation could well be a tactical maneuver in the game of diplomacy. But his keen interest in Western knowledge, especially Western medicine, was unmistakable.

Little evidence is available to suggest whence and from whom Krom Luang Wongsa learned the new medicine. Existing documents, however, clearly show that he was one among the group of Siamese elites who went to Dr. Samuel R. House and Rev. Jesse Caswell to feed off their curiosity for the new science. His espousal of Western medicine was, however, already evident when he invited Dr. Dan Beach Bradley to inoculate children in his palace against smallpox in March 1840.[31] And his favorable reception of Western medicine probably steadily increased when, in 1852, one of his wives had a difficulty delivering a baby, House and Bradley were promptly invited to help. Bradley's journal reads,

> The case of Krom Luang Wongsa Sanit's wife has proved to be a severe one. The prince felt that neither himself [sic] nor any other Siamese physician was able to do anything for her. There was no prospect that she would ever be delivered without instrumental aid. Hence I performed the operation for cephalotamy as we had good evidence to believe that the child was dead . . . we were all night in close attention upon the poor woman and did not complete our operation till after daylight. It is quite remarkable that almost the first case of mid-wifery among the Siamese committed entirely to our care from before the period of parturition should have been in the family of one of the highest princes in the Kingdom and the wife of confessedly the most learned and skillful physician in the land. The Lord, we trust, intends to bring great good out of this circumstance. May we grace to be his servants.[32]

In the same year (1852), Bradley moved his residence to the area of Klong Bang Luang, next to the old palace where Krom Luang Wongsa resided. Some writers suggest that the close proximity would have allowed the two to meet more often, and Krom Luang Wongsa must have learned a good deal from being closely acquainted with Bradley.[33]

It was said that Krom Luang Wongsa's expansive knowledge of Western medicine earned him a certificate from New York Academy of Medicine. He was even invited to be a fellow of the institute. Sir John Bowring's journal of his visit to Krom Luang Wongsa's residential palace on April 10, 1855, provided the evidence,

> At six, went with Keane, H. S. P., J. C. B., and Bell, to visit Prince Pra Chau Nong Ya Ter Krom Hluang Wongsa Dhiraj Snidh, the King's brother, who has an excellent reputation for good sense and honesty. We found, at the entrance to his palace, an American *medical* diploma given to his Royal Highness, pictures of English race-horses, and other adornings of European origin.[34]

William Maxwell Wood, the fleet surgeon of the East India Squadron aboard the USS San Jacinto, who came to Siam and took part in negotiating an American treaty with the King of Siam in 1856, also mentioned Krom Luang Wongsa as being a fellow of the New York Academy of Medicine in his book.[35] His mastery of modern medicine was further confirmed by Townsend Harris, who mentioned that when Prussian envoy Max Von Brandt visited Siam in 1861, he saw a medical certificate from Philadelphia hung in Krom Luang Wongsa's drawing room.[36,37] The *Syllabus of the Course of Lectures on the Principles and Practice of Surgery* also mentioned that Krom Luang Wongsa was one of the corresponding fellows of the New York Academy of Medicine in 1858.[38]

Bowring's journal suggests that Krom Luang Wongsa acquired the certificate from the New York Academy of Medicine before 1855. To master the art of modern medicine to the point that such a prestigious certificate was granted took not only perseverance but also time. His interest in modern medicine must have stemmed from as early as 1852, for an official archive described an incident in which Krom Luang Wongsa was requested to provide medical care for Queen Somanass Waddhanawathy of the reigning King Rama IV thus:

> That same night her Majesty became worse, and vomited so frequently she almost died from the attack. The Siamese official physicians tried to revive her, but they could not succeed to stop the painful vomiting even for half an hour. His Royal Highness the Prince Krom Hluang Wongsa Dhiraj Sniddh administered some homeopathic medicine, from the effect of which her majesty's frequent vomiting was relieved, and she had the happiness to have a good sleep, at four or five o'clock, A M.[39]

Krom Luang Wongsa must have been practicing this Western science to the extent that he was confident in using it to treat the queen. The story, however, not only reveals that Krom Luang Wongsa was capable of administering homeopathic medicine but also predicates the influence Bradley had on him. Bradley's acknowledgement of his own conversion to homeopathy could be found in his 1849 journal:

The first breach occurs when Dr. Lane looked into the box of homeopathic medicines that Dr. Ball of New York City had provided for my use in Siam. . . . Dr. Ball, knowing that I had a convert to homeopathy had drawn up a subscription to present to homeopathic physicians in New York, soliciting books and medicine for my personal use in the Kingdom of Siam.[40]

Krom Luang Wongsa not only learned the techne of Western medicine, but also endeavored to localize Western episteme in indigenous system of medical knowledge. His attempt to compose a textbook on folk *materia medica* was nothing but an Aristotelian undertaking.[41] Contrary to the convention of collecting medical recipes consisting of formulae of various herbs and other remedies, Krom Luang Wongsa's pharmacopoeia not only compiled but also divided, classified, and categorized. One by one, plants were divided into parts, each with descriptions of specific pharmaceutical effects:

Speaking of the properties of cardamom, the leaves have the effect of moving the wind below, repelling discomfort in the throat, relieving fever, and remedying phlegm; the seeds are for dissipating blood, phlegm, and wind; flowers are for diseases arising from rotten eyes; the bark is for fever stemming from eating improper food; the outer skin is for effecting all kinds of blood; the stem is for dissipating poison; the root is for killing off coagulated blood inside the stomach. Such are the brief properties of cardamom.[42]

The manner in which Krom Luang Wongsa composed his *materia medica,* in which medicinal plants were divided into parts, each with specific properties, use, and effect, bears traces of influence from Western pharmacological studies of plants. He also wrote a Thai-language pharmacopoeia of Western *materia medica* including forty-two medicines; all the English and Latin names of which were transliterated into Thai. The text has been recognized as the first textbook on pharmacognosy in the Thai language.[43] Examples of transliterated entries include camphor water, phosphoric acid, liquor arsenicum, arnica, cantharis, cinchona, ignatia, opium, coffee, and Merccurius Dulcis.[44]

Krom Luang Wongsa's enthusiastic acceptance and adoption of Western medicine was ahead of his time. The general public had not yet come to accept the efficacy of Western medicine. When dispensing quinine pills, an effective Western antimalarial medicine, to patients, Krom Luang Wongsa came up with a trick of concealing the quinine pellet inside his large medicinal bolus. As Prince Damrong described,

When quinine was first introduced in Thailand during the Third Reign, Krom Luang Wongsa Dhiraj Snid, who was knowledgeable on Thai medicine, was the first to test and appreciate the medication. But he could not use it openly. When I was ordained as a novice, I heard from Krom Somdet Phra Pawares Wariyalongkorn that every single pill of Krom Luang Wongsa's well-respected antipyretic drug was cut in half and "the farang white pill" (quinine) enclosed inside.[45]

Within two decades after the arrival of American missionaries, the chief of the royal physicians had already inoculated his children against smallpox, allowed a Western doctor to cut open the skull of his dead baby inside his pregnant wife, prescribed homeopathy to the queen, rewritten folk *materia medica* in conformity with Western pharmacopoeia, and approvingly enclosed pellets of Western medicine within his own large pills. His enthusiastic espousal and eclectic attitude toward Western knowledge has left some historians seeking a satisfactory explanation.

Changing Contexts and the New Knowledge

Western knowledge was favorably accepted in nineteenth century Siam not simply out of the Siamese elites' curiosity, nor because of its pragmatic utilities. Sociopolitical development since the reign of King Rama I had already paved the way for the Siamese elites' reception of modern knowledge. The fall of Ayutthaya and the attempt to establish the new capital in Thonburi contributed greatly to the growing tribute trade system between Siam and China. The flourishing trade with China continued into the First Reign of the Chakri Dynasty of Bangkok. The new commercial opportunities created a new elite stratum consisting of the king and his courtiers, nobilities, and Chinese mercenaries. A new class, whose members possessed superior intellectual or socioeconomic status and were open and receptive to changes, had emerged.[46] A new worldview was also in the making. Nidhi examines the changing literary style in the early Rattanakosin era and finds that the old romantic style of writing had been replaced with a more realistic genre. The traveling troubadour's agonizing feelings of longing for loved ones was superseded by the naturalistic depiction of what the authors had encountered on their journeys. It was no coincidence that "Klong Nirat Phra Prathom," one of the works in the new literary style, was composed by Krom Luang Wongsa himself in 1834.[47]

The characters in classical literature were also transformed into what Nidhi calls "humanistic" personae. Human actors were portrayed in Rattanakosin literature more as subjects acting according to their circumstances. The characters in literature of Ayutthaya era, on the contrary, mostly bore magical powers bestowed upon them by supernatural beings. Otherwise they would acquire special protection from deities or become the avatars of Boddhisatvas to defeat demons.[48] Buddhist teaching in the early Rattanakosin also inclined towards a more rationalistic overtone. King Rama I himself was known to reject superstitious and ritualistic practices, preferring more experiential and empirical modes of religious conduct.[49] The result was nothing less than a new worldview among the Siamese elites, a worldview imbued with the intertwining traits of realism, humanism, and rationalism.

The level of favorable reception was evident not only among enthusiasts of Western knowledge such as Vajirayan Bhikkhu (who later became King Rama IV), Prince Chutamani (Chao Fa Noi), and Jamuen Wai Woranat (Chuang Bunnag); even King Rama III (Phra Bat Somdet Phra Nangklao Chao Yu Hua), who was considered to be exceptionally conservative, still expressed his appreciation of Western knowledge.[50] John Crawfurd, the British envoy who came to Siam in 1822 during the reign of King Rama II, noted his impressions after he had an audience with Kromma Muen Jessadabodindra, who later became King Rama III:

> The impression which his conversation throughout the night made upon us was favourable, and he seemed certainly to maintain the character assigned to him in public estimation, of being the most intelligent of all the princes and chiefs of the Siam Court. The Portuguese Consul afterwards told me an anecdote respecting him, which showed that he was not insensible to deeds of high renown, or unacquainted with the great events which had recently passed in Europe. Mr. De Silverio stated that the prince had frequently expressed to him his admiration of the great achievements of the Emperor Napoleon; and that he had at last offered him a handsome sum of money, if he would translate from French into the Portuguese language a history of his wars, for the purpose of being rendered into Siamese through the Christian interpreters.[51]

The prevalence of epidemic outbreaks, especially smallpox and cholera, also made the social environment conducive to the introduction of modern medicine. Dan Beach Bradley, upon his arrival in Bangkok in 1835, noted in his journal, "Mister Hunter, The British merchant, came to the house with a message from Phrya Sri pipat, requesting me in the name of the King to go immediately and try my skill on a company of slaves who were sick of the small pox and cholera."[52]

Bradley's account suggested an unbearable situation and the recklessness on behalf of the court physician to seek a way out for the epidemic:

> Phra Nai Wai remarked that the King did not care much for the people we were going to see and therefore, he had chosen to try me first upon them; and if I should prove myself skillful he would employ me among the great men. . . . My host wished to know if I could not always cure the small pox and cholera. When I told him that I could not, he asked me if I could tell by looking at a sick person whether he would die of the disease or not. When I told him that I could not certainly predict in such cases, he seemed to think that I was not as great doctor as I had been reported to be.[53]

Cholera and smallpox posed atrocious threats to Siamese authority. An outbreak could bring a death toll of more than ten thousand at a time. During the Second Reign, for instance, cholera spread to the whole kingdom and caused roughly thirty thousand deaths.[54] In 1838, Bradley proposed to write a textbook on smallpox vaccination for the royal court. Upon learning that Bradley had successfully vaccinated the children of a missionary against smallpox, court physicians were dispatched to learn this skill from Bradley, and a score of slaves were also readily sent to serve as subjects for the physicians to practice on. *Treatise on Vaccination Comprising a Narrative of the Introduction and Successful Propagation of Vaccine in Siam 1840 & 1844* was subsequently published and distributed among those who came to learn about vaccination. The achievement earned Dr. Bradley a prize from King Rama III.

The interest in the new science lay, however, not in ideology but in the intriguing science of the concrete. Samuel Reynolds House was another influential missionary doctor who advocated modern science among Siamese elites. He was well acquainted with Vajirayan Bhikkhu. House knew that Vajirayan Bhikkhu had asked Rev. Jesse Caswell, another American missionary, to teach him English in exchange for the permission to use his temple to preach the gospel.[55] In his conversation with House, Vajirayan Bhikkhu told him that he was not interested in Christianity at all, but very much interested in Western science—especially astronomy, geography, and mathematics.[56] Dr. House described Vajirayan Bhikkhu's room in Wat Bovornives as follows: "I looked around the room; Bible from A.B. Society, and Webster dictionary stood side by side on shelf of his secretary, also a Nautical Tables and Navigation. On the table a diagram of the forthcoming eclipse in pencil with calculations, and a copy of the printed chart of Mr. Chandler."[57]

To feed the curiosity of the elites, in 1847 House arranged for series of lectures at his office. He gave the introductory outlines and Rev. Jesse Caswell gave the lectures. House also demonstrated the experiments with all the necessary equipment and materials such as chemical substances, magnets, globes, physiological and hygienic charts, as well as some anatomical models. It is worth noting that Krom Luang Wongsa, who was a court physician at the time, was also invited by Vajirayan Bhikkhu to attend the lectures and observe the experiments.[58]

The scientific method of inquiry was also advocated by Dan Beach Bradley through the publication of scientific articles, for instance, on chemistry, oxygen, and the physiology of human heart, in *The Bangkok Recorder,* the newspaper he published in 1865.[59] His familiarity with the Siamese elites led Bradley to the impression that

> Prince Mongkut's party had a strong interest in bringing about reforms in the teaching and practice of the Buddhist religion in Siam. He told Caswell, for instance, of the substance of a conversation held one evening at the palace of the Foreign Minister. One of those present enquired in the playful way, who in the company had joined the missionaries, meaning by the question, who were believers in the spherical shape of the earth? Mongkut replied that he had joined them fifteen years ago, before they came here. Phra Nai Wai stated that he had joined them thirteen years ago, while his brother, Phra Nai Si, said that he had become a disciple only a year before, when he had read Caswell's tract on astronomy. Whereupon Phya Sripipat, the Foreign Minister's brother, replied impatiently that he was no believer at all: he never had been and never would be.[60]

The espousal of modern knowledge was never without controversy. And nowhere was such controversy more in evidence than in the struggle over women's bodies.

Midwifery and the Contested Domain

Interest in the Western practice of midwifery had already surfaced when the Second King still assumed the title of Prince Chutamani. The Prince asked Bradley to look after his wife, who had just delivered her first baby. Bradley stated, "The Prince was anxious to have the *farang* doctor convince the women of the palace that the ancient custom of lying-by-the-fire was useless and cruel, because he wished to spare his wife that terrible ordeal."[61] Bradley tried his best to convince the ladies, but to no avail:

> With all the reasoning and eloquence that I could employ both through Prince Chutamani and speaking directly to them, I could not persuade the women that it would be prudent to suspend their practice even for the night, so that the sufferer might have quiet rest on her bed. They said that the plane of treatment that I proposed was entirely new to them and also that I was a stranger, and that it would not do at all to expose so honorable a person to the dangers of an experiment.[62]

Years later, Bradley was asked to take care of a wife of King Rama IV. He went with Samuel Reynolds House into the inner chamber of the palace in January 1852:

> At His majesty's request—the prince physician desiring it, Dr. Bradley was summoned to take charge of one of the royal ladies who had been confined but a few days before of a princess—His Majesty's first begotten since his accession. . . . Never before had any foreign physician been within the forbidden precincts of the harem of the royal palace. His Majesty, like a good husband anxious for his young wife, desired Dr. Bradley to invite me to accompany him as counsel in the case. . . . Dr. Bradley had got the fire by which she was lying extinguished (custom required "lying by the fire"), had put her on close diet and other treatment.[63]

The treatment successfully saved the life of the king's young wife. The king sent a letter of appreciation as well as some tokens of gratitude to Bradley and House. In the letter, he affirmed his confidence in Western midwifery: "I trust(ed) previously the manner of curing in the obstetric of America and Europe, but sorry to say I could not get the same lady to believe before her approaching (threatening) death, because her kindred were many more who lead her according to their custom. Your present curing, however, was just now most wonderful in this palace."[64]

The death of Queen Somanass Waddhanawathy in 1852 after she gave birth to her son had pressed King Rama IV to seriously abolish "the senseless and monstrous crime of having lying-in women smoked and roasted from 15 to 30 days." The King declared that "he would effect reform in his own families on the subject."[65] It was, however, not until the reign of King Rama V, some thirty-seven years later, that the practice of lying by the fireplace came to an end. When Queen Saovabha Phongsri became feverish after giving birth to a son, Krom Muen Prap Porapuk explained to the queen the benefit his wife derived from Western obstetric practice. The queen was instead put under the care of Dr. Peter Cowan. The practice of lying by the fire was abolished in the royal court, and more and more nobles came to give up the practice.[66] The incident eventually led to the abolishment of the same practice in the state hospital.[67]

Changes in practice entailed changes of ideas and vice versa. Before the abolition of such practice, Malcolm Smith, physician to Queen Saovabha Phongsri, deplored that the king's women did not accede to the king's desire to get rid of the practice of lying by the fire, "[b]ut the women would have nothing to do with his new ideas. They were having the babies they said, not the King. They refused to change their ways. They preferred the frying pan that they knew, with all its discomforts, to the fire of the unknown. It would let loose the evil spirits (pi) they said."[68]

Scientific disenchantment with the sacred allowed for radical changes, and also threatened the legitimacy and power of the divine monarch. The new knowledge had proven to be an influential force, while the English language had increasingly become the lingua franca of the new power.[69] Siamese elites were ready to adapt to the new reality; they were keen to adopt what they deemed far removed from what they once held as ultimate reality.[70]

King Rama IV seemed willing to accept this new power. In 1849, when still ordained as Vajirayan Bhikkhu, he explained to his European acquaintances how Siamese intellectuals readily espoused the new ideals:

> Here are many gentlemen who formerly believed in the cosmogony [sic] & cosmography according to Brahmanical works which the old ancient Buddhist authors of book have adopted to their system without hesitation. They took contrary contest with many subjects of European or enlightened Geography, astronomy, Horology, navigation chemistry & c. on their first hearing or receipt. they thought that such the system & knowledges were but the influence of imagination of heathen nation or propounded subject from the Christ and his disciples. afterward [sic] they have examined accurately & exemplified with many reason, arguments & circumstands. now the skilful gentlemen & wise men of our country generally believed all foresaid sciences & pleased with them much so that a few of them including myself endeavored to study language of English proposing the knowledge of reading & persuing their book of scientific action or arts to be immated & introduce to our country whatever would come under their power.[71]

Krom Luang Wongsa was obviously one among these gentlemen. Caught in the winds of change, Krom Luang Wongsa's medical practices juggled the knowledge he inherited and the new knowledge he learned. This transitional practice he passed on to members of his family, the House of Snidvongs, first to one of his beloved sons, His Highness Prince Sai Snid Wongse (or Prince Sai), and, later, to his grandson, M. R. Suvabhan Sanitwongsa.

Transformation of Knowledge:
Changing Medical Tradition in the House of Snidvongs

Prince Sai was born in 1845. Although his father, Krom Luang Wongsa, begat some fifty-two sons and daughters, Prince Sai was one of his most beloved children.[72] Krom Luang Wongsa imparted to him both traditional and modern medical knowledge.[73] After he was bestowed the title "Phra Ong Chao" in 1872 during the reign of King Rama V, Prince Sai became court physician and was in charge of the Department of Royal Physicians.[74] Modern medicine had already become mainstream in the Royal Court of Siam. He recruited Peter Cowan, a Scottish doctor who would later become the supervisor of the first public hospital in Siam.[75] Inheriting an eclectic and pragmatic trait from his father, when a cholera outbreak occurred in 1881, Prince Sai endeavored to apply Western pharmaceutical techniques to develop a new cure.[76]

Although not trained as a modern physician, Prince Sai's commitment to Western medicine was unmistakable; his eldest son, M. R. Suvabhan Sanitwongsa was the first Siamese to earn a degree in Western medicine. It was Peter Cowan who suggested the idea of having Siamese students learn medicine in Europe and come back to work for the government, and Prince Sai proposed it to the king. Convinced by the idea, King Rama V purposely chose M. R. Suvabhan for the task, hoping that he would learn and return to carry on his family's tradition of practicing medicine. It seemed that the medical tradition to be carried on was no longer the traditional Thai medicine long practiced by his family.

M. R. Suvabhan Sanitwongsa acquired his Bachelor of Medicine from Edinburgh University in Scotland and returned to Bangkok in 1884. Upon his return, he worked mostly to assist his father, as there were only two Western-trained Siamese physicians serving in the court at the time. As the role of traditional doctors in Siamese court dwindled, Prince Sai's traditional medical knowledge became increasingly irrelevant. He had become more and more involved in other public administrative affairs as well as building his private enterprises. In 1888 Prince Sai set up the Siam Canals Land and Irrigation Company and was granted the concession to dig canals, which have become known as Klong Chao Sai, in Rangsit.[77] When Prince Sai became sick, M. R. Suvabhan stepped in and took over the responsibility of running the enterprise. He continued to dispense his medicine not at the royal court, but mostly for the sick local people in the precinct of Klong Luang, Rangsit District, where he managed his company.

After M. R. Suvabhan, direct descendants of the Snidvongs lineage neither passed on the family's traditional medical knowledge nor served as court physicians. One of his nephews, Prince Jainad (or Somdej Phra Chao Boromawogse Ther Krom Phraya Jainad Narendhorn), who was educated in Germany, became the director of the Royal Medical College. He also served as the director general of the Public Health Department, which later became the Ministry of Public Health. Prince Jainad has been recognized as the founder of the Ministry of Public Health. Under his leadership, the medical school was transformed in various regards. The curriculum was modernized. Between 1915 and 1917, traditional medicine, which had been taught and practiced alongside modern medicine in the medical school, was abolished.

In 1922, King Rama VI approved Prince Jainad's idea to solicit Prince Song-khla's help to secure the Rockefeller Foundation's assistance in upgrading the medical school to meet international standards. The promulgation of a new medical practice bill requiring traditional practitioners to pass a licensing examination dealt another blow to traditional medicine. A great number of traditional practitioners gave up practicing because they were fearful of the new law. It was as if Prince Jainad put the last nail on the coffin of Thai traditional medicine. Yet it was Prince Jainad who in 1917 delivered a copy of *King Narai's Medical Treatise* to Prince Damrong.[78] The discovery and deliverance of this significant textbook brought a remarkable reprieve for traditional medicine. The text was reprinted many times and has become an essential pharmacopoeia for the study of Thai traditional medicine. The reprieve came, however, with an ironic twist, for this very book contained entries on Western medicine, formulae of ointments proffered to King Narai by his Western court physician. As Prince Damrong himself observed, the ointment was still being used by Portuguese immigrant communities residing in Siam—250 years after it was prescribed for King Narai.[79]

Conclusion

During the reign of King Rama V (1868–73) Siam was transforming itself into a modern nation-state. Sanitation management was implemented. Hospitals, a medical school, as well as midwifery and nursing colleges were built. Traditional medicine, on the other hand, became increasingly neglected and irrelevant. Traditional medicine was no longer deployed in the royal court and the teaching of traditional medicine in medical school was eventually abolished. Within these changing contexts, many prominent families of traditional practitioners were affected and needed to adapt to the new circumstances. The family history of Krom Luang Wongsa shows the dynamic adaptation and the transformation of traditional medical practices in changing circumstances.

Political and social changes in the early Rattanakosin era ushered in a new worldview, one which favored a more realistic, humanistic, and rationalistic way of seeing, knowing, and acting. Within these contexts, traditional doctors in the royal court faced an immense challenge and had to adapt their practices. Krom

A Historical Overview of Traditional Medicine in Cambodia
Sokhieng Au

On April 29, 2009, the first official school for Khmer Practitioners of Traditional Medicine opened in Phnom Penh.[1] In reality a short training program run through the National Center for Traditional Medicine, its creation was funded by the Japanese Nippon Foundation in cooperation with the Cambodian Ministry of Health, an initiative that was in line with the 2008 World Health Organization Beijing Declaration on Traditional Medicine.[2] The WHO definition of traditional medicine, "the sum total of knowledge, skills and practices based on the theories, beliefs and experiences indigenous to different cultures that are used to maintain health, as well as to prevent, diagnose, improve or treat physical and mental illnesses," is sweeping in its scope, and hinges on the idea of "indigenous" knowledge and practices.[3]

In the case of Cambodia—and most of Southeast Asia—what was 150 years ago simply medicine has been corralled into the category of traditional medicine under the processes of colonialism, modernization, and westernization.[4] In the end, the term "traditional medicine" is used almost casually in much social science literature to note anything health-related that does not fit into the biomedical paradigm. What I am calling traditional medicine (TM) in Cambodia will be the institutions, theories, and practices related to sickness and healing that have roots predating the colonial period, even if they have evolved in the last 150 years.[5]

Institutionally-based medicine in Cambodia has perhaps an older documented record than any in Southeast Asia, thanks to Jayavarman VII. King at the height of the Angkorean period, Jayavarman VII ordered the construction of 102 hospitals in his realm. The founding stelae of certain of these hospitals reveal that they were not the equivalent of modern hospitals in terms of purpose and ideals, but rather more like contemporary almshouses of Europe, places for the poor to find shelter, food, and some care.[6] These hospitals disappeared at the end of the Angkorean period, marking the end of state-supported medical care until the arrival of the French colonial period. Under the colonial period, the French medical establishment largely ignored TM as it undertook various state-sponsored medical programs.[7] However, institutional support of TM continued within the religious realm. Until recently, the strongest organized base for TM was the

Theravada Buddhist *sangha;* monks were and are frequently known as healers, although more often the *achaar* (roughly, the lay abbott) is attributed healing powers. Beyond the *sangha,* healers existed in all ranks of Khmer society, and varied in their specialties and skills from spirit medium to simple herbalist. The majority of today's recognized traditional medicine practitioners (TMPs) likely derive from learned practitioners (*kru khmer*) who used palm-leaf manuscript recipes for medicines.[8]

In common with most of Southeast Asia, the evolution of medical theories in Cambodia reflects the syncretic nature of the local cultures. Contemporary traditional medical theories derive from various external influences, as well as local knowledge. Changes in learned medical theories can be traced to waves of influence from cultures of the north and east. For example, court medicine prior to the Angkorean period was strongly influenced by Hindu-based Ayurvedic theory from India, and the highest doctors of the royal court were Brahmins.[9] By the era of Jayavarman's 102 hospitals (1181–1200 CE), Mahayana Buddhism had been introduced into Cambodia and integrated into indigenous medical theory.

Influences as wide-ranging as Ayurveda, animism, and Theravada Buddhism are still integral to TM today. If one considers also the variety of ethnic groups in Cambodia, this picture becomes more complicated. For example, the Cham are strongly influenced by Islamic medical theories, while the Sino-Khmer and Vietnamese populations rely more upon Traditional Chinese Medicine. The general understanding of the human spirit reflects this dual local and foreign nature of medical theory. A human being has 19 *praluung* (vital spirit or consciousness) and four *cato phut* (major essence). The theory of *praluung* appears to be autochthonous to the region, while the *cato phut* are likely derived from Ayurveda.[10] These elements of the human spirit, particularly the *praluung,* can wander off or be lured away from their host. Their extended absence will lead to illness in the host, requiring a ritual ceremony to recall the vital spirit to its owner.[11] Other prevailing concepts that have both local and foreign aspects include the theory of *kchaal* (wind) in the body; the physiological balance of hot and cold, and "roasting" postpartum women.[12]

In the same vein, TM practices are also eclectic. Ritual, tattooage, herbal medicines (naturopathy), taboos, massage, coinage, moxibustion, and totems (lustral water, amulets) are all used in Khmer TM, most in some combination.[13] Ill health can have both natural and supernatural causes, thus treatment is often multifaceted as well. For example, a cold may be caused by a problem of *kchaal* brought about by wrong behavior. Coinage or moxibustion would be required to correct the imbalance of *kchaal*, while an offering to a guardian spirit or some other ritualistic atonement would be an additional treatment to efface the wrong behavior. In the past few decades, more intangible and supernatural practices are being marginalized in favor of herbal medicine and physical manipulation of the body (massage and moxibustion), aspects of TM more complementary to the empirical basis of western medicine and the funding practices of international public health organizations.

The value of a locally-derived medical knowledge and practices is fiercely defended in post-colonial nations world-wide, and Southeast Asia is no exception. While TM practitioners in Cambodia have been collecting and publishing their knowledge for the last twenty years, the founding of a program supported by the state and foreign government funding marks a new level in the search for recognition and indeed survival by TM in the modern world of international public health. However, these changes are accompanied by a fundamental restructuring and redefinition of Cambodian TM, as TMPs attempt to gain wider legitimacy and professional status. It remains to be seen if Khmer health-seeking behaviors will follow.

Notes

1. The Nippon Foundation, "Program List for Asia," available at http://www.nippon foundation.or.jp/ eng/worldwide/program/region_asia.html (accessed August 30, 2012).

2. World Health Organization, "Beijing Declaration," available at http://www.who.int/medicines/areas/traditional/congress/beijing_declaration/en/ (accessed August 28, 2012). As the Declaration illustrates, the WHO and its member nations have become increasingly cognizant of the importance of traditional medicine in many cultures of the world. The Declaration encourages nation-states to protect and promote traditional medicine as part of a national healthcare agenda.

3. World Health Organization, "Traditional Medicine," available at http://www.who.int/mediacentre/factsheets/fs134/en/ (accessed August 28, 2012).

4. This, too, has been parsed out and disputed within medical anthropological literature, where there was an effort to distinguish organized medical systems in Cambodia from folk practices. M. Piat, "Médecine Populaire au Cambodge," *Bulletin de la Sociéte des Etudes Indochinoises* 40 (1965): 1–15, M. A. Martine, "Elements de Medicine Traditionnelle Khmer," *Seksa Khmer* 1, no. 6 (1983): 135–70.

5. Even with this broad definition, we must make exceptions for practices and substances borrowed from western medicine but used outside the biomedical paradigm, such as injections and many pharmaceutical drugs. For a public health review, see S. Vong, J. F. Perz, S. Sok, S. Som, S. Goldstein, Y. Hutin and J. Tulloch, "Rapid assessment of injection practices in Cambodia, 2002," *BMC Public Health* 5 (2005): 56, available at http://www.biomedcentral .com/1471-2458/5/56. For a historical review of injection practices in Indochina, see A. Guénel, "La Lutte Antivariolique en Extrême-Orient: Ruptures et continuité," in *L'Aventure de la Vaccination*, ed. A. M. Moulin (Paris: Fayard, 1996), 82–94.

6. B. Menaut, *Matière Médicale Cambodgienne. Indochine Française. Section des Services d'Intérêt Social. Inspection Générale des Services Sanitaires et Médicaux de l'Indochine, editor. Exposition Coloniale Internationale* (Hanoi: Imprimerie d'Extrême–Orient, 1931). According to the stelae of Say Fong, two doctors at each hospital were assisted by a staff of over a hundred assistants, guards, supplicants, and cooks. See also George Coedès, "Les hôpitaux de Jayavarman VII," *BEFEO* 40 (1940): 344–47, and C. Jacques, "Les édits des hôpitaux de Jayavarman VII," *Etudes Cambodgiennes* 13 (1968): 14–17.

7. S. Au, *Mixed Medicines: Health and Culture in French Colonial Cambodia* (Chicago: University of Chicago Press, 2011).

8. M. Piat, "Médecine Populaire au Cambodge," *Bulletin de la Sociéte des Etudes Indochinoises* 40, no. 4 (1965): 1–15. M. A. Martine, "Elements de Medicine Traditionnelle Khmer," *Seksa Khmer* 1 (1983): 135–70. Most medical texts were written on palm-leaf manuscripts (a subset of *kbuon*). They serve mostly as compilations, seemingly in hodge-podge order, of medical recipes. In last twenty years, traditional medical practitioners have published several collections of such recipes in an attempt to preserve and promote their beliefs. Also in the post-UNTAC period, public health NGOs have been active in collecting such information.

9. R. Chhem entry on Yajnavaraha in W. F. Bynum, H. Bynum eds., *Dictionary of Medical Biography*. Vol. 5 (Westport: Greenwood Press 2007), 1331–32.

10. A. Choulean, "Apports Indiens à la Médecine Traditionnelle Khmère," *Journal of the European Ayurvedic Society* 2 (1992): 101–13.

11. P. Bitard, *Le Monde du Sorcier au Cambodge* (Paris: Editions du Seuil, 1966); E. Porée-Maspero, "La Cérémonie de l'Appel des Esprits Vitaux Chez les Cambodgiens," *BEFEO* 45, no. 1 (1951): 145–83.

12. M. A. Martine, "Elements de Medicine Traditionnelle Khmer," *Seksa Khmer* 1 (1983): 135–70; M. Muecke, "An Explanation of 'Wind Illness' in Northern Thailand," *Culture, Medicine and Psychiatry* 3, no. 3 (1979): 267–300; P. White, "Heat, Balance, Humors, and Ghosts: Postpartum in Cambodia," *Health Care for Women International* 25, no. 2 (2004): 179–94.

13. E. Aymonier, *Notes Sur les Coutumes et Croyances Superstitieuses des Cambodgiens*. (Paris: Centre de Documentation et de Recherche sur la Civilisation Khmere, 1984); O. Chan, "Contribution à L'étude de la Therapeutique Traditionnelle au Pays Khmer: These pour le doctorate en medicine," (M.D. thesis, Faculte de Médecine de Paris; 1955); R. K. Chhem, "Medicine and Culture in Ancient Cambodia," *The Singapore Biochemist* 13 (2000): 23–27; A. Forest, *Le*

Culte des Genies Protecteurs au Cambodge: Analysis et traduction d'un corpus de textes sur les neak ta (Paris: Harmattan; 1992); B. Menaut, "Matière Médicale Cambodgienne," in *Exposition Coloniale Internationale,* ed. Indochine Française. Section des Services d'Intérêt Social. Inspection Générale des Services Sanitaires et Médicaux de l'Indochine (Hanoi: Imprimerie d'extrême-orient, 1931); A. Souyris-Rolland, "Les Procédés Magiques d'Immunisation Chez les Cambodgiens," *Bulletin de la Sociéte des Etudes Indochinoises* 26 (1951): 175–87.

Luang Wongsa, the chief of royal physicians was not only enthusiastic about learning new science, but eager to experiment and use it in his practice. As the efficacy of Western medicine was increasingly apparent in vaccination against smallpox, treatment of cholera, in obstetrics and postpartum care, as well as in surgery, the Siamese elite quickly understood the inevitability of change and the necessity of learning new science. Traditional medical knowledge long passed down by the House of Snidvongs had been abandoned by the third generation, when Krom Luang Wongsa's grandson earned his medical degree from Europe and embarked upon a new career in modern medicine. Thus ended the knowledge tradition once carried on through the members of the House of Snidvongs.

Notes

1. Craig A. Lockard, "'The Sea Common to All': Maritime Frontiers, Port Cities, and Chinese Traders in the Southeast Asian Age of Commerce, ca. 1400–1750," *Journal of World History* 21, no. 2 (2010): 228; and Anthony Reid, *Southeast Asia in the Age of Commerce 1450–1680,* vol. 2, *Expansion and Crisis* (New Haven, CT: Yale University Press, 1993), 64–67.

2. David K. Wyatt, *Thailand: A Short History,* 2nd ed. (Bangkok, Silkworm, 2003), 98–104; Rong Syamananda, *A History of Thailand,* 2nd ed. (Bangkok: Thai Watana Panich, 1973), 71–83; Leonard Y. Andaya, "Interactions with the Outside World and Adaptation in Southeast Asian Society, 1500–1800," in *The Cambridge History of Southeast Asia,* vol. 1, *From Early Times to c. 1800,* ed. Nicholas Taring (Singapore: Cambridge University Press, 1992), 345–401; Chatichai Muksong and Komatra Chuengsatiansup, "Medicine and Health in Thai Historiography: From an Elitist View to Counter-Hegemonic Discourse," in *Global Movements, Local Concerns: Medicine and Health in Southeast Asia,* ed. Laurence Monnais and Harold J. Cook (Singapore: NUS Press, 2012), 226–45.

3. For more information about Phaulkon, see George A. Sioris, *Phaulkon: The Greek First Counsellor at the Court of Siam: An Appraisal* (Bangkok: The Siam Society, 1998).

4. Dhiravat Na Pombejra, *Siamese Court Life in the Seventeenth Century as Depicted in European Sources,* International Series 1 (Bangkok: Faculty of Arts Chulalongkorn University, 2001), 169. See also Dhiravat Na Pombejra, "Ayutthaya as a Cosmopolitan Society: A Case Study of Daniel Brochebourde and His Descendants," in *Kham yok yon khong pra wat ti sat pi pit ni pon ched chu kiet sat tra jan mom chao Subhasdis Diskul* [Problems in Thai history: Essays in honor of HSH Prince Subhasdis Diskul on the occasion of his seventy-second birthday anniversary], ed. Winai Pongsripian (Bangkok: n.p., 1994), 294–310.

5. Adrien Launay, *Pra wat mit sang krung siam* [originally published as *Histoire de la mission de Siam, 1662–1811: Documents historiques*], trans. Paul Xavier (Bangkok: Bangkok Archdiocese, 2003), 23.

6. Somrat Charuluxananan and Vilai Chentanez, "History and Evolution of Western Medicine in Thailand," *Asian Biomedicine* 1 (2007): 98.

7. Simone de La Loubère, *A New Historical Relation of the Kingdom of Siam* (Kuala Lumpur: Oxford University Press, 1969), 62. (Quoted as it appears in the original.)

8. Launay, *Pra wat mit sang krung siam*, 59.

9. Somdet Krom Praya Damrong Rajanuphap, preface to *Tam ra phra o-sot phra narai* [King Narai's Medical Treatise], somdet pra barom rachininat prod kao hai pim pra rat cha tan nai ngan sop phrayapaetpongsa (nak rotchanaphaet) peemaseng pho sor 2460 (Bangkok: Sophonpipatthanakan, 1917), (2)–(4); *Tam ra phra o-sot phra narai* [King Narai's Medical Treatise], pim pen a nu son nai ngan pra rach than ploeng sop ngang khai sri thongthio na meru wat Makutkasatriyaram wan athit thi 29 karakadakom 2533 (Bangkok: n.p., 1990), 7–8.

10. Chayan Pichiensoonthorn, Manmaas Chawalit, and Wichien Jeerawong, *Kham a thi bai tam ra phra o-sot phra narai* [Explanation of King Narai's Medical Treatise] (Bangkok: Amarin, 2001).

11. Prateep Chumpol, *Pra wat sart kan pat pan thai: kan suk sa jak tmara ya* [History of Thai traditional medicine: Study from Medical Treatise], (Bangkok: Odain Store, 2011), 49–50.

12. Chaophraya Thiphakonrawong (Kham Bunnag), *Phra rat cha pong saw a dan krung rattanakosin rat cha kan thi 1 cha bab chao pra ya thip pha kon ra wong cha bab tua khian* [Chronicle of Rattanakosin in the reign of the King Rama I in the edition of Chao Phaya Thiphakorawong manuscript edition], duplicate of original manual script, Naruemon thirawat, ed. Nidhi Eoseewong (Bangkok, Ammarin Vichakarn, 1996), 210.

13. Royal Physicians Department, *Tam ra pra osot krang rat cha kan thi song* [Treatise of medicine in the reign of King Rama II] (Bangkok: Sophonpipatthanakorn, 1916); see also Prateep Chumpol, *Pra wat sart kan pat pan thai: kan suk sa jak tmara ya* [History of Thai Traditional Medicine: Study from Medical Treatise], (Bangkok, Odain Store, 2011), 82–83.

14. William Lee Bradley, *Siam Then: The Foreign Colony in Bangkok before and after Anna*. (California: William Carey Library, 1981), 46.

15. Piyanat Bunnag, Waraporn Chiochaisak, Sunant Anchaleenukun and Nawawan Wutthakun, *200 pi pra chao barom wong ther Krom Luang Wongsa Dhiraj Snid: Pra dam ri lae kor ra nee ya kit tor pra thet chat* [200 Years of Krom Luang Wongsa Dhiraj Snid: Thoughts and works for his country], chut pim nueng nai ngan cha long 200 pi wan khai wan pra sut pra chao barom wong ther Krom Luang Wongsa Dhiraj Snid (Bangkok: Committee of Books and Souvenirs, 2008), 21.

16. Piyanat Bunnag et al., *200 pi pra chao barom wong ther Krom Luang Wongsa Dhiraj Snid*, 23.

17. Orawan Sapploy, *Phra baromwong ther Krom Luang Wongsa Dhiraj Snid prat pu pen kam lang khong phan din* [Krom Luang Wongsa Dhiraj Snid: Sophist of the nation] (Bangkok: Sangsan Book, 2009), 17–20.

18. Orawan Sapploy, *Phra baromwong ther Krom Luang Wongsa Dhiraj Snid*, 25.

19. Piyanat Bunnag et al., *200 pi pra chao barom wong ther Krom Luang Wongsa Dhiraj Snid*, 29.

20. Yuwadee Tapaneeyakorn, "Wi watt ha na kan khong kan pat thai tang tae sa mai ruem ton chon thueng sin sud rat cha kan pra bat som det phra chun la chom kao chao yu hau" [The evolution of Thai medicine from its beginning until the end of the reign of King Chulalongkorn] (MA thesis, Chulalongkorn University, 1979), 54–65.

21. Piyanat Bunnag et al., *200 pi pra chao barom wong ther Krom Luang Wongsa Dhiraj Snid*, 30.

22. Monsignor Jean-Baptiste Pallegoix, *Description of the Thai Kingdom of Siam: Thailand under King Mongkut*, trans. Walter E. Tips (Bangkok: White Lotus, 2000), 180.

23. Orawan Sapploy, *Phra baromwong ther Krom Luang Wongsa Dhiraj Snid*, 32.

24. *Bot la kon rueng phra ma hle the thai rueng a nu rut roi rueng rueng ra den lan dai klon pleng yao rueng mom ped sa wan rueng pra a kan pra chuan khong krom muen apson su da thep* [Anthology of plays: *Phra ma hle the thai, 100 story of Anurut, Ra den Lan dai, Poem on Mom ped sa wan,* and *Poem on account of HRH Krom Muen Apson Suda Thep's illness*], 2nd ed. (Bangkok: Silpabannakan, 1971), 143–45.

25. *Bot la kon rueng*, 166.

26. Orawan Sapploy, *Phra baromwong ther Krom Luang Wongsa Dhiraj Snid*, 34–35.

27. The full name of Krom Luang Wongsa is spelled differently by different authors. In this article, spellings from different sources were kept as they appeared in the original texts.

28. "Krom Hluang Wongsa Dhiraj Snid," *Illustrirte Zeitung* 960 (November 23, 1861): 376–77, trans. Chanthima Kroegsuwannachai in *Pra Ong Nuam chad chan ka wee: pra chum pra nip on pra chao barom wong ther Krom Luang Wongsa Dhiraj Snid* [Prince Nuam, the versed poet: Collected works of Krom Luang Wongsa Dhiraj Snid], ed. Wilaiwan Somsopon (Khon Kaen: Phra ma ha cha nok Funds, Khon Kaen University), (9)–(12). (Translation ours.)

29. John Bowring, *The Kingdom and People of Siam; with a Narrative of the Mission to that Country in 1855* (London: John W. Parker, 1857), 2:228–29.

30. Townsend Harris, *The Complete Journal of Townsend Harris, First American Consul General and Minister to Japan* (New York: Doubleday, Doran and Company, 1930), 112.

31. Dan Beach Bradley, *Abstract of the Journal of Rev. Dan Beach Bradley, M.D., Medical Missionary in Siam 1835–1973*, ed. George Haws Feltus (Cleveland, OH: Multigraph Department of Pilgrim Church, 1936), 67.

32. Bradley, *Abstract of the Journal of Rev. Dan Beach Bradley*, 148.

33. Orawan Sapploy, *Phra baromwong ther Krom Luang Wongsa Dhiraj Snid*, 109.

34. Bowring, *The Kingdom and People of Siam*, 2:293–94.

35. William Maxwell Wood, *Fankwei; or the San Jacinto in the Seas of India, China and Japan* (New York: S. Harper and Brothers, 1859), 150.

36. Harris, *The Complete Journal*, 113.

37. Max Von Brandt, *Dreiunddreissig Jahre on Ost-Asien. Erinnerungen eines deutshen Diplomaten*, vol. 1 (Leipzig: Georg Wigand, 1901).

38. Thomas D. (Thomas Dent) Mütter, *Syllabus of the Course of Lectures on the Principles and Practice of Surgery: Delivered in the Jefferson Medical College, Philadelphia* (Philadelphia: Barrett and Jones, 1846), 75. Also available at the U.S. National Library of Medicine website, collections.nlm.nih.gov/catalog/nlm:nlmuid-66841570R-bk.

39. "An Account of the Most Lamentable Illness and Death of Her Young and Amiable Majesty, the Queen Somanass Waddhanawathy, the Lawful Royal Consort of His Most Gracious Majesty somdetch Phra Paramender Maha Mongkut, the Reigning King of Siam," appendix 3 in Abbot Low Moffat, *MongKut, the King of Siam* (Ithaca, NY: Cornell University Press,1961), 213–14.

40. Bradley, *Siam Then*, 83–84.

41. Prachot Plengwithaya, *Phe sut cha kam haeng krung rat ta na ko sin nai rob 200 pi* [Pharmacy of Ratthanakosin era in the time of the bicentennial] (Bangkok: Faculty of Pharmaceutical Sciences Chulalongkorn University, 1983), 39. See more descriptions in Prateep Chumpol, *Pra wat sart kan pat pan thai*, 110–11, 119–28..

42. *Tamra sap pa kun ya cha bap khong Krom Luang Wongsa Dhiraj Snid* [Krom Luang Wongsa Dhiraj Snid's pharmacopoeia], in *Tamra pra o-sot pra narai* [King Narai's Medical Treatise], pim pen a nu son nai ngan pra rach than ploeng sop ngang khai sri thongthio na meru wat Makutkasatriyaram wan athit thi 29 karakadakom 2533 (Bangkok: n.p., 1990), 134. (Translation ours.)

43. Prachot Plengwithaya, *Phe sut cha kam haeng krung rat ta na ko sin nai rob 200 pi*, 139.

44. National Library, *Tamra Krom Luang Wongsa Dhiraj Snid* [Treatise of Krom Luang Wongsa Dhiraj Snid], manuscript, Medical Collection W no. 6. Quoted in Prachote plenwitthakom, *Phe sut cha kam haeng krung rat tan a ko sin nai rob 200 pi* [Pharmacy of Ratthanakosin era in the time of the bicentennial], 140–41.

45. Somdet Krom Praya Damrong Rajanuphap, *Nithan bo ran kha di* [Ancient tale] (Bangkok: Samakkhisan, 2000), 224–25. (Translation ours.)

46. Saichon Sattayanurak, *Put tha sas sa na kab naeo kit thang kan mueng nai rat cha sa mai pra bat somdet phra phuttha yod fa chula lok (phor. sor. 2325–2352)* [Buddhism and Political Thought in the Reign of Somdet Phra Phuttha Yod Fah Chula Lok (King Rama 1), 1782–1809 AD] (Bangkok: Matichon, 2003), 90–94.

47. Krom Luang Wongsa Dhiraj Snid, *Klong ni rat phra pra thom pra tone* [Poem on the journey to Phar Pra Thom Phra Pra Tone Chedi (Stupa)] (Bangkok: Sophonpipatthakorn, 1922); see also Nidhi Eoseewong, "Wat tha na tham kra dum phi kab wan na kam ton rattanakosin" [Bourgeois culture and early Bangkok literature], in *Pak kai lae bai rue ruam kham riang wa dua prawat ti sat lae wan na kam ton rattanakosin* [Pen and sail literature and history in early Bangkok] (Bangkok: Ammarin, 1984), 203.

48. Nidhi Eoseewong, "Wat tha na tham kra dum phi kab wan na kam ton rattanakosin," 205–6.

49. Saichon Sattayanurak, *Put tha sas sa na kab naeo kit thang kan mueng nai rat cha sa mai pra bat somdet phra phuttha yod fa chula lok*, 112.

50. Kriangsak Chetpatanavanich, "Pra wat mor bradley" [Biography of Dr. Dan Beach Bradley], in *Mor bradley kab sang kom thai* [Dr. Dan Beach Bradley and Thai society], Paper no. 57 for Thai Study Project Chulalongkorn University and Thai Study Institute Thammasart University Seminar, at Multipurpose Building Thammasart University, July, 16–17, 1985 (Bangkok: Thai Study Institute, Thammasart University, 1995), 8–9.

51. John Crawfurd, *Journal of an Embassy from the Governor-General of India to the Courts of Siam and Cochin China* (Singapore: Oxford University Press, 1987), 124.

52. Bradley, *Siam Then*, 24.

53. Bradley, *Siam Then*, 25.

54. Chaophraya Thiphakonrawong (Kham Bunnag), *Pra rat cha pong sa wa dan krung rattanakosin rat cha kan thi 2 cha bab chao pra ya thip pha kon ra wong cha bab tua khian*, [Chronicle of Rattanakosin in the reign of the King Rama II in the edition of Chao Phaya Thiphakorawong manuscript edition], duplicate of original manual script, Naruemon Thirawat, ed. Nidhi Eoowsriwong (Bangkok: Ammarin Vichakarn, 2005), 85–87.

55. George Haws Feltus, *Samuel Reynolds House of Siam, Pioneer Medical Missionary, 1847–1876* (Bangkok: White Lotus, 2007), 48.

56. Feltus, *Samuel Reynolds House of Siam*, 50.

57. Feltus, *Samuel Reynolds House of Siam*, 53.

58. Feltus, *Samuel Reynolds House of Siam*, 57–59.

59. *The Bangkok Recorder*, vol. 1, no. 10, July 22, 1865, in Office of His Majesty's Principal Private Secretary, *Nang sue chot mai het* [The *Bangkok Recorder*] (Bangkok: Office of His Majesty's Principal Private Secretary, 1994), 133.

60. Bradley, *Siam Then*, 49.

61. Bradley, *Siam Then*, 27.

62. Bradley, *Siam Then*, 27–28.

63. Feltus, *Samuel Reynolds House of Siam*, 114–15.

64. Feltus, *Samuel Reynolds House of Siam*, 115–16 (Quoted as it appears in the original.)

65. Malcolm Smith, *A Physician at the Court of Siam* (Kuala Lumpur: Oxford University Press 1982), 59.

66. Somdet Krom Praya Damrong Rajanuphap, *Nithan bo ran kha di*, 217.

67. Somdet Krom Praya Damrong Rajanuphap, *Nithan bo ran kha di*, 218.

68. Smith, *A Physician at the Court of Siam*, 59.

69. Nidhi Eoseewong, "Wat tha na tham kra dum phi kab wan na kam ton rattanakosin," 214–15.

70. Nidhi Eoseewong, "Wat tha na tham kra dum phi kab wan na kam ton rattanakosin," 214–15.

71. Phrabat Somdej Phra Chom Klao Chaoyuhua, Prince T. Y. Chaufa Monkut, to Mr. & Mrs. Eddy of New York, November 18, 1849, in *Pra rat cha hat tha le kha Phrabat Somdej Phra Chom Klao Chaoyuhua* [Collection of Letters of King Monkut], pim nai ngan cha long krop 84 pi ma ha monkut rat cha wit tha y alai nai pra ba rom ra chu pha tham 1–5 tu la kom 1978 (Bangkok: Mahamakut Buddhist University 1978), 12–13 (Quoted as it appears in the original.)

72. Orawan Sapploy, *Phra baromwong ther Krom Luang Wongsa Dhiraj Snid*, 353.

73. Somdet Krom Praya Damrong Rajanuphap, "Prawat nai phan tri M. R. Suvabhan Sanitwongsa" [Biography of Major M. R. Suvabhan Sanitwongsa], preface to *Rueng khao khong pra thet siam* [The rice of Siam], by M. R. Suvabhan Sanitwongsa, pimp nai ngan pra rat cha than ploeng sop nai phan tri mom rat cha wong Suvabhan Sanitwongsa Na Ayuthaya (Bangkok: Sophonpipatthanakon, 1927), (3)–(4).

74. Somdet Krom Praya Damrong Rajanuphap, "Prawat nai phan tri M. R. Suvabhan Sanitwongsa," (4).

75. Somdet Krom Praya Damrong Rajanuphap, "Prawat nai phan tri M. R. Suvabhan Sanitwongsa," (4)–(5).

76. Somdet Krom Praya Damrong Rajanuphap, *Kham song cham* [Memoir] (Bangkok: Matichon, 2003), 173.

77. Somdet Krom Praya Damrong Rajanuphap, "Prawat nai phan tri M. R. Suvabhan Sanitwongsa," (7)–(8).

78. *Tam ra phra o-sot phra narai* (Bangkok: n.p., 1990), 7.

79. *Tam ra phra o-sot phra narai* (Bangkok: n.p., 1990), 7.

PART II
HEALTH AND CRISIS

2 Pilgrim Ships and the Frontiers of Contagion

Quarantine Regimes from Southeast Asia to the Red Sea

Eric Tagliacozzo

Disease was an important yardstick in how Europeans conceptualized the rest of the world during the past several hundred years.[1] This was particularly so as the Industrial Age wore on, and definite links started to be established between sanitation and public health in the metropolitan capitals of the West.[2] Yet, as Myron Echenberg has shown to such devastating effect in his book *Plague Ports*, the industrialization of steam-shipping, increased transoceanic travel, and global commerce all went hand in hand, and in fact facilitated the spread of pathogens on a heretofore unparalleled scale.[3] Technology enabled the spread of virulent microbes in ways that previously would have taken much longer periods of time. The non-West may have been seen as filthy, diseased, and dangerous by Europeans, therefore, but in the very act of conquering the rest of the world with state-of-the-art technologies, the West also laid some of the preconditions necessary for a number of diseases to spiral out of control.

In this chapter, the nexus between the Hajj and health is examined, particularly through the lens of cholera (and other diseases) that traveled on the steamships that made the pilgrimage to Mecca possible from places like Southeast Asia. Hajjis made these journeys by ship during the colonial period in vast numbers, and the prospect of contagion traveling on the wings of the Hajj became one of the great health issues of the late nineteenth and early twentieth centuries. I analyze this state of affairs by providing a brief section of background on both cholera and on the structures that were put into place to try to control it, before narrowing the field of vision down to the Red Sea region, asking how a regime was enacted to deal with the disease as it spread every year on the myriad ships that pulled into Jeddah. Subsequent divisions in the essay then examine how the Middle Eastern theater of disease-control was mirrored in varied and either effective or ineffective ways in Dutch and British Southeast Asia, respectively. The fight against cholera on the Hajj became a global phenomenon, with the center of action remaining focused on the Red Sea, and important tendrils of prophylaxis stretching all the way to small villages in distant Muslim lands, such as parts of Southeast Asia. Yet this fight also became very much a European crusade as well, as the disease was terrifying in its outcomes and was acknowledged as all too penetrative to Western societies as well. For this reason a huge period literature is available to read in French, Dutch, Italian, and English, as the European powers sought to manage the Hajj on the grounds of global epidemiological survival, as well as a host of other related concerns.

Cholera and the Road to Ruin

There are, perhaps, few worse ways to die than through contracting cholera. The disease moves with astonishing swiftness: a healthy human being can contract cholera and be dead less than a day later. The primary symptom is a loss of the body's fluids: extreme diarrhea is accompanied with small white particles—which are actually parts of the intestinal lining literally peeling off of the afflicted body—floating in the victim's stool. Once the diarrhea starts, vomiting is never far behind, and the subject starts to lose at an alarming rate the 90 percent fluidity that makes up the substance of all human beings. The body begins to painfully cramp from the loss of water; eventually patients turn blue and sallow, the eyes sinking farther and farther into the skull (yet actually at the same time protruding) because the body itself is shrinking so quickly. Descriptions of people with cholera are horrific. Left untreated, close to 50 percent of cholera's victims succumb fatally to the disease. It is contracted by drinking the bacterium *Vibrio cholerae* in unclean water, almost always as a result of feces appearing in a common, public water supply. This fact was discovered by the German physician Robert Koch in 1883, but by that time cholera had already ravaged large swaths of the world for over half a century. It was first noticed in 1817 when it spread from the Gangetic plain in India and then started to move wherever Indian laborers were sent to perform manual labor as coolies. The pilgrimage to Mecca by sea was almost tailor-made for cholera to thrive and then spread: the disease found in the nineteenth-century Hajj the perfect vehicle to survive and imprint its misery on millions of human beings, all of them in perilously close contact in the holds of slow-moving ships.[4]

In 1821 cholera was found in Arabia for the first time, and it is likely that it came to the Arabian Peninsula from India via the Persian Gulf. Ten years later, in 1831, it was in the Hejaz, and after this date cholera became a mainstay on the pilgrimage routes, with the sea a particularly dangerous conduit because of the sanitation and close proximity of pilgrims on crowded vessels. The 1831 epidemic in the Hejaz killed twenty thousand people, and subsequent epidemics came to the region of the Holy Cities in 1841, 1847, 1851, 1856–57, and 1859. Cholera had entered Europe during the middle decades of the nineteenth century as well, although it likely came not through the Middle East but rather over the Eurasian steppe, from Russia eventually into Germany. However the 1865 epidemic was so powerful in the Hejaz and did such eventual damage not only in Europe but all the way west to the United States that the Hajj became a matter of international concern, and huge scrutiny. Fumigant devices, new disinfection techniques, and the distillation of water on a mass scale all were experimented with on a very short timeframe to try to combat the disease.[5] Yet cholera continued to plague the pilgrimage routes to Mecca, and there were further outbreaks of the disease in 1883, 1889, 1891, and 1893. The epidemic of 1893 was catastrophic in scale and in the impression it left on horrified European observers. After this time international arrangements to try to deal with the disease were rushed forward, when bickering and mistrust between the emerging European powers had been the rule before.[6] And it was not just cholera but also smallpox, malaria, dengue fever, and amoebic dysentery that were also in grim evidence during the annual months of the Hajj, ensuring that the pilgrimage and disease were manifestly equated with each other in the consciousness of the West at this time.[7]

The most obvious physical result of this history of infection and misery over several decades was the establishment of quarantine stations at several points in and around the Red Sea and the Holy Cities. Several of these stations were erected for land caravans, but the more important ones (from a numerical point of view given the steady stream of pilgrims passing through them) were on either side of the Red Sea waterway. The single most important station was on the barren, tiny island of Kamaran, not far off the Yemeni coast.[8] Kamaran became the central locus for trying to combat the effects of cholera and other diseases attendant on maritime Hajj traffic. It was particularly important for Southeast Asians, as almost all pilgrims from the "lands beneath the winds" came on ships passing through Kamaran. The bare spit of land had an embarkation jetty, a disinfection station, buildings for administration services, a bacteriological laboratory, campsites for pilgrims to stay by the thousands while they awaited "cleansing," a choleric hospital, and a few small villages of fisherfolk who eked out a living from smuggling, pearling, or fishing in the blazing heat of the Tihama.[9] Pilgrims had to stay in Kamaran for anywhere between ten and fifteen days while the colonial or Ottoman authorities contented themselves that anyone sick with one of the more serious communicable diseases could be isolated (and hopefully cured, although many people who were sick enough after the long voyage from Southeast Asia never made it off the island alive). Kamaran had no banking facilities, and all pilgrims had to pay dues for the sanitary processes that were enforced on the island, so the entire procedure was cumbersome and rather inefficient.[10] In addition to this, there was constant wrangling between the various powers and Muslim interests in the Red Sea region as to who was to control Kamaran, its operations, and its revenues, a fact that receives almost as much ink in the period sources as the care of the countless pilgrims for whom the station was constructed.[11] This was the reality of the Hajj: pilgrimage, politics, disease, and revenue all were part of the same sprawling system.

Kamaran and the other quarantine stations in the Red Sea had been set up as part of the larger rubric of the sanitary conventions, a series of large-scale international meetings held to deal primarily with the threat of cholera (although other contagious diseases that were judged to be dangerous were also debated at these gatherings). The first of these meetings was held at Constantinople in 1866, and it eventually became known simply as "the cholera conference," because this pandemic was in fact the one on everyone's minds. Subsequent meetings were held every few years in Dresden (in 1883), in Venice (in 1892) and in Paris (in 1894), the latter of these coming about so soon after the Italian meeting because of the devastations wrought by cholera during the 1893 Hajj.[12] The substance of the sanitary regimes may have been epidemiological, but the mechanics of policy and enforcement were always going to be political in an era of rapidly expanding and aggressive imperial states. Some of this political maneuvering was between Europeans themselves, who saw the Middle East (and the Red Sea waterway in particular, especially after Suez opened in 1869) as part of the great game of international politics. Yet there was also a sense of playing the politics of the Hajj vis-à-vis the Muslim world as well, as the European powers tried to show Muslim populations who were increasingly restive (both in the Middle East, and in places like Southeast Asia) that the West held their best interests at heart. The emplacement of Muslim pilgrimage officers (who sometimes doubled as medical personnel) for each of the European powers in Jeddah in the 1920s was part of this general trend, although there were other reasons besides politics why these moves made good sense.[13] Yet politics as a rule was never very far away from the medical situation of the Hajj in the Hejaz, and this continued throughout the colonial period from the late nineteenth into the early twentieth century.

These are all bird's-eye, systemic visions of the pilgrimage and health maintenance in the age of cholera; it would be wrong to finish this subsection without a glance at how these matters operated at ground level, too. For this we can hope for no better source than the memoirs of doctors who were attendant on the Hajj in the Red Sea, either as medical professionals in situ or as members of epidemiological study tours, often under the patronage of the sanitary conventions themselves.[14] Of the spread of these examples perhaps no study is as useful as a social and epidemiological document as the memoir of Dr. M. Carbonell.[15] Carbonell saw the Hajj up close as a doctor in the Hejaz in the first decade of the twentieth century: his published memoir (recently rereleased out of Avignon) contains horrendous descriptions of the overcrowding, dirt, disease, and suffering of the ethnically mixed choleric populations of Arabia during that time. The disease was on the road to really being mapped and understood as a plague to humanity at this juncture, but the abilities of both the local Muslim governments and the European powers were not yet developed enough at the moment of his writing to fully eradicate cholera as a ghostly presence hovering over the global pilgrimage. Carbonell's account does stand out as a scientific and moral document, however, in a landscape of lower-class despair and rapidly shifting politics during the fin-de-siècle period. One gets a sense by reading through its pages that a corner was being turned in efforts against the disease. This does not mean that ignorance and superstition of cholera as a danger to the Hajj (and to Europe, ultimately) had disappeared—far from it. In the decades on either side of 1900 there was still plenty of misconception about the best way to tackle the nightmare of plagues such as this one.[16] But there was a growing sense that the problem could be examined, both in the laboratory and out in the field among the believers, and that the disease could be halted. This would not happen quickly, but by the end of the colonial period in the mid-twentieth century, cholera was a far less threatening problem than it had been for a century previously, even if the disease had not yet disappeared from the face of the earth.

The Dutch Connection: The Indies to the Desert

Very large numbers of the pilgrims who sailed into the Red Sea came from the Dutch East Indies, so knowledge and cognizance of the health situation in the Hejaz was a matter of yearly concern in Indonesia, despite these islands being half a world away from Arabia. We have very little knowledge of how cholera was dealt with by Indies populations (and indeed by Southeast Asians as a whole) before the advent of colonial record keeping. The *Koloniaal Verslag* (or Colonial report) for each year that was published in the Indies makes careful mention that chiefs of residencies were responsible for letting indigenes within their administrative orbits know the state of cholera in Mecca. This information included the charges for sanitary control in the Red Sea, as well as the possibility in certain years that Indies pilgrims would not be allowed in the Hejaz at all.[17] Yet what happened in the Indies themselves was one thing; regulating affairs from a health perspective on the long voyages across the Indian Ocean was quite another. This was the incubation chamber, as it were, for the worst of the infections to spread, as the pilgrims were cramped together into huge rusting steamships that crawled across the surface of the sea. For this reason strict care was paid to a number of details that might affect the health of those making the long voyages. Doctors were put aboard the pilgrim ships, and these men needed to have certain qualifications and experiences, by Indies law.[18] The decks of the steamships were to be made of wood or iron or steel, too, and the upper decks needed to be covered so as to ensure that pilgrims were not overexposed to the ferocious sun.[19] Adequate provisions also had to be reckoned for the whole voyage, not just the roughly three weeks that it took to get across the ocean, but also the ten days to two weeks that pilgrims could expect to be in quarantine, where they also needed to eat and drink (canned foods such as sardines and salmon were favored, as were dry goods such as biscuits, which did not go off in the heat of the Red Sea.[20] Medicines down to individual dosages and chemical minutae of prophylaxis and drug treatments were also legislated, so that outbreaks of infection could be dealt with quickly and efficiently by trained medical personnel on board.[21] Finally, a system of flags was instituted as well, so that any ship approaching port (or other vessels) flying a yellow flag was an immediate sign for caution. The flag meant that cholera or some other virulent, contagious sickness was on board—and that everyone should maintain a strict distance, on pain of the spread of the disease.[22]

When the Dutch ships finally pulled into Kamaran, most of the pilgrims were exhausted—they had been out at sea for weeks by this time, living in very close quarters and mostly at the mercy of the elements (and each other). Although every care was put forward to try to protect the passengers against epidemic, quite often the ships pulled into port with a number of sick people on board. The Dutch consul at Jeddah spent time at Kamaran during the pilgrimage seasons, and he made careful notes of the ships coming in, one by one, from the huge expanse of the Indian Ocean. Just one of these reports, from January 1938, gives an idea of the kind of reportage desired of this official. The *Clytoneus* arrived from Singapore on January 1 from Singapore; we know the tonnage, the number of passengers subdivided by gender and age (there were 680 in total), and the number of sick on board, as well as the nature and outcomes of the sicknesses. The *El Amin,* a much smaller ship, arrived the next day from Aden, and the *Buitenzorg* arrived on January 4 from Batavia, again with several deaths reported.[23] The entire system of Kamaran and its health procedures for Southeast Asian (and other) pilgrims became public knowledge and an issue debated in print, with a number of authors (writing in Dutch, French, and English, primarily) all giving window into how this vast medical apparatus stretched its radials of surveillance, maintenance, and care across the oceans.[24] Yet it is only by reading the detailed autobiographical accounts of some of these travelers, such as the Indies regent of Bandung, Raden Adipati Aria Wiranata Koesoma, that we get a more human sense of the scope of Kamaran and its operations. He finished his narrative of travels through Kamaran with the notice of two Indies children who died en route to Mecca, and who were buried in Jeddah, only a few miles from the destination they had traveled so far to see.[25]

Jeddah became the most important stopping point for the Dutch Indies pilgrims to organize themselves before they disappeared into the interior: it was a crucial way station for the Hajj, both for arriving and for leaving, and especially from a medical point of view. Because of this fact the Dutch spent a fair bit of time trying to decide on who would be their medical representatives in the city—the appointment was an important one, and officials from many levels of government seemed to have understood this very clearly. The portfolio was a large one and the responsibilities, given the seriousness of cholera in particular, were huge: during the month of Ramadan in 1933 more than five hundred patients passed through the Dutch clinic in the city, many of them sick with a number of debilitating diseases.[26] The Dutch medical facility was only one among four there: there was also an Arab station, a Russian station, and an English one, the latter staffed with a British-Indian (Muslim) doctor.[27] The Dutch establishment in the city had somewhere between sixty and one hundred beds, depending on whose letters we can believe, but even this was very limited, as the patients' families needed to provide for their loved ones (the Dutch gave the afflicted only small quantities of bread and milk).[28] The Dutch clinic did have a drug dispensary, however, and it ended up giving out medicines not only to Dutch subjects, but to a number of poor Arabs as well.

From Jeddah the Indies pilgrims would finally wind their way into the desert itself, and toward Mecca, Medina, and the other holy sites that made up the religious stations of the Hajj. The Dutch consul in Jeddah knew that realistically his facility was the last one where the pilgrims under his charge could expect to receive any real standard of care, as the medical stations farther on into the interior were less modern than his own. These latter facilities were staffed by Middle Eastern Muslim doctors as a rule because of religious prohibitions; the dispensary in Medina had an Egyptian doctor, for example, the one in Yambo was staffed by an Ottoman Turk, while the three in Mecca were all run by Syrian doctors.[29] In a report from November 1936 the Dutch consul told the Minister for Foreign Affairs in The Hague the kinds of diseases he was treating as the Hajj season progressed; he had just seen over one hundred patients, who had a variety of ailments ranging across the spectrum of disease (malaria, influenza, amoebic dysentery, gonorrhea, rheumic disease, lymph disease, laryngitis, acute bronchitis, bronchopneumonia, bronchial asthma, dental disorders, diarrhea, menstrual problems, and abscesses, etc.).[30] He tried to provide for their immediate needs, he explained, but also tried to give them things that they would likely need for the journey once they were out of his reach.[31] In this we can see something of the confluence of philanthropy and epidemiological self-interest of the Western regimes now firmly ensconced in the Hejaz, as they attempted to regulate the massive flood of pilgrims upon whose continuing health so much had come to depend.

The British Connection: The Malay Peninsula to the Holy Cities

In terms of health maintenance, the British Hajj from Southeast Asia mirrored the Dutch regime in many ways, although there were places in which the two projects differed. By the 1880s bills of health were being issued to pilgrim ships sailing from Singapore's harbor, and it is clear that part of the reason for this move was London's worried eye on Mecca, where plague was reported in the years before.[32] Singapore was expressly tasked to ensure its ships were cholera free, although the regulations were nowhere near foolproof at this date.[33] Corruption and avarice conspired to make this the case, the British Consul at Jeddah reported, and in an exasperated letter to his administrative superiors in Asia he expressly singled out shipping companies in Singapore for their negligence in allowing too many pilgrims on board in that port.[34] Many peasants in British Southeast Asia continued to avoid inpatient care in Western hospitals when possible, too, and preferred exposure to disease (often brought to the *desas* by pilgrims returning from the Hajj) to undergoing inoculations and prophylaxis.[35] In 1899 an entire company of British troops even stormed a Malay village with fixed bayonets, as the peasantry refused to allow a diseased body (and the corpse's house) to be fumigated and then burned.[36] The British in Southeast Asia only "bore the burden" of the Hajj because they felt they had to, although there was a concerted sense in local colonial circles that the entire exercise was much more trouble than it was worth, both from political and public health points of view. The High Commission in Malaya seems to have continued these attitudes (and practices) after the turn of the twentieth century in the high colonial era, when the health of pilgrims was still seen as a lodestone of sorts around the proverbial neck of Malaya's colonial overlords.[37]

Once the ships left British Southeast Asia and reached the high seas, many of the same issues were in play as with Dutch ships, which were paralleling the British-flagged ones across the Indian Ocean. Overcrowding was the serial killer of the vessels: a handwritten letter from the Dutch Consul in Jeddah to the Foreign Office in London described how captains turning a blind eye to extra pilgrims could quite literally net themselves small fortunes considering the scale of the voyages (only one hundred extra Hajjis would easily pay off any fine if the captain was caught overcrowding his ships, but since many of these vessels were several hundred souls over capacity, the lure of serious profits were on offer—and this was assuming the ship was caught at all, which many vessels were not).[38] The British colonial administration in Singapore fought a long battle with the steamship companies, and particularly the Alfred Holt line, to ensure that qualified doctors were on board every ship, though the doctors' salaries and any enforcement against overcrowding cut into the companies' profits.[39] As with the Dutch ships, everything from the number of passengers, the amounts of space each was to have, provisions for food and water, search procedures and fines were all laid out in meticulous detail.[40] Yet the imperfect understanding of how cholera and other infectious diseases spread still made the regulations (and enforcement) difficult, even as a fuller cognizance of containment regimes developed and was instituted in various ports along the international seaways. Fighting cholera even on British ships, the "best vessels in the world," took time: it was not a zero-sum outcome that was achieved in a day.

At Kamaran there were more ships flying British flags than of any other nation on earth. Many of these were from British Southeast Asia, and this was reflected in the fact that signs posted on the island often had Javanese or Malay inscribed upon them, since many Indies pilgrims chose to make their journeys via Penang or Singapore in British-owned bottoms.[41] The report of the civil administrator of Kamaran in 1939 even specified diseases that were particularly common among the "Malay races" coming to the island: paralysis, furunculosis, bronchopneumonia, and gangrene, in addition to the more common epidemic sicknesses.[42] The flow of ships from Straits Settlements and the Malay Peninsula was fairly relentless in the end, and the sanitary board on Kamaran made large sums of money from their taxes, which were well instituted into the system as part of the entire pilgrimage regime by the early twentieth century.[43] In the fin-de-siècle period the laws and acts enforcing the *cordon sanitaire* before the Holy Cities even stretched into gendered terms, with regulations spelling out how female passengers were to be searched, since many women were hidden away from the public by the older male members of their families.[44] In the years before the outbreak of World War II the payment of dues at Kamaran by Malayan pilgrims coming from the peninsula ended up totaling a very large amount of money—a sum that seems all the greater considering from how far away these Straits dollars had come. There were few competitors who could rival this Southeast Asian combination of cash and religiosity.[45]

In Jeddah, as was the case with Hajjis coming from the Dutch sphere of Southeast Asia, the British in Singapore and Malaya kept a close eye on disease vis-à-vis the health of their own pilgrims. The British in the tropics monitored the hospital situation for their charges from afar, noting down how many Hajjis were in formal medical care and what ailments they possessed while they were being treated in Jeddah's facilities.[46] Those Malay pilgrims who died in Jeddah had to be buried and their affairs arranged; one of the most important issues stemming from this situation (which did not happen infrequently) was that family members wished to get a refund on the Hajji's return ticket's passage, which was often considered a lot of money to many poor Malays. Only in the 1920s were procedures set up to amend existing shortcomings in this system, so that the half of the non-used ticket could be repatriated as a bank draft back to the deceased's family.[47] The confluence of health and financial concerns became more and more important, and this was especially so in wartime (for both World Wars), when the imperial powers—and particularly Britain—took extra steps to try to win over the "hearts and minds" of Southeast Asian pilgrims through programs such as these.[48] Jeddah became the clearing port, therefore, both for epidemiological matters and attendant administrative issues, both of which needed to be dealt with together.

The last step in this medical journey was the Holy Cities themselves, and here, too, the authorities in British Southeast Asia kept vigil on what was going on, despite the fact that nonbelievers were not even allowed into Mecca and Medina. Singapore knew very clearly when there was cholera in Mecca, not just in

Jeddah or Kamaran—reports circulated back and forth with the Foreign Office in London at such times, as they did with other outposts of the British Empire.[49] Right after the end of hostilities in World War I the British began to prepare detailed reports on individual diseases circulating in the holy sites, with separate folders on cholera, plague, typhus, and epidemic influenza, which had become a new nightmare after the pandemic of 1918.[50] Similarly, when World War II ended new energies could be spared for disease control again with regards to the Hajj, and new reports were commissioned on protecting Mecca and Medina by land nonbelievers quarantine, as well as by air quarantine.[51] The British High Commissioner in Kuala Lumpur engaged in discussions at this time with the British consul in Jeddah as to how to reduce the amount of time that Malay pilgrims might spend in the Hejaz—partially for political reasons, but also very much as an epidemiological precaution after a particularly grim death toll in the Hajj of 1951.[52] The confluence of health and the Hajj stretched even into the age of decolonization, therefore, and became an old issue facing a new world of independent Muslim states whose policies had been decided for them for decades by the imperial powers.

Conclusion

Diseases have often been ascribed to individual countries or races as a kind of national disgrace (the "English sweat"; the "Danish disease" (scurvy); the *morbus hungaricus*; the *plica polonica*).[53] One of the reasons that cholera is so interesting—and why it was also so exceedingly dangerous in the eyes of late-nineteenth- and early-twentieth-century humans—was that it was not identifiable with any particular group: it killed indiscriminately. Cholera may have had its origins in India, but the pilgrimage routes to and from Mecca were one of the main arteries that spread the disease. Although Western and Muslim societies had rather different concepts of what contagion might actually be at this time, it became clear that the most important task at hand was stopping cholera before it literally spiraled out of control and massacred entire civilizations.[54] Theories of how infection worked gradually progressed in Europe during the middle decades of the nineteenth century, and by the second half of the 1800s cholera itself was being used as a tool for social and economic analysis, propagating a number of conclusions that were reasonably correct about how cleanliness and physical proximity conspired to get people sick.[55] The medical pluralities that existed in places like the Ottoman world of this time made it difficult to enforce sanitary regimes, however, and increasingly European governments took it upon themselves to guarantee the overall health of the Hajj on a large, systems-wide basis.[56] This was accomplished as part of only a very slow process, however, with the very real difficulties of politics, nascent epidemiology, and enforcement militating against the saving of many thousands of lives. Cholera for many decades was an inescapable component of the Muslim pilgrimage; in other words, many people (both

Muslim and Western) were fatalistic about this, and the graves of members of both of these groups still litter the Hejaz as testament to this fact.

The transmission of cholera along the transoceanic pilgrimage routes in the late nineteenth and early twentieth centuries effectively rendered the Hajj as a dangerous institution, and perhaps a fatal one not only to the community of believers practicing its rites (the *umma*), but also to Westerners in general. Because of this the maintenance of public health measures as part of the global pilgrimage became a matter of pressing concern to the expanding imperial powers— and never more so than after years of particularly serious epidemic, such as 1831, 1865, and 1893. These three dates, roughly thirty years apart across the breadth of the nineteenth century, reminded all parties involved in the Hajj how serious the consequences of inaction really were, and attempts were increasingly made through the twentieth century to ameliorate the situation. Legislation was passed in the various colonial empires to try to rationalize shipping, and to maintain clean and adequate water supplies, as well as a modicum of space for individual pilgrims. Sanitary conventions were also held on a grand and repeated scale, giving rise to large public documents (and even larger reams of correspondence) as to how to control the radials of the Hajj from an epidemiological point of view. Finally, even land itself was commandeered for the purpose of quarantine stations, set up at semi-regular intervals wherever caravans (or caravans of ships) might pass into the Red Sea region and disgorge thousands upon thousands of pilgrims into the religious cities of the Hejaz. Stations like Kamaran became emblematic of the possibilities of the age: bacteriological laboratories, docking complexes, and limed-in gravesites all appeared within a few hundred meters of each other, and the ships in port flew the flags of many nations. In some ways this confluence suggests best the nature of the medical mountain that was there to climb, as the living, the sick, and the dead all passed through the same roads, on their way in or on their way out from the cities of the Prophet.

Notes

1. David Arnold, "Disease, Medicine and Empire," in *Imperial Medicine and Indigenous Societies,* ed. David Arnold (Manchester: Manchester University Press, 1988), 7.

2. Jean-Pierre Goubert, *The Conquest of Water: The Advent of Health in the Industrial Age* (Princeton, NJ: Princeton University Press, 1989), 58–67.

3. Myron Echenberg, *Plague Ports: The Global Bubonic Plague of 1906* (New York: New York University Press, 2007). For a review that puts this book into context with the rest of the Indian Ocean world, see Eric Tagliacozzo, "Underneath the Indian Ocean: A Review Essay," *Journal of Asian Studies* 67, no. 3 (2008): 1–8.

4. Period journal articles preserved in the New York Academy of Medicine's library are very useful in getting a sense of how cholera was appraised at the high point of the epidemic period. Some of the more important articles include S. W. Johnson, "Cholera and the Meccan Pilgrimage," *British Medical Journal* 1 (1895): 1218–19; A. Proust, "Le cholera de la Mer Rouge

en 1890," *Bulletin de l'académie de médecine* 3S 25 (1891): 421–45; "Cholera on Pilgrim Steamers at Camaran," *Lancet* 2 (1912): 913; "Small-pox and Cholera in the Pilgrimage," *Lancet* 1 (1910): 1792; "Cholera at Jiddah and Mecca," *US Public Health Report* 23, no. 1 (1908): 289; E. Rossi, "Il Hedjaz, il Pellegrinaggio e il cholera," *Gior. D. Soc. Ital. ig.* 4 (1882): 549–78; R. Bowman, "Cholera in Turkish Arabia," *British Medical Journal* 1 (1890): 1031–32; and "Cholera, the Haj and the Hadjaz Railway" *Lancet* 2 (1908): 1377. This is by no means an exhaustive list; there are dozens upon dozens of period sources available here.

5. C. Izzedine, *Le cholera el l'hygiene a la Mecque* (Paris: A. Maloine, 1909), 30–36.

6. D. Oslchanjetzki, "Souvenirs de l'epidemie de cholera au Hedjaz en 1893," in *Le pelerinage de la Mecque*, ed. F. Daguet (Paris: n.p., 1932), 297.

7. Izzedine, *Le cholera*, 9–11.

8. For an interesting history of this station, see Nigel Groom, "The Island of Two Moons: Kamaran 1954," *British-Yemeni Society Journal* 10 (2002): 29–37.

9. Rapport de la Commission des Lazarets Presente Au Conseil Superieur de Sante le 23/24 Aout 1896, Plan General des Lazarets de Camaran et Abou-Saad (Mer-Rouge) avec Planches, 1.2.4 Medische Aangelegenheden, Fiche #155: following page 15, ARA, Djeddah Archives.

10. See Colonial Secretary, Singapore to Government of India Department of Education, Health and Lands, 26 January 1928, #1202, in IOR/L/E/7/1513/File 4070, India Office Records, British Library.

11. Inter-Departmental Pilgrimage Quarantine Committee, 25 July 1922, E7501/113/91 in IOR/L/E/7/1908/File 7376, India Office Records, British Library.

12. For the details on these conferences, see William Roff, "Sanitation and Security: The Imperial Powers and the Nineteenth Century Hajj," *Arabian Studies* 6 (1982): 143–160.

13. See Government of India, Foreign and Political Department, to UK Consul, Jeddah, 25 January 1926, #482E, in "Kamaran: Establishment of Pilgrimage Officer" (1926), IOR/R/20/A/4121, India Office Records, British Library.

14. A list of just a few of the studies that I have found helpful in this respect are as follows: Dr. B. Schnepp, *Le pelerinage de la Mecque* (Paris: n.p., 1865); Dr. P. Remlinger, *Police sanitaire: Les conditions sanitaires du pelerinage musulman* (Paris: n.p., 1908); Dr. F. Duguet, *Le pelerinage de la Mecque au point de vue religieux, social et sanitaire* (Paris: n.p., 1932); and L. Couvy, *Le cholera et le pelerinage musulman au Hedjaz* (Paris: n.p., 1934).

15. Marcelin Carbonell, *Relation médicale d'un voyage de transport de pèlerins musulmans au Hedjaz 1907–1908* (Aix-en-Provence: Publications de l'Université de Provence, 2001).

16. See, for example, "Travaux originaux: Epidemiologie," *Gazette hebdomadaire de médecine et de chirurgie*, September 18, 1873, #38, 604; also "Sociétés savantes: Académie des Sciences," *Gazette hebdomadaire de médecine et de chirurgie*, 14 November 1873, #46, 734.

17. *Koloniaal Verslagen* 1872, 98; *Koloniaal Verslagen* 1875, 122.

18. *Bijblad* #11018, 1926, 362.

19. *Staatsblad* #557, 1912, 3; *Staatsblad* #507, 1937, 3.

20. Inspector for NEI to Captains of Pilgrimships of the Rotterdamsche Lloyd, 30 Jan. 1922, 1.2.4 Medische Aangelegenheden, Fiche #156, ARA, Djeddah Archives.

21. *Staatsblad* #597, 1923, 4–5.

22. *Staatsblad* #208, 1911, 1–2.

23. Maandrapport, Dutch Consul in Jeddah, Kamaran, January/February 1938, 1.2.4 Medische Aangelegenheden, Fiche #157, ARA, Djeddah Archives.

24. J. Eisenberger, *Indie en de Bedevaart naar Mekka* (Leiden: M. Dubbeldeman, 1928), 103–11.

25. G. A. van Bovene, *Mijn Reis Naar Mekka: Naar het Dagboek van het Regent van Bandoeg Raden Adipati Aria Wiranata Koesoma* (N.p.: n.p., 1924), 38.

26. Medical Service of the Dutch Consulate, Mecca, to Dutch Consulate, Jeddah, 31 December 1933, #5, 1.2.4 Medische Aangelegenheden, Fiche #158, ARA, Djeddah Archives.

27. Medical Service of the Dutch Consulate, Mecca, to Dutch Consulate, Jeddah, 15 December 1933, 1.2.4 Medische Aangelegenheden, Fiche #158, ARA, Djeddah Archives.

28. Dutch Consul to MvBZ, 5 January 1934, #33, 1.2.4 Medische Aangelegenheden, Fiche #163, ARA, Djeddah Archives.

29. Dutch Consul to MvBZ, 5 January 1934.

30. Vice-Consul, Dutch Consulate, Jeddah, to MvBZ, 11 November 1936, #896, 1.2.4 Medische Aangelegenheden, Fiche #159, ARA, Djeddah Archives.

31. Vice-Consul, Dutch Consulate, Jeddah, to MvBZ, 2 February 1936, #93, ARA, 1.2.4 Medische Aangelegenheden, Fiche #159, Djeddah Archives.

32. Because the volume of correspondence is so large in this series, and would take up far too much space here, in this subsection of the chapter I provide only rubrics for the CO/273 series which can then easily be consulted by subsequent researchers. For this citation, see CO 273, 142/12072, 8 January 1886, Public Record Office, London.

33. See the correspondence in CO 273, 53/11250, 14 October 1871, Public Record Office, London.

34. UK Consul, Jeddah to Sec. of Gov't, Bombay, 30 April 1875, FO 78/2418, in *Records of the Hajj: A Documentary History of the Pilgrimage to Mecca* (Chippenham, UK: Archive Editions, 1993), 3.07.

35. J. M. Gullick, *Malay Society in the Late Nineteenth Century: The Beginnings of Change* (Singapore: Oxford University Press, 1987), 259.

36. *Malay Mail*, March 23, 1899. An incident along these lines happened in Parit Buntar, Perak.

37. ARNEG, High Commission, #1305/1928.

38. UK Consul, Jeddah, to Foreign Office, London, 20 August 1875, FO 78/2418, in *Records of the Hajj*, 3.07.

39. See CO 273/396/28656, 22 July 1913; CO 273/402/26309, 30 July 1913; CO 273/408/35816, 19 September 1914; CO 273/418/34307, 9 September 1914; and CO 273/418/38345, 5 October 1914, Public Record Office, London.

40. *Straits Settlements Government Gazette* 1867, #31; 1868, #12; 1890, #7.

41. Note from Col. E. Wilkinson to the Committee, 15 December 1919, in "Peace Conference (1919)," FO 608/275/1, Public Record Office, London.

42. Report of the Civil Administrator and Director, Kamaran Quarantine Station, 1939, in "Health and Sanitary (1939–40)," CO 323/1699/14, Public Record Office, London.

43. See CO 273/256/11913, 24 March 1900; CO 273/264/4246, 7 Feb 1900; CO 273/264/13611, 2 May 1900, Public Record Office, London, for some of the details.

44. *Straits Settlements Government Gazette* 1897, #16; see clause 34, "Medical inspection of women"—the inspection of women was, as far as possible, to be carried out by women officers.

45. ARNEG, High Commission, #187/1936.

46. See CO 273/501/50389, 16 September 1920; CO 273/505/37352, 27 July 1920, Public Record Office, London.

47. "Report on the Pilgrimage of 1923, Eastern Confidential E 25/11/91," IOR/R/20/A/4347, File 44/1, India Office Records, British Library.

48. Confidential Memo from W.H. Lee-Warner, c/o UK Consul Batavia, 11 October 1918, #6115 (Prop. 21/18), Sanitary and Destitute Pilgrims, 1920–23, T161/1086, Public Records Office, London.

49. See CO 273/209/11948, 9 July 1895 and CO 273/491/21684, 5 April 1919, Public Records Office, London, as only two examples.

50. "Report by the Delegate of Great Britain on the Autumn Session of the Committee of the Office International d'Hygiene Publique, Paris 1919," Peace Conference 1919, FO 608/275/1, Public Records Office, London.

51. "Report of Dr. N. I. Corkill on the Jeddah Quarantine and Certain Related Matters as Seen During the 1948 Mecca Pilgrimage, 25 November 1948," Anti-Cholera Certificate: Report and Correspondence, 1937–55, MH 55/1888, Public Records Office, London.

52. UK Embassy, Jeddah, to High Commissioner, Federation of Malay, 17 January 1952, #1784/3/52, Arrangements of Pilgrimages to Mecca from Southeast Asia, 1952–53, CO 1022/409, Public Records Office, London.

53. Vivian Nutton, "The Contact Between Civilizations," in *The Great Maritime Discoveries and World Health,* ed. Mario Gomes Marques and John Cule (Lisbon: Escola Nacional Saude Publica Ordem dos Medicos, 1991), 77.

54. For the Greco-Roman and Classical Muslim worldviews, respectively, as bases for later thought, see Saul Jarcho, *The Concept of Contagion in Medicine, Literature, and Religion* (Malabar, FL: Krieger, 2000), 1–20, 21–26.

55. For the period 1830s to the 1870s, see J. K. Crellin, "The Dawn of Germ Theory: Particles, Infection and Biology," in *Medicine and Science in the 1860s,* ed. F. N. L. Poynter (London: Wellcome Institute, 1968), 61–66; see also Charles Rosenberg, *Explaining Epidemics and Other Studies in the History of Medicine* (Cambridge: Cambridge University Press, 1992), 109.

56. See Yaron Perry and Efraim Lev, *Modern Medicine in the Holy Land: Pioneering British Medical Services in Late Ottoman Palestine* (London: Tauris, 2007); and Bridie Andrews and Mary Sutphen, "Introduction," in *Medicine and Colonial Identity,* ed. Mary Sutphen and Bridie Andrews (London: Routledge, 2003), 5.

3 The Influenza Pandemic of 1918 in Southeast Asia

Kirsty Walker

THE INFLUENZA PANDEMIC of 1918 has been described as the worst demographic disaster of the twentieth century. It traveled insidiously across the globe in a series of waves, decimating many of the populations it encountered, and claiming an estimated worldwide mortality of up to fifty million.[1] It was ruthlessly transnational, traveling surreptitiously through quarantine systems and across state borders. As news of a relatively mild but widespread flu epidemic in parts of Europe and the United States began to be reported, the virus reached Southeast Asia, and from June 1918 it spread across Malaya, the Dutch East Indies, the Philippines, Burma, and Indochina with fearsome speed. By October, the virus had mutated into something more vicious and had penetrated virtually every corner of the region. Official returns of morbidity and mortality were woefully incomplete and imprecise due to non-registration of deaths, missing records, and misdiagnosis, and the death toll has crept steadily higher as demographers have revised their judgments in the years following the pandemic. But even the tentative figures that do exist indicate that the demographic impact was significant. At least 1.5 million died in the Dutch East Indies.[2] In Burma, studies have estimated that the flu claimed as many as four hundred thousand lives, equating to between 2 and 3 percent of the population.[3] Over eighty-five thousand died from influenza in the Philippines.[4] Malaya had at least thirty-five thousand victims.[5] Between September and December 1918 alone, over a million people fell ill, and almost thirty thousand died in Siam.[6] In Vietnam, Cambodia, and Laos, morbidity in some areas reached 50 percent. There were around thirteen thousand recorded deaths, and in areas outside French administrative control, many more went unrecorded.[7]

Fear and uncertainty gripped Southeast Asia as the flu infiltrated the lives of millions. Fragments of many dramatic, tragic stories emerge from underused sources. Within the records of the Coroner's Court in Singapore is the death of Tan See Yok, a Hokkien speaker, who cut his own throat with a piece of glass while delirious with what was likely to be influenza-induced pneumonia in October 1918.[8] A newspaper report recording the experiences of survivors in Malaya, recounted the tale of one unconscious Tamil mine worker who was thought to be dead, lying among hundreds of other sleeping victims, finding himself consigned to the mortuary when he regained consciousness.[9] Harrowing stories abound from all over the region of orphaned children starving, of people dying by the side of the road, and of corpses improperly buried or cremated as established customs and rituals fell by the wayside. At the local level, the impact of the pandemic proved unequivocally devastating in some areas. In parts of Siam, over 70 percent of the population fell ill.[10] Countless families were obliterated. At the peak of the pandemic, one family of five in Cochinchina suffered the deaths of four of its members within twelve days of each other.[11] Although the impact of the flu pandemic was variable, mild cases and survival were often forgotten. Its swiftness and severity came to be integrated into local folklore, as powerful oral histories can attest. In parts of Java, survivors remembered that a common saying at that time of crisis was "pagi sakit, sore meninggal; sore sakit, pagi meninggal," meaning "sick in the morning, dead by evening; sick in the evening, dead by morning."[12] The flu had a profound effect on individuals, families and communities across the region, who remembered and misremembered it in turn.

Despite its profound impact on the history of Southeast Asia, the flu pandemic remains a conspicuous gap in our knowledge of the region. A handful of important studies have focused on the impact of the flu in individual countries.[13] Yet by nature the pandemic was transnational, continuously traveling, and crossing borders. Global approaches have tended to focus on its devastating demographic consequences, but the impact of the flu went far beyond its death toll.[14] By taking a comparative, connective approach, this chapter will explore the many meanings of this moment of crisis for the states and societies of Southeast Asia.

Epidemic Disease in Southeast Asia

As Eric Tagliacozzo's chapter in this volume has made clear, the control of epidemic disease was central to the colonial enterprise in Southeast Asia. The dramatic increase in trade, commerce, and the movement of people across the region resulting from British, Dutch, and French imperial expansion over the course of the nineteenth century, was inevitably accompanied by the increased movement of diseases across borders. Illness traveled with traders, migrant laborers, and pilgrims from India and China, which had long been the sources of epidemic diseases in Southeast Asia—including bubonic plague, smallpox, and cholera—and the Indian Ocean quickly became a site of epidemiological exchange.[15]

Sanitary regimes and quarantine systems designed to prevent the spread of disease were integral mechanisms of Southeast Asia's colonial states. In the Straits Settlements, quarantine provisions had been in place since the mid-nineteenth century, enforcing sanitary regulations for all ships entering the ports, as well as measures for the surveillance of contagious diseases, though the efficiency of the system continued to be a subject of debate.[16] In the Philippines, quarantine stations had been established in Mariveles, Cebu, and Iloilo at the start of the American occupation, and inspection stations were introduced at the other ports. The American colonial obsession with contagion made the control of disease a central feature of its civilizing mission.[17] At the same time, measures were introduced to control the spread of disease already existent in the country. In Cambodia, a list of epidemic diseases requiring declaration to the authorities had been decreed in 1902, and outbreaks were controlled in standardized, prescriptive ways: namely notification, containment, and disinfection.[18] But despite this elaborate apparatus, nowhere in colonial Southeast Asia was influenza considered dangerous enough to be a notifiable contagious disease.

Centers for scientific research around the region were tasked with understanding the epidemiology of disease. In Saigon, the Pasteur Institute had been established in 1891 to develop treatments for rabies and smallpox, and it became one of a network of centers in Indochina for developing public health programs and research into contagious and non-contagious diseases, including bubonic plague, cholera, and cancer.[19] In Kuala Lumpur, the Institute for Medical Research had been founded at the turn of the century to investigate the causes, treatment, and prevention of tropical diseases, and by 1918 it had made significant advances toward the treatment of beriberi and malaria.[20] At the same time, the presence of international organizations in Asia made scientific research a transnational affair. The Rockefeller Foundation supported innovative research and public health schemes through its International Health Board. In the years preceding the flu pandemic, it sponsored research into hookworm and malaria in Java and Malaya.[21] By 1918 an elaborate infrastructure of official, voluntary, and philanthropic agencies sought to understand and control endemic and epidemic diseases. Through these efforts a hierarchy of disease emerged, in which influenza justifiably ranked very low. The flu lacked the immediate horror of cholera, or the prolonged misery of malaria. It should be no surprise, then, that in 1918 influenza slipped so effortlessly into Southeast Asia.

Itineraries of Disease

Although generally an innocuous seasonal virus, the influenza of 1918 was markedly different in its intensity, rapidity, and immunity to treatment. It was characterized by a sudden onset, high fever, and severe headache, usually with a sore throat and hacking cough as well as aching, stiffness, and exhaustion. Severe cases were often accompanied by nausea and vomiting, bleeding from the nose and coughing up blood. The fatal cases developed pulmonary and respiratory complications within a few days of its onset, often pneumonia. For them, death was swift. In other victims the flu exacerbated existing illnesses, like malaria or dysentery, and led eventually to the same demise.

The first cases appeared almost simultaneously in countries across the region in June 1918. Although the route of the flu pandemic across Europe and America has been well mapped out, its journeys through Southeast Asia are less well understood. The itinerary of the disease revealed the embedded transnational connections which linked an increasingly modern Southeast Asia to the wider world. It traveled along the paths of war and demobilization, on oceanic sea lanes and trading routes, and along the railways and other conduits of communication and migrant labor. Coastal areas, port cities, and urban centers were the disease entrepôts, the main points of entry and spread.[22] Contemporaries in Malaya speculated that the flu had been imported from Manchuria and Vladivostok via Hong Kong, following the route of the Trans-Siberian Railway and a well-established migration flow.[23,24] Another argued that it had accompanied migrant laborers from Ceylon and from India, where the flu had "assumed the proportions of a national calamity."[25] Other sources maintained that it had come from Spain via the Philippines where many, quite wrongly, believed it had originated. It spread rapidly from Singapore to the rest of Malaya and to British North Borneo, rampaging across and beyond the peninsula "with great fury," and acquiring a multitude of appellations as it did so.[26] In Penang it was "Singapore Fever," in Singapore the name "knock me down fever" was recycled from earlier, milder influenza epidemics, while in Kedah, the flu was known locally as *demam Khamis,* or "Thursday fever," as many of its victims were believed to have fallen ill on Thursdays.[27,28,29] Although it affected all classes and ethnic groups, Indian migrant populations in Malaya were disproportionately susceptible to the flu. The October wave proved fatal to vast numbers of Tamil estate laborers, whose health had long been a matter of concern.[30] The conclusions reached by the press and by contemporary scientific research revealed the ingrained assumption that race was a major influence on individual immunity to disease, as it was suggested that an inherent "racial weakness," as well as poor hygiene and diet were to blame.[31]

Soon after it appeared in the Straits Settlements, it was reported to have reached the Dutch East Indies at Pankattan in eastern Sumatra, spreading to Java and Kalimantan by the end of July.[32] As people instinctively responded to the crisis by *pulang kampung* (returning to their home villages), by the time the second, more deadly wave of flu struck in October, the disease had spread far and wide across the archipelago. At the same time as influenza was making its presence felt in Malaya and the Dutch East Indies, it appeared in the Philippines, and was known locally as *trancazo,* meaning "a blow from a heavy stick."[33] Although the outbreak of influenza in Manila in June seemed to be of local origin and relatively mild, as it was elsewhere, with the arrival of ships from infected countries the virus assumed a more severe form.[34] By October, all provinces were affected. Mobilization of troops in a camp on the outskirts of Manila in anticipation of their participation in World War I in September provided a breeding ground for the spread of the virus; at the peak of the pandemic, 650 cases were reported at the camp in a single day.[35] Unlike in the Dutch East Indies, where most deaths occurred among the very young and the very old, in the Philippines, able-bodied young adults were worst affected.[36]

The flu reached Rangoon by ship in late June, and within three months it had spread to the whole country as troops and military police carried the infection to various military headquarters, as pilgrims attending the Mahumuni festival at Mandalay returned home with the virus, and as infected migrants from Calcutta spread the disease through the transport network to Lower Burma.[37] As in Malaya, Indian migrant populations were decimated by the virus. Children, too, were particularly badly affected: in 1918 childhood mortality rose by 100 percent.[38] Women were also noted to have had a higher registered mortality in Burma, as pregnancy rendered them particularly vulnerable.[39] Reports confirmed that the flu had reached French Indochina in July, appearing simultaneously in Tonkin and in Cochinchina, where it had arrived by ship from Shanghai and Hong Kong. It spread quickly via the Mekong to Laos and Cambodia, where it was reported for the first time in the country's history.[40] By the end of August, the virus had spread to all areas under French control in Cambodia.[41] In Laos, the villages of the interior were worse affected than urban areas.[42] The more severe wave in October was believed to have been introduced by Indian migrants to Saigon, and it was spread by the panicked exodus of people away from the epicenter of the disease, ultimately invading all provinces.[43] The October wave reached Siam, too, when Bangkok was reported to be besieged by *kai wat yai,* or "the great cold fever."[44]

Health Responses

At this time of crisis, people were desperate for measures to prevent and cure the virus. This was a moment when it became clear how ideas about illness and disease were formed, and how people negotiated these understandings between colonial and indigenous structures of power. Explanations for the pandemic were sought in predetermined laws of nature and their binding covenants of moral behavior. In the Dutch East Indies some ascribed the causes of the epidemic to the inevitable workings of *hukum kodrat* (natural law). Death from the disease was viewed as punishment for immorality and gluttony, and it was believed that the epidemic would only be brought to an end through moral and physical purification.[45] Many sought solutions in religion, making efforts to appease the deity responsible. Muslims in Klang held a week of special prayers in the local mosque, while Hindus in Kuala Lumpur organized a procession of the silver chariot around town, followed by prayers for the swift recovery of all those suffering from influenza.[46,47] Some understood the flu to be a product of transactions within the spirit world. In Pahang, the outbreak was attributed to the "evil influence of earth spirits and 'djinns' [Islamic concept of spirit beings]," countered by prayers, incantations, and offerings rather than treatment by disinfection and quarantine.[48] Others pinned its origins on more earthly causes: hygiene, diet, and overcrowded urban conditions. In Singapore, it was even suggested that eating durians rendered one susceptible to the flu.[49] And indeed, the marketplace probably did become a site for the exchange of disease as well as commodities.

Many turned first to traditional remedies to alleviate their physical symptoms. Some looked to the extensive network of Chinese medicine, and its theories of harmonious balance of elements and essential energy.[50] Others sought out Ayurvedic practitioners, who fused elements of European medicine with humoral theory, folk remedies, and spiritual healing.[51] In Malaya and the Dutch East Indies, many turned to the indigenous traditions of healing offered by the *bomoh* or *dukan,* who dealt primarily with the illnesses attributed to the actions of supernatural beings, offering protection as well as cure through taboos and talismans, but also performing medical procedures.[52] In the Dutch East Indies, where the majority of people did not have access to Western medicine, available remedies included a poultice of lime juice, ginger, and red onions ground into a paste and mixed with local vinegar; and a drink made from an extract of cloves, the number of cloves matching the age of the patient in years.[53] People moved between multiple medical worlds. One flu victim in Malaya was taken by his mother to European doctors, Chinese druggists, and Siamese *bomohs* in search of a cure.[54] Colonial medicine was evidently just part of a rich and diverse landscape of healing specialists.

The colonial state in Malaya repeatedly dismissed such traditional medical practices as primitive native superstition, criticizing those who had invented ineffectual cures and prayed on the vulnerable. Yet the treatments offered by Western medicine were equally ineffective in the face of the virus. Contemporary understanding of the epidemiology of influenza located the cause in a bacterium known as Pfeiffer's Bacillus. In fact, the flu was caused by a virus, only correctly identified by scientists in 1933.[55] Preventative vaccines were prepared in Kuala Lumpur and in the Philippines, with equivocal results.[56] In Indochina, Malaya, the Dutch East Indies, and elsewhere quinine—usually used against malaria— was used to treat mild cases, but this had no effect beyond alleviating the fever and headache. In fact, colonial medical officials were reluctantly forced to concede that "no treatment appeared to be of the slightest avail."[57]

Across the region, public health services were overwhelmed. The authorities in Burma set up emergency hospitals, temporary dispensaries, and transport for the seriously ill, but facilities were sparse outside the major towns.[58] In Selangor, wards were set aside to accommodate flu victims, and closed cinemas were transformed into hospitals.[59] Efforts were made to make medicines as widely available as possible, and they were distributed by village headmen, schoolteachers, and the local police.[60] The flu pandemic brought many people into contact with the state and its medical infrastructure for the first time. Pamphlets—printed in Malay, Chinese, Tamil, and English to cater to the multiethnic population—warned of the dangers of congregating in public places.[61] In Indochina, prophylactic measures included isolation of the sick, the restriction of public gatherings, and disinfecting the floors of public establishments and houses with lime water.[62] The infected military camp in Manila and the surrounding area were effectively quarantined to prevent further spread. The authorities held lectures on preventative measures, conducted weekly inspections of public schools, disinfection of wells, and the poisoning of stray dogs, among other measures.[63] This went beyond the immediate needs of the crisis. In using the opportunity to enforce the American sanitary order, the influence of military models of disease control on colonial public health became strikingly clear.

Despite these efforts, there was much criticism of the belated attempts of medical departments to halt the spread of the disease. The Colonial Office did not dispatch a circular on influenza prevention until November 1918, when the pandemic was well underway.[64] There were even murmurings of nationalism in the criticism. In the Dutch East Indies, Abdul Rivai, a Netherlands-trained doctor and Minangkabau intellectual, argued in the People's Council that the Civil Medical Service was effectively allowing Javanese people to die, as they made far less effort to reduce the mortality rate in Java than they had in Europe.[65] Rivai was one of many Western-trained Asian nationalists who united medicine and health with political power, as described by Rachel Leow in this volume. Efforts to replace indigenous systems of healing with Western medicine had limited success, particularly in remote rural areas. Many distrusted Western medicine, and were wary of hospitals, finding their impersonal care and isolation from family entirely alien. Medical reports in Malaya frequently complained that Chinese patients were brought into hospitals in such a moribund state that there was often little that could be done for them.[66] Similarly, many Indonesians refused to accept Dutch remedies even when they were offered them for free.[67]

The impact of the pandemic in Southeast Asia went far beyond health. It effectively brought everyday life to a complete halt. In Indonesia, shops, offices, and schools were closed and markets deserted. In Manila, transpacific ships were delayed in sailing, and several newspapers suspended publication.[68] Across the region, schools, cinemas, and theaters were closed to prevent the gathering of people and therefore the spread of the virus. In Malaya, work in many estates came to a standstill. Inevitably, the flu had longer-term effects on colonial economies, and was undoubtedly a factor in the more general decline of rural economies between the wars.[69] Soaring rice prices in Burma in 1920 and 1921 were believed to be a consequence of the disturbances to planting and harvesting caused by the epidemic.[70] Other economies were able to withstand the disruption rather better. In the Dutch East Indies the area under smallholder food cultivation was actually higher in 1919 than in 1917.[71] But the pandemic did affect the strategic choices of agricultural cultivators, as the figures reveal a preference for dry-season crops and sacrifice of those which were less valuable while the flu was ongoing.[72] At the level of the household economy it was evidently a time of deep anxiety for some. Increased use of credit institutions like the Government Pawnshop Service and village grain banks in the Dutch East Indies suggested a more subtle impact of the flu at the household level.[73] The flu also had a wider impact on society. It coincided with an upsurge in violence, robberies, and murders in parts of the Dutch East Indies. It was also responsible in part for provoking an anti-Chinese riot in Kudus, in central Java, in November. Clashes occurred when the owners of a local Chinese cigarette company sponsored a festival intended to banish the pandemic, and an insult to Islam was believed to have occurred; fifty houses were burned down, eight Chinese were killed and two thousand fled to Semarang. The flu was the catalyst to the eruption of local economic and religious tensions already deeply embedded in the area.[74] But alongside these discordant social effects were communal efforts to provide assistance to the victims of the epidemic. Committees of local notables—which played an important role in fundraising, disseminating information and medicine, providing practical assistance, and relief work—formed in Penang, Selangor, Perak, and Surakarta.[75]

The influenza pandemic began to peter out by the end of 1918. It was over in Cochinchina by the end of December, although elsewhere in French Indochina it continued until April 1919.[76] By the end of January it had come to an end in the Dutch East Indies, although localized outbreaks continued to be reported for the rest of the year.[77] Contemporary writers quickly began its memorialization. In Singapore, where the impact of the flu had been comparatively mild, it was remembered as "the great epidemic of influenza in 1918, when sickness and death seemed to reign supreme."[78] Beyond its obvious imprint on public and personal memory, many practical lessons were learned. Across the region, influenza was made a notifiable disease, empowering colonial authorities to control its spread. But, more importantly, it brought health to the forefront of the colonial agenda. In Malaya, it stimulated an invigorated official interest in health and medical infrastructure into the 1920s.[79] It led to a more centralized, more transnational disease information network in the form of the Eastern Bureau of the League of Nations Health Organization, established in Singapore in the 1920s, which collected and disseminated information regarding infectious disease in the ports and countries of the region.[80] Although studies of health and medicine in empire have tended to focus either on the development of European medicine in the colony, or on medicine as a tool of empire with its own colonizing power, the history of the flu pandemic in Southeast Asia does not fit easily into either framework. Rather, this was a moment of vulnerability which exposed the impotence of colonial power in the face of a virus which had total disregard for geopolitical borders. It revealed the many different ways in which people made sense of illness and death, and the diverse, overlapping systems of medicine and healing to which they turned in times of crisis. The flu pandemic of 1918 seems to belong at the intersection of histories of health and medicine, and histories of the transnational interactions and connections which characterized early-twentieth-century Southeast Asia.

Notes

1. N. P. A. S. Johnson, J. Mueller, "Updating the Accounts: Global Mortality of the 1918–1920 "Spanish" Influenza Pandemic," *Bulletin of the History of Medicine* 76 (2002): 105.

2. C. Brown, "The Influenza Pandemic of 1918 in Indonesia," in *Death and Disease in Southeast Asia: Explorations in Social, Medical and Demographic History*, ed. Norman G. Owen (Singapore: Oxford University Press, 1987), 235.

3. J. Richell, *Disease and Demography in Colonial Burma* (Singapore: NUS Press, 2006), 203.

4. *Report on the Pandemic of Influenza, 1918–19* (London: His Majesty's Stationery Office, 1920), 386.

5. K. K. Liew, "Terribly Severe Though Mercifully Short: The Episode of the 1918 Influenza in British Malaya," *Modern Asian Studies* 41 (2007): 222.

6. "Influenza in Siam," *Singapore Free Press*, March 12, 1919, 4.

7. M. le Dr Garnier, "L'épidemie d'influenza de 1918–1919 dans les colonies françaises," *Annales de médecine et de pharmacie coloniales* 20 (1922): 44.

8. *Coroner's Inquiries and Views 1918*, 279/10/18, National Archives of Singapore. Thanks to Gayne Lim for her assistance in locating this reference.

9. "Dead Men Stories," *The Times of Malaya*, November 7, 1918, cited in Liew, "Terribly Severe Though Mercifully Short," 221.

10. "Influenza in Siam."

11. "L'épidemie d'influenza de 1918–1919," 49.

12. Brown, "The Influenza Pandemic of 1918 in Indonesia," 253.

13. Brown, "The Influenza Pandemic of 1918 in Indonesia," 235–56; Liew, "Terribly Severe Though Mercifully Short," 221–52; F. A. Gealogo, "The Philippines in the World of the Influenza Pandemic of 1918–1919," *Philippine Studies* 57 (2009): 261–92.

14. K. D. Patterson and G. F. Pyle, "The Geography and Mortality of the 1918 Influenza Pandemic," *Bulletin of the History of Medicine* 65 (1991): 4–21; Johnson and Mueller, "Updating the Accounts," 105–15.

15. D. Arnold, "The Indian Ocean as a Disease Zone, 1500–1950," *South Asia: Journal of South Asian Studies* 14 (1991): 1–21.

16. L. Manderson, *Sickness and the State: Health and Illness in Colonial Malaya, 1870–1940* (Cambridge: Cambridge University Press, 1996), 45.

17. W. Anderson, *Colonial Pathologies: American Tropical Medicine, Race and Hygiene in the Philippines* (Durham, NC, and London: Duke University Press, 2006).

18. S. Au, *Mixed Medicines: Health and Culture in French Colonial Cambodia* (Chicago and London: University of Chicago Press, 2011), 100.

19. A. Marcovich, "French Colonial Medicine and Colonial Rule: Algeria and Indochina," in *Disease, Medicine, and Empire: Perspectives on Western Medicine and the Experience of European Expansion*, ed. R. Macleod and M. Lewis (London and New York: Routledge, 1988), 103–17.

20. The Institute for Medical Research, *The Institute for Medical Research, 1900–1950* (Kuala Lumpur: Government Press, 1951).

21. Rockefeller Foundation, International Health Board, Report of the Uncinariasis Commission of the Orient, 1915–1917, *Hookworm and Malaria Research in Malaya, Java and the Fiji Islands; Report of Uncinariasis Commission to the Orient, 1915–1917* (New York: Rockefeller Foundation, International Health Board, 1920).

22. Arnold, "The Indian Ocean as a Disease Zone, 1500–1950," 10.

23. On routes of transmission into Malaya, see Liew, "Terribly Severe Though Mercifully Short," 226.

24. A. McKeown, "Global Migration, 1846–1940," *Journal of World History* 15 (2004): 158–59.

25. Sanitary Commissioner with the Government of India, *A Preliminary Report on the Influenza Pandemic of 1918 in India* (Simla: Government Monotype Press, 1919), 1.

26. "The Influenza," *Singapore Free Press*, October 15, 1918, 5.

27. R. Collier, *The Plague of the Spanish Lady: The Influenza Pandemic of 1918–1919* (London and Basingstoke: Macmillan London, 1974), 82.

28. L. Nurenee, "A Plague o' Both Your Houses: Medicine, Power and the Great Flu of 1918–1919 in Britain and Singapore" (master's thesis, National University of Singapore, 2011), 74.

29. Liew, "Terribly Severe Though Mercifully Short," 226.

30. G. W. Scott, "Epidemic Pneumonic Influenza as Seen in Malaya," *British Medical Journal* 1 (1919): 305; A. Kaur, "Indian Labour, Labour Standards and Workers' Health in Burma and Malaya, 1900–1940," *Modern Asian Studies* 40 (2006): 425–75; L. Brennan and R. Shlomowitz, "Mortality and Indian Labour in Malaya, 1877–1933," *Indian Economic and Social History Review* 29 (1992): 57–64.

31. For a summary of these arguments, see Liew, "Terribly Severe Though Mercifully Short," 236–38.

32. Brown, "The Influenza Pandemic of 1918 in Indonesia," 236.

33. Gealogo, "The Philippines in the World of the Influenza Pandemic of 1918–1919," 286.

34. A. F. Coutant, "An Epidemic of Influenza at Manila, P.I.," *Journal of the American Medical Association* 71 (1918): 1566.

35. Gealogo, "The Philippines in the World of the Influenza Pandemic of 1918–1919," 283.

36. Gealogo, "The Philippines in the World of the Influenza Pandemic of 1918–1919," 281; Brown, "The Influenza Pandemic of 1918 in Indonesia," 242.

37. Richell, *Disease and Demography in Colonial Burma*, 204.

38. Richell, *Disease and Demography in Colonial Burma*, 203.

39. Richell, *Disease and Demography in Colonial Burma*, 204–5.

40. "L'épidemie d'influenza de 1918–1919," 48, 52.

41. "L'épidemie d'influenza de 1918–1919," 52.

42. "L'épidemie d'influenza de 1918–1919," 55.

43. "L'épidemie d'influenza de 1918–1919," 44, 48.

44. *Singapore Free Press*, October 26, 1918, 5; Collier, *The Plague of the Spanish Lady*, 82.

45. Brown, "The Influenza Pandemic of 1918 in Indonesia," 246.

46. *Straits Times*, October 25, 1918, 8.
47. "The Influenza."
48. "Influenza Spreads in the F.M.S.," *Singapore Free Press*, October 10, 1918, 228.
49. Nurenee, "A Plague o' Both Your Houses," 74.
50. S. Cochran, *Chinese Medicine Men: Consumer Culture in China and Southeast Asia* (Cambridge, MA: Harvard University Press, 2006).
51. F. Colley, "Traditional Indian Medicine in Malaysia," *Journal of the Malaysian Branch of the Royal Asiatic Society* 51 (1978): 84.
52. R. Werner, *Bomoh/Dukun: The Practices and Philosophies of the Traditional Malay Healer* (Berne: University of Berne, Institute of Ethnology, 1986).
53. Brown, "The Influenza Pandemic of 1918 in Indonesia," 245.
54. Liew, "Terribly Severe Though Mercifully Short," 248.
55. H. Van Epps, "Influenza: Exposing the True Killer," *Journal of Experimental Medicine* 203 (2006): 803.
56. The Institute for Medical Research, *The Institute for Medical Research 1900–1950*, 57; Gealogo, "The Philippines in the World of the Influenza Pandemic of 1918–1919," 284.
57. Scott, "Epidemic Pneumonic Influenza as Seen in Malaya," 306.
58. Richell, *Disease and Demography in Colonial Burma*, 205.
59. Manderson, *Sickness and the State*, 52.
60. Manderson, *Sickness and the State*, 52.
61. Manderson, *Sickness and the State*, 52.
62. "L'épidemie d'influenza de 1918–1919," 45.
63. Gealogo, "The Philippines in the World of the Influenza Pandemic of 1918–1919," 284.
64. D. Killingray, "The New 'Imperial Disease': The Influenza Pandemic of 1918–19 and Its Impact on the British Empire," *Caribbean Quarterly* 49 (2003): 33.
65. Brown, "The Influenza Pandemic of 1918 in Indonesia," 243.
66. Manderson, *Sickness and the State*, 69.
67. Brown, "The Influenza Pandemic of 1918 in Indonesia," 244.
68. Coutant, "An Epidemic of Influenza at Manila, P.I.," 1567.
69. C. Baker, "Economic Reorganization and the Slump in South and Southeast Asia," *Comparative Studies in Society and History* 23 (1981): 325–49.
70. Richell, *Disease and Demography in Colonial Burma*, 213.
71. Brown, "The Influenza Pandemic of 1918 in Indonesia," 249.
72. Brown, "The Influenza Pandemic of 1918 in Indonesia," 251.
73. Brown, "The Influenza Pandemic of 1918 in Indonesia," 251.
74. Kuntowidjojo, "The Indonesian Muslim Middle Class in Search of Identity, 1910–1950," in *Comparative History of India and Indonesia*, vol. 1, *India and Indonesia from the 1920s to the 1950s: The Origins of Planning*, ed. L. Blusse (Leiden: Brill, 1987), 184.
75. Brown, "The Influenza Pandemic of 1918 in Indonesia," 249; Liew, "Terribly Severe Though Mercifully Short," 248–50.
76. "L'épidemie d'influenza de 1918–1919," 44, 47.
77. Brown, "The Influenza Pandemic of 1918 in Indonesia," 252.
78. "Dr. Malcolm Watson and Ross Institute," *Straits Times*, November 1, 1923, 9.
79. N. J. Parmer, "Health and Health Services in British Malaya in the 1920s," *Modern Asian Studies* 23 (1989): 49–71.
80. L. Manderson, "Wireless Wars in the Eastern Arena: Epidemiological Surveillance, Disease Prevention and the Work of Eastern Bureau of the League of Nations Health Organization, 1925–1942," in *International Health Organizations and Movements, 1918–1939*, ed. P. Weindling (Cambridge: Cambridge University Press, 1995), 109–33.

4 Disaster Medicine in Southeast Asia

Greg Bankoff

SOME OF THE most notorious natural disasters of the past two centuries have taken place in Southeast Asia. Even if death tolls have been greater in other events, the eruption of Krakatoa in 1883 and the Indian Ocean Tsunami of 2004 have come to be widely seen as symbolic of the power of nature and the unpredictability of human existence. Southeast Asia is often depicted as the "Ring of Fire," the arc of active volcanoes that run through Indonesia and the Philippines; or "Typhoon Alley," the area between the Philippines and southern Japan where tropical storms usually form before heading westward to wreak their destructive paths across the region. Although danger is no stranger to the lives and lifestyles of the peoples of Southeast Asia and recognition is accorded to their resilience and the varied ways and means by which they have learned to deal with the constancy of threat, little attention has been paid to "disaster medicine," the system of medical practice primarily associated with emergency medicine and public health during a disaster.

"Disaster medicine" is a relatively new term, dating from the 1980s, although the practice has its roots in the system of triage developed and implemented during the Napoleonic wars by Baron Dominique Jean Larrey.[1] A disaster is defined in specifically medical terms as when the number of patients presenting within a given time period are such that an emergency department cannot provide care for them without external assistance.[2] Disaster medicine, then, is the study and collaborative application of various health disciplines to "the prevention, preparedness, response and recovery from the health problems arising from disasters."[3] The emphasis, too, on public health interventions and preventative services challenges mainly Western-derived medical practice that is focused on the clinical demands of the individual patient. Pre-hospital triage procedures, for instance, are designed to deploy emergency care to the greatest effect for the largest number of people. Patients with the most severe injuries who are deemed to have only a minimal chance of survival are designated as "expectant" by black tags and are not transported to medical facilities until all those with a greater chance of survival have been evacuated.

Studies of communities in developing countries indicate that more than 80 percent of individuals have been exposed to severe trauma.[4] This trauma can be both immediate and physical or more long-term and mental. It can be caused by human-induced disasters such as wars and revolutions, by natural hazards such as earthquakes and tsunamis, or by a combination of both (complex emergencies). Despite the fact that four out of five people in developing countries have personal experience of such events, most research to date on the broader medical impact of disasters has been on Western case studies. This chapter examines disaster medicine in an Asian—more specifically, Southeast Asian—context. It explores the role of medicine in treating both the physical and the mental impact of disasters caused by natural hazards. As in many other aspects of disaster risk reduction (DRR) and emergency management procedures, Western concepts and norms have been largely imposed upon local practice with often unforeseen results. In fact, culture is revealed to be an important determinant in defining both how trauma is defined and treated during a disaster.

"Natural" Disasters in Southeast Asia

There are no such things as "natural" disasters. The term, however, is widely and popularly used to refer to those disasters triggered by natural, physical hazards—such as earthquakes, volcanic eruptions, typhoons, and tsunamis—in order to differentiate those caused by human error, such as technological failures or accidents. In reality, all disasters are human induced to some degree, as a natural hazard remains nothing more than a physical event unless it interacts with a human population that is vulnerable to precipitate a disaster.[5] For most people in Southeast Asia, these natural disasters are a frequent life experience. Rather than regarding them as abnormal occurrences, departures from the normal routine of daily living as they are usually depicted through the epistemological lens of Western social sciences, it is more productive to consider them as normal everyday events—events, moreover, that people at the level of both society and community have had to live with on a recurring basis.[6] Of course, not everybody in Southeast Asia is exposed to the same degree of hazard, but the region as a whole has been historically disaster prone. There are many relative factors to consider in establishing whether one part of the globe experiences more disasters than another area, but Asia is considered to be a particularly hazard prone continent, and within Asia, Southeast Asia has suffered a disproportionate number of hazards per unit of surface area. The region may amount to only 3 percent of the world's total landmass, but it accounted for 11.5 percent of all recorded hazards and nearly 5 percent of all those affected by disasters since 1900.

Table 4.1. Southeast Asia compared to world disasters, 1900–2009

Factors	SEA	World	%
Hazards	815	7,075	11.5
Deaths	142,252	31,306,783	0.45
Affected	193,819,528	3,986,368,414	4.9

Source: Emergency Disaster Database, Centre for Research on the Epidemiology of Disasters, www.emdat.be.

A closer examination of the figures by decade, however, reveals some very clear trends. On the one hand, the global share of the number of disasters caused by natural hazards that the region accounts for remains fairly constant—at least since the 1950s, when statistics are more robust. On the other hand, the percentage of deaths from disasters in Southeast Asia has risen sharply, especially over the last two decades. In the first decade of the twenty-first century, in fact, the region accounted for 41 percent of all those who died in disasters caused in this manner. Although over half the fatalities died in just one event, the Indian Ocean Tsunami of December 26, 2004, the upsurge in mortality since 1990 is still quite evident. These figures are in sharp contrast to the dramatic decrease in the number of deaths worldwide from disasters since the 1920s and the generally declining decadal mortality rate (see table 4.2). That is to say, people in the region appear to be increasingly vulnerable to disasters, even considering the greater reliability of more recent data, the undoubted advances in forecasting and DRR, and the one-off effect of very infrequent, major events.

In one respect, of course, this increased vulnerability may simply be a matter of larger populations, denser urban areas, and more costly infrastructure than ever before. However, there are also indications that human activity has affected the magnitude and frequency of such phenomena, that it is adversely altering climate, and that it poses a serious threat to the environment—and especially agriculture—in the region.[7] Parts of Southeast Asia—particularly the Philippines and, to a lesser extent, Vietnam—have always been susceptible to the ravages of tropical storms, but flooding has now emerged as a major hazard in Indonesia and Thailand. Severe floods during the monsoon season of 2011 caused sixty-five of Thailand's seventy-seven provinces to be declared disaster zones, damaging over twenty thousand square kilometers of farmland. In all, storms and floods accounted for 861 events, or 67 percent of all disasters in Southeast Asia between 1950 and 2009.[8] Volcanic eruptions are confined only to Indonesia and the Philippines. Two of the largest seismic events in the last century, the eruption of Mount Pinatubo in 1991, the second-largest such event of the twentieth century, and the Indian Ocean earthquake and tsunami of 2004 also originated in the region.

Table 4.2. Southeast Asia compared to world disasters by decade, 1900–2009

Decades	Total disasters			Deaths			Affected		
	SEA	World	%	SEA	World	%	SEA	World	%
1900–09	5	72	6.9	6,780	4,497,847	0.15	N/A	240,000	
1910–19	6	71	8.5	21,455	3,326,492	0.64	N/A	5,667,000	
1920–29	5	97	5.2	3,611	8,726,265	0.041	N/A	44,146,000	
1930–39	16	101	16	5,539	4,700,954	0.12	N/A	10,089,500	
1940–49	6	142	4.2	1,588	3,871,695	0.041	14,000	2,804,475	0.5
1950–59	24	294	8.2	6,934	2,127,116	0.33	60,000	18,858,421	0.3
1960–69	64	582	11	24,951	1,750,440	1.4	5,948,962	189,709,572	3.1
1970–79	138	910	15	19,367	986,867	2	34,819,984	528,381,821	6.6
1980–89	212	1,831	12	17,746	793,746	2.2	61,666,025	1,228,362,067	5
1990–99	339	2,975	11	34,281	525,361	6.5	91,310,557	1,958,109,558	4.7
2000–09	516	4,501	12	342,341	839,555	41	119,094,307	2,323,389,426	5.1

Source: Emergency Disaster Database, Centre for Research on the Epidemiology of Disasters, www.emdat.be.

Finally, the climate of much of Southeast Asia is influenced by the El Niño Southern Oscillation (ENSO), the seesaw fluctuation in atmospheric pressure between the Western and Eastern Pacific that gives rise to periodic droughts and floods with devastating effects on agriculture and human health, most notably in 1877–78, 1899–1900, 1940–41, 1982–83 and 1997–98.[9]

Disaster Medicine in Southeast Asia

Disasters have the most impact in developing countries that have been historically poorly equipped to deal with their aftermath. The International Federation of Red Cross and Red Crescent Societies, in fact, reports that states undergoing rapid development are most at risk with medium and low human development countries accounting for 64 percent of the total number of natural disasters, 92 percent of all those reported killed in such events, and 97 percent of all those reported affected by them in the decade between 1999 and 2008.[10] Although DRR has greatly improved in Southeast Asia over recent decades and some states, like Singapore, have facilities and emergency services the equal of any in the world, the rapid expansion of informal settlements in urban areas and the increasing degradation of land and livelihoods in rural ones places much of the region's population at risk. Emergency medical services (EMS) are a critical component of effective disaster management. Disaster medicine emerged as a distinct discipline in the 1980s, building on the greatly improved casualty survival rates of soldiers wounded in World War II, the Korean War, and the Vietnam War who underwent the three major phases of initial mass casualty care: triage, evacuation, and definitive medical management. As such, disaster medicine has two quite distinctive components: the more immediate physical injuries inflicted on persons caught up in the actual event, and the often longer-term mental disorders that may affect a much wider circle of people who have lost property, homes, or even loved ones.

EMS and Physical Injuries

One of the unexpected side effects of the Indian Ocean Tsunami of 2004 was to focus attention on EMS in developing countries. The sheer scale of the death toll, the geographical extent of the disaster affecting an usually large number of countries and cultures, and the scope of the media coverage paid to the event focused attention on the public health systems concerned—as well as inevitably invited comparisons between them. Prior to this event, little notice had been paid to disaster medicine in developing countries, where the main emphasis was more on extending a primary health care system to include all within the national boundaries. In particular, greater recognition was accorded to the special circumstances that often accompany the impact of a disaster in a developing country.

Although disaster medicine has never been solely about providing EMS to people involved in disasters caused by natural or technological hazards, these—along with traffic accidents—are the main health concerns in Western countries. Emerging infectious diseases, complex humanitarian emergencies (CHE or intertwined issues of government instability, macroeconomic collapse, civil-military violence, population displacement, and the collapse of public health infrastructure), and terrorism and weapons of mass destruction are perceived as threats, but ones that originate externally, and contingency measures vary accordingly.[11] Monitoring, surveillance, and quarantine are the main focus.[12] Such is not the case in many developing countries, where CHE may elevate the rates of mortality as high as sixty times over the baseline due to a combination of disease, malnutrition, and violent trauma.[13] Disasters are always political events as well as public health emergencies. Relief and recovery efforts following the Indian Ocean Tsunami, for example, cut across two civil wars (against the Free Aceh Movement in Indonesia and the Liberation Tigers of Tamil Eelam in Sri Lanka) and a political crisis in the Maldives.[14] Internal conflicts present difficulties for the international community to provide humanitarian assistance if for political reasons national governments or separatist authorities fail to cooperate with the relief efforts, as happened in East Timor (Timor-Leste) prior to 1999.

In one important way, disaster medicine runs contrary to the normative ethos of Western practice. It prioritizes the allocation of limited resources under emergency conditions to provide the greatest health benefit to the greatest number of people. Emphasis is placed on disease prevention and health promotion, and relatively low priority is given to curative care. High mortality rates are most rapidly reduced through the implementation of six main public health interventions: the provision of food, water, sanitation, shelter, measles vaccinations, and basic medical care. Between 60 and 90 percent of all deaths in Asia during the emergency phase of a disaster can usually be attributed to one of five main preventable diseases: diarrhea, acute respiratory infections, measles, malaria, and malnutrition.[15] As circumstances usually preclude the provision of basic medical care to all victims on a timely basis, disaster triage is employed to determine the allocation of limited resources. The philosophy of the health care provider changes from a policy of providing high-intensity care to the sickest victims to one of doing "the greatest good for the greatest number."[16] Pre-hospital triage sorts patients into four categories designated by a color: red for patients whose injuries are critical but who can be cared for with only minimal time and resources and who have a good prognosis for survival; yellow for patients whose injuries are significant but are able to tolerate a delay in their care without the risk of substantial morbidity; green for the walking wounded, or patients whose injuries are minor enough that they can wait for treatment; and black for those whose injuries are so severe that they have only a minimal chance of survival even if significant resources are expended. Care in the latter circumstances is only palliative.

Some kinds of hazards, however, create their own particular signature. Major earthquakes usually provoke a substantial number of crush casualties. The collapse of multistoried and/or poorly constructed buildings especially in urban areas traps many survivors in the rubble. Many of the badly injured will develop crush syndrome or traumatic rhabdomyolysis, a medical condition caused by the compression of body extremities (predominantly legs and feet) trapped under fallen masonry that leads to muscle swelling and/or neurological disturbances in the affected areas of the body. For example, it is now estimated that some 2 to 5 percent of those injured in the 1976 Tangshan earthquake (China), in which an estimated 242,769 people died, suffered crush syndrome.[17] While crush syndrome affects many organs, the most common complication is acute kidney injury (AKI). AKI is often fatal if untreated but one of the few life-threatening conditions that is reversible if appropriate medical treatment, fluid resuscitation, and/or dialysis are applied. While the condition was first recognized during the London Blitz in World War II, the first recognized catastrophe of epidemic dimensions only occurred in the aftermath of the Armenian earthquake in 1988.[18] Problems arise, firstly, as many health care professionals are insufficiently versed in the pathophysiology, complications, and treatment of AKI and, secondly, because there are insufficient dialysis units in local hospitals to treat the sudden spike in demand. Survival of those affected primarily depends, therefore, on rapid evacuation to healthcare facilities in unaffected areas. It is estimated that many survivors of the massive Sumatra-Andaman earthquake of December 2004

(<9.1 on the Richter scale) suffered crush syndrome, but their bodies were swept away in the ensuing tsunami.

Mainly, however, EMS is concerned with primary care and public health issues. Many injuries in the aftermath of a disaster are caused by sharp and blunt trauma. Although these wounds are often not serious in themselves, adequate cleansing of lacerations and abrasions is difficult given the disruption to clean water supplies and sanitation systems. Wounds often become grossly contaminated with soil, sewerage, or seawater—leading to polymicrobial infections such as staphylococcal and streptococcal pathogens, tetanus, melioidosis, mucormycosis, and bacteria associated with fecal material.[19] The most immediate public health issue following a large disaster is the disposal of the dead, and the fear that the bodies of victims can cause epidemics among surviving populations. This sometimes leads to the hurried and often inappropriate burial of cadavers. While there may be a strong aversion to the dead and a natural instinct to protect oneself against disease, empirical evidence suggests that infectious diseases are no more likely to be present in disaster victims than in the general population. In fact, the opposite may be the case, as pathogens are unable to survive long in the human body following death and survivors may "present a much more important reservoir for disease."[20] Clearly, disasters with large numbers of fatalities may require a temporary workforce composed of military personnel, rescue workers, and volunteers for the collection, transportation, storage and disposal of the dead. There is no reason to suppose, however, that despite their prior lack of experience in handling cadavers that the risk of infection is any higher than that of public safety workers in general.[21] In particular, the risk of infection during flood-related events—the most frequent type of disaster in Southeast Asia—arises mainly from the transmission of disease through lack of access to clean water and sanitation and to the outbreak of vector-borne and/or rodent-borne diseases, and not from dead bodies.[22]

EMS and Mental Health Disorders

Mental health spending is less than 1 percent of the health budget in many developing countries, and over 30 percent of countries have no separate mental health budget and few mental health professionals.[23] Although Southeast Asia has experienced more than its fair share of major hazards in recent decades, few studies have been done on the mental health of trauma victims or the psychosocial issues of disaster survivors in the region. Until recently, the main focus of such research has been on the mental health problems and post-traumatic stress disorder (PTSD) resulting from human-induced disasters, more particularly on Vietnam veterans and Indochina refugees.[24] After thirty years of chronic warfare, it was generally felt that human-induced disasters tend to cause more psychosocial trauma than natural ones.[25] In fact, studies on survivors of disasters research

show that around 50 percent will suffer from mental health difficulties and between 5 and 10 percent will require psychiatric attention.[26] This general lack of
data on mental health disorders in the region is mainly attributed to limitations
in knowledge and practice among disaster victims as well as the lack of medical
and paramedical staff. Culture is also considered to be an important determining
factor (see below).

Exposure to trauma is a common human condition; community studies suggest that 80 percent of individuals have been exposed to severe trauma at some
point in their lives.[27] Estimates for untreated serious mental disorders in developing countries run as high as 85 percent, according to the WHO.[28] Difficulties
arise in determining the early phase of post-disaster psychopathology in traumatized survivors. The two most widely applied diagnostic systems, diagnostic
and statistical manual of mental disorders, *DSM-IV* and *ICD-10* include acute
stress disorder (ASD) and PTSD with inconclusive studies indicating that those
persons subject to the former are more likely to develop the latter.[29] ASD sufferers are further classified into three groups: probable ASD, early traumatic stress
response (ETSR), and no acute diagnosis. A study of those directly affected by
the eruption of Mount Pinatubo in June 1991 found major depression and anxiety
disorders the most frequent diagnosis.[30] However, individual responses to trauma cover a large spectrum including disassociation, somatization, and emotional
dysregulation as well as PTSD. In fact, there is an ongoing debate as to whether
PTSD is a diagnostic construction of Western origin to medicalize normal distress.[31] Some groups, too, tend to be more vulnerable to mental health disorders—including women, children, the elderly, those with learning disabilities,
the physically frail, and those with existing mental illnesses. The latter, especially
in developing countries are at particular risk from lack of access to necessary psy-
chotropic medication, disruption of appropriate psychological support, the scar-
city of mental health workers in general, as well as the trauma experience itself.[32]

Psychosocial interventions during a disaster seek to promote "the restoration of social cohesion and infrastructure as well as the independence and dignity of individuals and groups."[33] Psychosocial support has been categorized into
four phases that mirror the disaster management cycle. The "heroic," or rescue,
phase immediately after an event evokes a high degree of altruism as people work
together to prevent further loss of life or property. This is followed by the relief phase in the first six weeks to two months after the event; it is also known
as the "honeymoon phase" because of the optimism generated by the influx of
relief supplies and support from both national and international sources. The
next phase, however—that of rehabilitation—is characterized by disillusionment
and skepticism as promises are not kept or fall short of expectations, and may
last from one to two years. The final, or rebuilding phase, is a time of emotional
reconstruction in which individuals and communities work together to reestab-

lish normal functioning. It may last for years, or even decades, and involves an acceptance of the disaster and coming to terms with its aftermath.[34] It took a disaster of the scale and magnitude of the Indian Ocean Tsunami, however, to force governments to rethink their neglect toward mental health interventions in such situations and to develop national guidelines as a preparatory measure.[35]

Culture, Disaster, and Medicine

Not all scholars, however, emphasize only the negative side of trauma. There has been greater recognition that trauma often affects communities as well as individuals. As Peter Suedfeld shows, not all traumatic stress is "so overwhelming that neither at the micro- nor at the macro-level can people withstand its negative effects or deal with it in healthy ways."[36] He argues that there are both positive and negative aspects of stress, that they may be either pathogenic or salutogenic (or both at the same time)—what he calls distress and eustress. While the distress manifests itself in mental health disorders, eustress focuses on the impact disasters can have on improving social organization and leadership, personal coping and adaptation, emotional and cognitive resilience, and the allocation of coping resources in the community.[37] Suedfeld's work raises the question of culture as a variant in determining how societies deal with trauma, in that disaster not only affects individuals put at risk because of a particular social structure but also communities embedded within a specific culture. More to the point, do people respond to disasters in the same way across cultures, and in what ways do the differences that arise affect disaster medicine?

Culture is recognized as an important variant in dealing with trauma. For example, the exceptionally low suicide rate among traumatized populations in contemporary Afghanistan is attributed to the strong Islamic injunctions against taking one's own life.[38] Likewise, the infrequency of PTSD diagnoses among disaster victims in China is ascribed to the reluctance in that culture to express psychological stress.[39] As might be expected, very little has been written about the subject in Southeast Asia. Some few studies, however, have explored the notion of cultural responses to disaster from a Sri Lankan perspective. Sri Lanka shares with Thailand, Myanmar, Cambodia, and Laos a deeply held Theravada Buddhist tradition, so that it may be possible to extrapolate to some extent from one to the other. Research on the aftermath of the Indian Ocean Tsunami in Sri Lanka suggests an important role for religion in dealing with and understanding the effects of disaster. On the physical injuries side of EMS, it was noted that numerous Buddhist monks and laypersons in the affected areas lent immediate help and support to survivors by providing shelter and food in temple compounds or their own homes. While Buddhism, perhaps, is little different from other major religions in this respect, the psychological support from its religious teachings was credited with explaining the remarkable resilience of the population to the disaster that had engulfed them. In particular, the key concept of *anicca,* that everything is impermanent, has been credited with helping survivors to frame the event within their daily lives; the notion of *kamma,* or reaping the consequences of one's actions, made them better able to accept the losses. The therapeutic value of *bhāvanā* (meditation), too, in coping with depression, anxiety, and pain has been recognized in psychological practice.[40] In Thailand, where Buddhism is also widely adhered to, the resilience shown by people in the aftermath of the tsunami has been noted.[41]

A better understanding that custom, tradition, and religious beliefs constitute an important variant in EMS also highlights the question of culturally insensitive psychosocial interventions. To what extent is EMS as presently envisaged constructed according to Western norms and practices? Does this model encourage the view that trauma responses are "entirely universal and fixed"?[42] One inherent danger of importing healers and healing strategies is the possibility of the unnecessary medicalization of normal human reactions because they are outside the accepted clinical model.[43] By medicalizing suffering and labeling it as a disorder (through the use of concepts such as PTSD and other similar definitions), a community may be led to invalidate their own culturally accepted methods.[44] An alternate approach suggests that while trauma causes distress, not all distress is pathological and emphasizes, instead, resilience and "planful problem-solving."[45] Although disasters may be a frequent life experience in Southeast Asia, the cultural resilience shown by its peoples and the evolving practice of EMS there has implications far beyond the region.

Notes

1. F. Burkle, *Disaster Medicine: Application for the Immediate Management and Triage of Civil and Military Disaster Victims* (New York: Medical Publishing Co., 1984); K. Kennedy, R. Aghababian, I. Gans, and C. Lewis, "Triage: Techniques and Applications in Decision Making," *Annals of Emergency Medicine* 28 (1996): 136–44.

2. D. E. Hogan and J. Burstein, "Basic Physics of Disasters," in *Disaster Medicine* (Philadelphia: Lippincott Williams and Wilkins, 2002), 3–9.

3. A. Bradt, K. Abraham, and R. Franks, "A Strategic Plan for Disaster Medicine in Australasia," *Emergency Medicine* 15 (2003): 271–82, quotation on 272.

4. D. Stein, S. Seedat, A. Iversen, and S. Wessely, "Post-traumatic Stress Disorder: Medicine and Politics," *Lancet* 369 (2007): 139–44.

5. B. Wisner, P. Blaikie, T. Cannon, and I. Davis, *At Risk: Natural Hazards, People's Vulnerability, and Disasters* (New York: Routledge, 2003).

6. G. Bankoff, "Cultures of Disaster, Cultures of Coping: Hazard as a Frequent Life Experience in the Philippines, 1600–2000," in *Natural Disasters, Cultural Responses: Case Studies Toward a Global Environmental History,* ed. C. Mauch and C. Pfister (Lanham, MD: Lexington Books, 2009), 265–84.

7. G. Bankoff, "Environment, Resources and Hazards," in *The Southeast Asian Handbook*, ed. P. Heenan and M. Lamontage (London and Chicago: Fitzroy Dearborn, 2001), 179–92.

8. Emergency Disaster Database, Centre for Research on the Epidemiology of Disasters website, www.emdat.be.

9. R. Kovats, "El Niño and Human Health," *Bulletin of the World Health Organization* 78 (2000): 1127–35; P. Boomgaard, *South East Asia: An Environmental History* (Santa Barbara, CA, Denver, CO, and Oxford: ABC Clio, 2007).

10. *World Disaster Report 2009* (Geneva: International Federation of Red Cross and Red Crescent Societies, 2009).

11. G. Bankoff, "Rendering the world unsafe: 'vulnerability' as Western discourse," *Disasters* 25 (2002): 19–35.

12. Bradt et al., "Strategic Plan."

13. R. Brennan and R. Nandi, "Complex Humanitarian Emergencies: a Major Global Health Challenge," *Emergency Medicine* 13 (2001): 147–56.

14. I. Kelman, "Acting on Disaster Diplomacy," *Journal of International Affairs* 59 (2006): 216–40.

15. Brennan and Nandi, "Complex Humanitarian Emergencies," 153.

16. Hogan and Burstein, "Basic Physics of Disasters," 11.

17. M. S. Sever, R. Vanholder, and N. Lameire, "Management of Crush-Related Injuries after Disasters," *New England Journal of Medicine* 35 (2006): 1052–63.

18. R. Vanholder, A. van der Tol, M. De Smet, E. Hoste, M. Koç, A. Hussain, S. Khan, and M. S. Sever, "Earthquakes and Crush Syndrome Casualties: Lessons Learnt from the Kashmir Disaster," *Kidney International* 71 (2007): 17–23.

19. P. Lim, "Wound Infections in Tsunami Survivors: A Commentary," *Annals of the Academy of Medicine* 34 (2005): 582–85.

20. O. Morgan, "Infectious Disease Risks from Dead Bodies Following Natural Disasters," *Pan-American Journal of Public Health* 15 (2004): 307–12.

21. Morgan, "Infectious Disease Risks," 308.

22. M. Ahern, R. Sari Kovats, P. Wilkinson, R. Few, and F. Matthies, "Global Health Impacts of Floods: Epidemiologic Evidence," *Epidemiologic Reviews* 27 (2005): 36–46.

23. S. Saxena, M. Van Ommeren, and B. Saraceno, "Mental Health Assistance to Populations Affected by Disasters: World Health Organization's Role," *International Review of Psychiatry* 18 (2006): 199–204.

24. L. August and B. Gianola, "Symptoms of War Trauma Induced Psychiatric Disorders: Southeast Asian Refugees and Vietnam Veterans," *International Migration Review* 21 (1987): 820–32.

25. M. Ganesan, "Psychosocial Responses to Disasters—Some Concerns," *International Review of Psychiatry* 18 (2006): 241–47.

26. H. Ghodse and S. Galea, "Tsunami: Understanding Mental Health Consequences and the Unprecedented Response," *International Review of Psychiatry* 18 (2006): 289–97.

27. Stein et al., "Post-traumatic Stress Disorder."

28. Saxena et al., "Mental Health Assistance," 199.

29. American Psychiatric Association, *Diagnostic and Statistical Manual of Mental Disorders: DSM-IV* (Washington, DC: American Psychiatric Association, 1994); World Health Organization, The *ICD-10 Classification of Mental and Behavioural Disorders* (Geneva: World Health Organization, 1992).

30. W. Howard, F. Loberiza, B. Pfohl, P. Thorne, R. Magpantay, and B. Woolson, "Initial Results, Reliability and Validity of a Mental Health Survey of Mount Pinatubo Disaster Victims," *Journal of Mental and Nervous Disease* 57 (1999): 661–72.

31. M. Kokai, S. Fujil, N. Shinfuku, and G. Edwards, "Natural Disaster and Mental Health in Asia," *Psychiatry and Clinical Neurosciences* 58 (2004): 110–16.

32. Ghodse and Galea, "Tsunami," 291–92.

33. K. Rao, "Psychosocial Support in Disaster-Affected Communities," *International Review of Psychiatry* 18 (2006): 501–5.

34. Rao, "Psychosocial Support."

35. P. Udomratn, "Mental Health and the Psychosocial Consequences of Natural Disasters in Asia," *International Review of Psychiatry* 20 (2008): 441–44.

36. P. Suedfeld, "Reactions to Societal Trauma: Distress and/or Eustress," *Political Psychology* 18 (1997): 849–61, quotation on 849.

37. Suedfeld, "Reactions to Societal Trauma."

38. A. Wardak, "The Psychiatric Effects or Stress on Afghan Society," in *International Handbook of Traumatic Stress Syndromes*, ed. J. Wilson and B. Rafael (New York: Plenum Press, 1993), 349–64.

39. X. Wang, L. Gao, N. Shinfuku, H. Zhang, C. Zhao, and Y. Shen, "Longitudinal Study of Earthquake-Related PTSD in a Randomly Selected Community Sample in North China," *American Journal of Psychiatry* 157 (2000): 1260–66.

40. P. De Silva, "The Tsunami and its Aftermath in Sri Lanka: Explorations of a Buddhist Perspective," *International Review of Psychiatry* 18 (2006): 281–87.

41. F. Van Griensven, M. Chakkraband, W. Thienkrua, B. Cardozo, P. Tantipiwatanaskul, P. Mock, S. Ekassawin, A. Varangrat, C. Gotway, M. Sabin, and J. Tappero, "Mental Health Problems among Adults in Tsunami-Affected Areas in Southern Thailand," *Journal of the American Medical Association* 296 (2006): 537–48.

42. Stein et al., "Post-traumatic Stress Disorder," 139.

43. D. Bhugra, "The Asian Tsunami," *International Review of Psychiatry* 18 (2006): 197–98.

44. Ganesan, "Psychosocial Responses to Disasters," 245.

45. Suedfeld, "Reactions to Societal Trauma," 853.

PART III
UNEVEN TRANSITIONS

5   The Demographic History of Southeast Asia in the Twentieth Century

Peter Boomgaard

FROM THE MIDDLE of the twentieth century, Southeast Asia witnessed a rapid fall in mortality, inaugurating a fundamental demographic transition. By 1945, the very high mortality from infectious diseases in Southeast Asia—detailed in the chapters by Eric Tagliacozzo, Kirsty Walker, and Mary Wilson—had yielded to improved sanitation and the gradual improvement of health facilities and the availability of antibiotic drugs. This chapter considers Southeast Asia's demographic transition in long historical perspective, providing the demographic background to this volume's consideration of the politics of health and crisis. It shows, too, that significant underlying drivers of Southeast Asia's population (and population health) were often invisible to contemporary observers. In the 1950s and 1960s, mortality decline in Southeast Asia provoked alarm as much as relief. Scholars and others were getting worried about high population growth rates. While death caused by starvation had disappeared in most of Europe and North America ("the West"), such was not the case in many Third World countries, then called Underdeveloped Countries (UDCs). In these countries, recurrent famines and high birth rates were not seldom to be found in each other's company.

A description of this trend, and a classic of its kind, is Paul Ehrlich's *The Population Bomb,* originally published in 1968.[1] He showed how the populations of UDCs like Indonesia and the Philippines doubled every twenty to twenty-five years or so, while the doubling times of what he called the Overdeveloped Countries (ODCs) tended to be in the fifty- to two-hundred-year range. These industrialized countries had undergone the so-called demographic transition—a transition from high to low population growth rates. According to Ehrlich, this was still a "catastrophic population growth" rate. And there were no signs, so he went on, of a demographic transition in the UDCs.

Writing more than forty years later, we know that there were two developments Ehrlich had not foreseen: East and Southeast Asia were starting on the path of demographic transition even when he was writing, and many Western countries would soon reach much larger doubling times, occasionally approaching or even attaining zero population growth (and therefore stopped growing or even experienced negative growth).

The point I am trying to make here is not that Ehrlich was terribly wrong in 1968—high rates of population growth (or even low ones) cannot be sustained indefinitely, and should be lowered sooner rather than later. Even with much lower growth rates nowadays in many regions, experts are still alarmed that we are heading towards a global food crisis.[2,3] The point is that population growth rates are notoriously fickle entities that can change almost overnight, and that even experts can miss the signs of what is going on under their very noses, issues to which I will return.

Very Low to Low Growth

Around 1600, some twenty-five million people lived in Southeast Asia, a figure that had increased to thirty-five million by around 1800, and to eighty-five million by 1900. By the year 2000, Southeast Asia had a population of more than five hundred million.[4]

These figures show that the average rate of population growth was very low between 1600 and 1800, clearly higher between 1800 and 1900, and much higher during the last one hundred years. Prior to circa 1800, the average annual rate of natural increase (births minus deaths) in Southeast Asia was close to zero—probably somewhere between 0.1 and 0.2 percent per year. In the nineteenth century the average annual growth rate jumped to almost 1 percent, to almost 2 percent between 1930 and 1960, and peaked at 2.2 percent on average between 1960 and 1990. Then the growth rate started to drop, a process that is still going on, reaching 1.3 percent during the period 2000–5, and it is expected to come down to an estimated 1.1 percent for the years 2010–15.[5] To account for these changes over time, we must look at the basic demographic components: mortality, fertility, and migration.

Prior to 1800, in most societies across the world, deaths and births were often roughly in balance. Mean annual population increase was therefore usually close to zero, and occasionally even negative. Nevertheless, there were differences between regions. So it would appear that the average annual growth rate of the population of Southeast Asia between 1600 and 1800, estimated at around 0.17 percent per year, was of the same order of magnitude, but perhaps slightly larger than the growth rate of India (0.14 percent). The average annual growth rates of China and Europe during this period have been estimated to be roughly double those percentages (0.30 percent). This—sometimes called homeostatic—mechanism started to change in a few regions in the eighteenth century, and on a much larger scale in the nineteenth century.

There are indications that in some Southeast Asian regions, notably Java and parts of the Philippines, population growth also accelerated during the eighteenth century. In both cases, the relative absence of wars might have been the main cause, implying that it was largely a matter of decreasing mortality. The absence of war has been called *pax imperica* ("imperial peace"), as the colonial powers, although occasionally waging war themselves, stopped indigenous states and villages from doing so.[6,7]

During the nineteenth century, the annual rate of population growth increased significantly in Southeast Asia as a whole, although not everywhere at the same time or to the same extent. Occasionally this trend was reversed, as happened in the Philippines during the later decades of the century, but that appears to have been exceptional.[8]

Part of this growth was caused by a slowly dropping death rate. The factors to which this drop in mortality has been attributed are the further spread of the *pax imperica,* the introduction of Western medicine (vaccination against smallpox, the use of quinine against malaria) and hygiene, the expansion of the areas under American food crops (corn/maize, sweet potato, cassava), improved communications and transportation, and, in some regions, increasing economic growth and income per capita. The improved transportation and communication, apart from being conducive to economic growth, was instrumental in preventing, or at least mitigating, famines. Annual quantitative (serial) information on agricultural production is weak or even absent for most Southeast Asian areas in the nineteenth century, but locally some growth (per capita) could be recorded, which must have contributed to lower levels of famine as well. Famine was often caused by weather anomalies (e.g., harvest failures due to droughts), but also by wars and epidemics (destruction of crops, lack of agricultural labor), which implies that the abovementioned spread of the *pax imperica* and medical progress also contributed to a reduced impact of famines. The drop in mortality during the nineteenth century as a cause (or even the main cause, depending on what one thinks about fertility) of higher rates of natural increase is now generally accepted, although occasionally a modern study appears to have missed it.[9]

There are also indications—although not as clear as those regarding dropping mortality—that the birth rate went up locally during the nineteenth century, but it is impossible to say by how much. This notion goes against current orthodoxy, which argues that in early modern Southeast Asia fertility was high across the board, as the female age at first marriage was low, and marriage was universal.[10,11] It is argued here that far from having natural or unchecked fertility, as was often assumed, Southeast Asia had many areas where the birth rate prior to, say, 1800, was rather low—at least compared to modern fertility figures from the 1950s—and where a considerable proportion of women married late or even stayed single. Birth rates were also kept low by prolonged breastfeeding (lactation periods of two years and up), birth spacing, various ways of preventing conception, plus abortion and infanticide. Fertility in Southeast Asia, it would appear, was not a natural given, but something that was manipulated according to the needs of the women concerned.[12,13,14,15]

Now manipulating the birth rate, can, of course, be done in two directions—down or up. Whereas prior to 1800, it would appear that in many regions of Southeast Asia low fertility figures obtained, partly thanks to family planning, to use a modern turn of phrase, during the nineteenth century women might have relaxed these birth control measures. The question is, of course, why this change in behavior or attitude occurred. The literature usually mentions one of two possibilities (or both), which are both related to a growing interest in a larger availability of labor.

The first factor is that there was a slow but perceptible shift from foraging and slash-and-burn agriculture (also called swidden or shifting cultivation) to permanent wet-rice agriculture. It is generally accepted that wet-rice agriculture is more labor intensive than other types of agriculture (even though foraging can be quite demanding, foraging women do not want to be burdened too often by young kids). It is usually assumed that increasing population density was driving this type of agricultural intensification.

The second factor is that due to the presence of the colonial state, demand for labor was increasing in many other branches of the economy. Some of this labor was compulsory, and therefore badly remunerated, but there are also examples of demand for labor—increasing due to the worldwide expansion of international trade—leading to higher income for the people concerned. As children started working at an early age, more children might be an interesting option. For obvious reasons, this has been called the demand-for-labor hypothesis.[16,17]

However, there are indications for (locally) dropping birth rates as well. This might have happened due to locally deteriorating economic circumstances in high–population density areas (density-dependent reaction). In the areas where the death rate was dropping, this influenced infant mortality as well, and with fewer deaths among breast-fed children, the average lactation period increased, thus influencing fecundity.[18] On balance and on average, there might still have been a slight increase in the birth rate in the region as a whole.

Finally, we must look at migration. Migration from Southeast Asia to other regions (emigration, in other words) prior to 1900 was insignificant, at least in terms of its possible contribution to population growth. Immigration, however, was of some importance. Around 1920, Chinese, Indians, and Europeans constituted in all probability between 4 and 5 percent of Southeast Asia's total population, a significant proportion of which had arrived prior to 1900. On balance, therefore, migration had made a positive contribution to population growth during the nineteenth century.[19]

Some Growth, but How and Why?

Average annual population growth between 1900 and 1950 was higher than the figure for the nineteenth century, but lower than the post-1950 figure. For those used to population statistics from Europe or the United States, it may sound unlikely, but even the post-1900 figures for Southeast Asia are not always reliable, and the margin of error, therefore, is rather large. Nevertheless, most historical demographers would agree that the average rate of growth of the population must have been around 1.5 percent.[20,21,22]

Mortality may have dropped somewhat, as the great medical discoveries of the late nineteenth century, which established the so-called germ theory as the new orthodoxy, were now being elaborated and applied to practical everyday "doctoring" (although not on the same scale as in the West) while nineteenth-century measures (vaccination against smallpox, quinine) were spreading to new areas. New drugs were introduced, like Salvarsan (1909) and the sulfa drugs (1930s). Some diseases—such as smallpox, cholera, and typhoid fever—thus became much less important. The improvement of transportation and communication continued, which led to higher food security.

However, there were also setbacks. The (bubonic) plague made for higher mortality in the early twentieth century, soon followed by the influenza pandemic of 1918, which, in Indonesia alone, probably killed at least 1.5 million people (compared to 215,000 victims of the plague in the same country during the entire period 1911–39).[23,24,25] Although the Great Depression of the 1930s was not as terrible for Southeast Asia's indigenous population as has sometimes been assumed, neither was it a period of mortality reduction. Higher mortality did obtain during the 1940s, during the Pacific War, when the Japanese occupation led to famines in various regions of Southeast Asia.[26,27]

As I said before, the figures are not always reliable or even available (and might never become available), but most historical demographers working on the region assume that the death rate went on decreasing during the period 1900–50, albeit not by much.

Uncertainty also governs the field of fertility, because the figures on births were probably even worse than the ones on deaths. Nevertheless, we can be sure that birth rates dropped during the 1940s, but regarding the other decades data are less clear, and regarding the entire fifty-year period there might not have been much change as compared to the nineteenth century, although a slight increase on balance is not out of the question.

Migration, finally, did not produce as large a positive balance as it did in the nineteenth century. The balance was no doubt positive between 1900 and 1929, but after 1929, with the onset of the Great Depression, many recent and even not so recent migrants left the region, and went back to their country of origin (or even that of their parents). It is less clear how many people left, as in most cases the censuses that should have been held in the 1940s never took place. A slightly positive balance for the entire period is not impossible.

The Demographic Transition

The most dramatic changes and the most astonishing acceleration and then deceleration of average annual growth rates occurred during the period 1950 to 2000.[28] This is the period of the so-called Demographic Transition, which is now sometimes called the Second Demographic Transition (the first one having occurred between 1800 and 1950). Because the figures first increased and then decreased, the mean annual growth rate for Southeast Asia for the entire period is not much above 2 percent (2.2 percent, to be precise), but that figure masks peaks of 2.5 and 2.6 percent between 1960 and 1980, and as low as 1.5 percent close to the year 2000. What happened between 1950 and 2000 is that first mortality figures started to drop, while the birth rate remained stable, but soon fertility figures started to drop as well, while the death rate no longer decreased much.

Therefore, when Paul Ehrlich wrote *The Population Bomb,* annual growth rates in Southeast Asia were indeed very high, but if you looked closer at specific countries, the first signs of lower rates were already visible, as was the case in Malaysia, the Philippines, and Singapore. We will now look at the developments in more detail.

Mortality rates started to drop faster after the Pacific War, because of the arrival in the region of the so-called miracle drugs (antibiotics). Other successes were due to measures in the preventive sphere, such as the spraying of dichlorodiphenyltrichloroethane (DDT) against the vectors of the malaria plasmodium, the *Anopheles* mosquitoes. Later on, when it was discovered that DDT was harmful to other life forms as well, it had to be abandoned, but it did bring down the incidence of malaria, and therefore the death rate. Steadily improving hygiene, primary health care, and many new drugs and treatments coming from the Western world ensured that mortality dropped slowly but surely. Thus the drop in the death rate accelerated from the 1950s.

Finally, the better quality of the diet of large sections of Southeast Asian populations from the 1970s, owing to sustained rates of economic growth per capita, did much to reinforce the downward trend of the mortality figures. Thus, while in the 1950s death rates of 20 to 30 per 1,000 had been the rule, by the year 2000, national mortality figures in Southeast Asia ranged between 5 and 15 per 1,000.[29]

Around 1960, rates of natural increase were very high in most developing countries. Rates from 2.5 to 3.5 percent per year—much higher than they had ever been in the developed world—were normal. In the 1950s, national birth rates in Southeast Asia varied from 40 to almost 50 per 1,000. Around 2000, the extremes varied from just over 10 to around 35, but most rates are now below 25 per 1,000.[30]

How did this amazingly rapid fertility transition come about? The so-called proximate factors behind the process are clear: women marry later, and their marital fertility is lower than it used to be because they are using methods of family limitation, now that reliable methods of birth control are available—including the Pill, condoms, sterilization, and intrauterine devices (IUDs). Singapore, Thailand, and Indonesia are good examples of countries where the acceptance of modern birth control methods has been increasing steadily; in Indonesia and Singapore this has been strongly stimulated by the state. In the Philippines, where the influence of the Roman Catholic Church is strong, antinatalist policies were and are not very popular. This is reflected in the Philippines' rather high total fertility rate (TFR, or average number of children per woman), which in the year 2000 stood at 3.24. Generally speaking, the increased use of modern methods of birth control in Southeast Asia is reflected in lower rates of marital fertility (and a lower TFR). Early termination of pregnancies (induced abortions) may play a role as well, as is shown in the case of Singapore, but in some countries, like Indonesia, the legal status of abortions is unclear, and a case study from Thailand shows how often young women, for various reasons, have recourse to unsafe abortions.[31,32,33,34,35]

The effects of family planning are reinforced by the increasingly higher age of women at first marriage, and the growing proportion of women who never marry. Around 1960 the percentage of women that had never been married in age group 25–29 varied between 7.6 and 19.5 in the Southeast Asian countries for which we have these data; around 2000 the percentage varied between 16.7 and 40.8. The proportion of women who never got married in the age group 45–49 varied in 1960 between 1.3 and 7.1, which came close to a situation of universal marriage; around 2000 this proportion varied between 2.0 and 12.5, which suggests a trend toward increasing non-marriage, although in the countries with the lowest proportions, like Indonesia, that trend is not very strong. If experiences in East Asia are anything to go by, the age at first marriage might continue increasing. Generally speaking, past experience has shown that a higher age at marriage leads to lower numbers of children per woman. Later age at marriage is generally assumed to be related to a drop in arranged marriages and to higher proportions of women being educated beyond primary school.

It is not clear what the influence is of changes in the divorce rate, or even what these changes are exactly. We do know that in the 1950s the divorce rate was very high among Muslims in Indonesia, Malaysia, and Thailand, and that at least in the major cities of Indonesia and Malaysia these rates were dropping during most of the period under discussion. However, among Muslims in Singapore, the divorce rate was slowly increasing, and it would appear that this also applies to Indonesia after 2003. It is less clear how the—usually low or moderate—divorce rate developed among other groups in Southeast Asia, let alone that we can generalize about the influence of the changing rates on fertility.[36,37]

Having discussed the proximate factors behind the rapid fertility transition, we should now look at the so-called ultimate or underlying factors. These are generally held to be *modernization, economic development,* and *mass communication.* Economic growth is probably the most important driving force of the demographic transition in Southeast Asia. Through better diet and better medical care, it was largely responsible for the lower rate of mortality, and it was also one of the main forces behind the fertility transition. Economic development implies urbanization. Southeast Asia, which was not very urbanized circa 1950, is now known for its so-called extended metropolitan regions—cities with many millions of inhabitants, such as Jakarta, Manila, and Bangkok. Urbanization, in turn, implies a shift from agriculture to industry and the service sector, with young women migrating temporarily to urban areas. This influenced the age of marriage and the arrival of a first child, as children could be combined with agricultural activities, but far less easily with working in the factory. Economic development also implies schooling.

Modernization followed in the wake of economic growth. Notions of individual choice and destiny, of better education, and higher aspirations, particularly for women, are all part of the so-called Western ideology that is more or less identical with the modern way of life, which went global during the last few decades.

The enormous impact of modernization and the rapid adoption of methods of birth control would have been unthinkable without the spread of radio and television. It would appear that this goes a long way toward explaining why the fertility transition could have taken place so quickly in a number of countries.[38]

Finally, we must look at migration. For the quarter century after the Pacific War, Southeast Asia experienced very little international migration. There was some outmigration of former immigrants or their children (European and Chinese) owing to decolonization, but as a percentage of the total population that did not amount to much (perhaps 1 per 10,000 per year during a decade).

However, from the 1970s, international migration of Southeast Asians between countries in the region and out of the region gained momentum. During the Vietnam War, Thai and Filipino workers came to work for the Americans in Vietnam. With the increase in oil prices beginning in 1973, migrants from the Philippines, Thailand, and later Indonesia flocked to Saudi Arabia and other oil-producing Middle Eastern countries, where a building boom had taken off. During the 1980s and 1990s, the scale of the migration flows increased, as did the number of countries involved, owing to labor shortages in Japan, Hong Kong,

Singapore, South Korea, and Taiwan. In recent years we have seen a growing trend of emigrants from Southeast Asia to Organisation for Economic Co-operation and Development (OECD) countries. Around 2000, there were already about four million Southeast Asians, mainly from the Philippines and Vietnam, living in high-income nations like the United States and various Western European countries. Of the more recent flows of out-migration, a considerable proportion consists of women, often nurses, caregivers or domestic servants in the employ of private persons. In the two major countries of origin, the Philippines and Indonesia, women outnumber men among official labor migrants. I have never seen data regarding the age of these women, but some of them are no doubt young, and in that case emigration might lead to postponement of marriage, and possible fewer children. But even if they are already married, prolonged absence might have the same ultimate effect—fewer children. To my knowledge, these effects have not been properly researched so far.

One thing is certain, and that is that the many millions who are thus absent from the region for many years (and some will never return) are not compensated for by immigrants to Southeast Asia, and on balance, therefore, the region has fewer inhabitants, and therefore lower population growth. The difference could be to the tune of about 2 percent of the total population of the region disappearing annually.

Singapore and Brunei are mainly immigration countries, whereas emigrants come predominantly from the Philippines, Indonesia, Vietnam, Myanmar [Burma], Cambodia, and Laos. Malaysia and Thailand have both significant immigration and emigration flows. Clearly, then, there are huge differences in the region regarding the demographic effects of out-migration. In Malaysia and Thailand the migration balance is probably close to zero, while in the Philippines there is a considerable negative balance.[39]

The way the contribution of international migration to the economy and society of the sending country has been judged has varied considerably. Although the effects were seen as beneficial at an early stage, later (often Marxist) studies were largely negative. However, more recently, the role of out-migrants in their country of origin has been seen in a more positive light, emphasizing the role remittances can and do play in economic development, even though the reason so many people have to migrate is, of course, a lack of economic development.[40]

However, while the effects for the society of origin might be positive—and generally speaking more economic development would mean more income per capita, which at low income levels would probably be spent on more and better food, resulting in better health—there are indications that the migrants themselves are often worse off in terms of health. Higher risks of contracting tuberculosis and malaria, as well as hepatitis, have been reported, while among specific, highly mobile groups higher risks of HIV/AIDS and other STDs prevail. However, there are also studies reporting better physical health among immigrants from Southeast Asia relative to a broad range of reference groups.[41]

Is it likely that the birth and death rates will continue to drop? We do not want to make the same mistake as Paul Ehrlich did in the late 1960s and miss the signs of change (provided, of course, there are such signs). So are there signs that fertility will not continue to decrease? If we look at UN tables with Southeast Asian total fertility rates, projected as far into the future as the year 2050, this does hardly seem to be the case. The TFR for the whole of Southeast Asia continues to drop gradually from 2.45 during the period 2000–5 to 1.83 for the years 2045–50. In only a few individual countries—Singapore, Thailand and Vietnam—is the TFR expected to go up a bit between 2025–30 and 2045–50. In all other countries it continues to decrease, so in most of these countries, the population is no longer expected to reproduce itself (the so-called replacement level) by the mid-twenty-first century or even earlier.

However, there are some signs in individual countries that present trends may not be continued. While the singulate mean age at marriage (SMAM), an indirect measure of marriage age, had been rising gradually across the board in Southeast Asia since 1960, it dropped in the Philippines and Singapore between 1990 and 2000, and in Indonesia between 2000 and 2010. Since decentralization, Indonesia's contraceptive service programs are under the management of local governments, and there are fears that it will be difficult to revitalize these programs if and when needed. We should probably not expect a baby boom any time soon, but a slowing down of the drop in fertility would not be out of the question.[42,43,44]

And what will the death rate do? As the Southeast Asian population gets a higher proportion of old people (the life expectancy at birth in Southeast Asia rose from 42.4 years in 1950–55 to 68.0 years in 2000–5), the drop in the death rate will inevitably slow down a bit. It is also likely that climate change (possibly leading to more cyclones, and certainly to the inundation of coastal zones) and pollution of land, air, and water will make for increased morbidity and mortality—or at least a weakening of the downward trend. But evidence for these phenomena—at least in so far as the influence the death rate on any scale—is still tentative.[45,46]

Therefore, on balance, it is possible that the birth rate and the death rate will start to drop more slowly than they have so far, and perhaps at lower rates than predicted. But even then the Demographic Transition in Southeast Asia could be called a miracle—even for the specialists it came unexpectedly, the drop was faster than in the West, and the death and birth rates fell deeper.

Notes

1. Paul R. Ehrlich, *The Population Bomb* (New York: Ballantine, 1968).
2. Tanya Nolan, "Population Boom Increasing Global Food Crisis," *The World Today*, May 4, 2011, www.abc.net.au/news/2011-05-04.
3. Lester R. Brown, "The World Is Closer to a Food Crisis than Most People Realize," *The Guardian*, July 24, 2012, www.guardian.co.uk/environment/2012/jul/24.
4. Peter Boomgaard, *Southeast Asia: An Environmental History* (Santa Barbara, CA: ABC-CLIO, 2007).
5. Charles Hirschman and Sabrina Bonaparte, "Population and Society in Southeast Asia: A Historical Perspective," in *Demographic Change in Southeast Asia: Recent Histories and Future Directions,* ed. Lindy Williams and Michael Philip Guest (Ithaca, NY: Southeast Asia Program Publications, Cornell University, 2012), 5–41.
6. Boomgaard, *Southeast Asia.*
7. Linda A. Newson, *Conquest and Pestilence in the Early Spanish Philippines* (Honolulu: University of Hawai'i Press, 2009).
8. Ken de Bevoise, *Agents of Apocalypse: Epidemic Disease in the Colonial Philippines* (Princeton, NJ: Princeton University Press, 1995).
9. Hirschman and Bonaparte, "Population and Society in Southeast Asia," 5–41.
10. Hirschman and Bonaparte, "Population and Society in Southeast Asia," 5–41.
11. Anthony Reid, *Southeast Asia in the Age of Commerce, 1450–1680,* vol. 1, *The Lands below the Winds* (New Haven, CT, and London: Yale University Press, 1988).
12. Newson, *Conquest and Pestilence in the Early Spanish Philippines.*
13. Reid, *Southeast Asia in the Age of Commerce.*
14. Peter Boomgaard, "Bridewealth and Birth Control: Low Fertility in the Indonesian Archipelago, 1500–1900," *Population and Development Review* 29 (2003): 197–214.
15. Judith Richell, *Disease and Demography in Colonial Burma* (Singapore and Copenhagen: NUS Press, NIAS Press, 2006).
16. Boomgaard, "Bridewealth and Birth Control," 197–214.
17. David Henley, "From Low to High Fertility in Sulawesi (Indonesia) during the Colonial Period: Explaining the 'First Fertility Transition,'" *Population Studies* 60 (2006): 309–27.
18. Peter Boomgaard, "Demographic Transition in Southeast Asia," in *Southeast Asia: A Historical Encyclopedia, from Angkor Wat to East Timor,* ed. Ooi Keat Gin (Santa Barbara, CA: ABC-CLIO, 2004), 414–18.
19. Boomgaard, *Southeast Asia.*
20. Boomgaard, *Southeast Asia.*
21. Hirschman and Bonaparte, "Population and Society in Southeast Asia," 5–41.
22. Boomgaard, "Demographic Transition in Southeast Asia," 414–18.
23. Norman G. Owen, "Toward a History of Health in Southeast Asia," in *Death and Disease in Southeast Asia: Explorations in Social, Medical and Demographic History,* ed. Norman G. Owen (Singapore and New York: Oxford University Press, 1987), 3–30.
24. Terence H. Hull, "Plague in Java," in *Death and Disease in Southeast Asia: Explorations in Social, Medical and Demographic History,* ed. Norman G. Owen (Singapore and New York: Oxford University Press, 1987), 210–34.
25. Colin Brown, "The Influenza Pandemic of 1918 in Indonesia," in *Death and Disease in Southeast Asia: Explorations in Social, Medical and Demographic History,* ed. Norman G. Owen (Singapore and New York: Oxford University Press, 1987), 235–56.
26. Paul H. Kratoska, ed., *Food Supplies and the Japanese Occupation in South-East Asia* (New York: St. Martin's Press, 1998).

27. Peter Boomgaard and Ian Brown, eds., *Weathering the Storm: The Economies of Southeast Asia in the 1930s Depression* (Singapore and Leiden: ISEAS, KITLV, 2001).

28. Boomgaard, "Demographic Transition in Southeast Asia," 414–18.

29. East-West Center, *The Future of Population in Asia* (Honolulu, HI: East-West Center, 2002).

30. *The Future of Population in Asia.*

31. Terence H. Hull and Henry Mosley, *Revitalization of Family Planning in Indonesia* (Jakarta: Government of Indonesia and United Nations Population Fund, 2009).

32. Iwu Dwisetyani Utomo and Peter McDonald, "Adolescent Reproductive Health in Indonesia: Contested Values and Policy Inaction," *Studies in Family Planning* 40, no. 2 (2009): 133–46.

33. Andrea Whittaker, ed., *Abortion in Asia: Local Dilemmas, Global Politics* (New York and Oxford: Berghahn, 2010).

34. Arunrat Tangmunkongvorakul, Cathy Banwell, Gordon Carmichael, Iwu Dwisetyani Utomo and Adrian Sleigh, "Birth Control, Pregnancy and Abortion among Adolescents in Chiang Mai, Thailand," *Asian Population Studies* 7, no. 1 (2011): 15–34.

35. Terence H. Hull, "Fertility in Southeast Asia," in *Demographic Change in Southeast Asia: Recent Histories and Future Directions*, ed. Lindy Williams and Michael Philip Guest (Ithaca, NY: Southeast Asia Program Publications, Cornell University, 2012), 43–64.

36. Gavin Jones, Terence H. Hull, and Maznah Mohamad, eds., *Changing Marriage Patterns in Southeast Asia: Economic and Socio-Cultural Dimensions* (London and New York: Routledge, 2011).

37. Gavin Jones and Bina Gubhaju, "Marriage Trends in Southeast Asia," in *Demographic Change in Southeast Asia: Recent Histories and Future Directions*, ed. Lindy Williams and Michael Philip Guest (Ithaca, NY: Southeast Asia Program Publications, Cornell University, 2012), 65–91.

38. Boomgaard, "Demographic Transition in Southeast Asia," 414–18.

39. Graeme Hugo, "Changing Patterns of Population Mobility in Southeast Asia," in *Demographic Change in Southeast Asia: Recent Histories and Future Directions*, ed. Lindy Williams and Michael Philip Guest (Ithaca, NY: Southeast Asia Program Publications, Cornell University, 2012), 121–63.

40. Hein de Haas, "Migration and Development: A Theoretical Perspective," *International Migration Review* 44, no. 1 (2010): 227–64.

41. Mark J. VanLandingham and Hongyun Fu, "Migration and Health in Southeast Asia," in *Demographic Change in Southeast Asia: Recent Histories and Future Directions*, ed. Lindy Williams and Michael Philip Guest (Ithaca, NY: Southeast Asia Program Publications, Cornell University, 2012), 165–84.

42. Hirschman and Bonaparte, "Population and Society in Southeast Asia," 5–41.

43. Hull and Mosley, *Revitalization of Family Planning in Indonesia.*

44. Hull, "Fertility in Southeast Asia," 43–64.

45. Boomgaard, *Southeast Asia.*

46. Sara R. Curran and Noah Derman, "Population and Environment in Southeast Asia: Complex Dynamics and Trends," in *Demographic Change in Southeast Asia: Recent Histories and Future Directions*, ed. Lindy Williams and Michael Philip Guest (Ithaca, NY: Southeast Asia Program Publications, Cornell University, 2012), 185–208.

6 "Rural" Health in Modern Southeast Asia

Atsuko Naono

Introduction

Over the course of the past century in Southeast Asia, the term "rural" received sometimes sporadic and sometimes considerable attention from colonial governments, postcolonial governments, and international and private organizations concerned with health—such as the League of Nations Health Organization (LNHO), the Rockefeller Foundation, the World Health Organization (WHO), and other non-governmental organizations (NGOs). When and how rural medicine began to be viewed differently from urban medicine, when colonial doctors began to see the medicine differently in rural space and urban space, and when the idea that the village was a place where health was dealt with differently from anywhere else, however, are all questions that have hardly been dealt with directly in the literature on the history of medicine in Southeast Asia. Government records do not make the task any easier. Colonial and postcolonial medical reports are rich in statistics on rural and urban areas, but this terminology is rarely defined. While we might easily define Bangkok, Jakarta, Manila, Saigon, or Singapore as urban areas, in the colonial period, just as today, no single definition of what a rural area constitutes has been agreed upon. During the colonial period, the government authorities identified the village as the major unit of rural society, giving the village an importance and attributing to it administrative functions that it probably never had. These views influenced scholarship on Southeast Asia into the 1980s. It has been only recently that scholars have tried to understand rural Southeast Asia from the inside.[1]

Substantial literature has long been forthcoming on the place of civilizational or cultural space in the meeting and negotiation of European and indigenous medicine, medical technologies, and concepts of health. Although it is very useful to an understanding the trajectory of the spread of Western medicine in the historiography on colonialism, this literature has been less inclined to place these meetings in the context of geographical or developmental spaces that are commonly used to characterize zones of medical and health activity today. Changing and conflicting perceptions of the rural landscape had an important historical relationship to the implementation of health projects, at least in Southeast Asia, although this relationship has not been well understood or much discussed in the prevailing literature on the history of medicine in the region.

In this chapter, I attempt to show how an understanding of so-called rural health in modern Southeast Asia can be helped by considerations not just of how health was changing outside of the cities and major towns, which is as precise a definition of rural as I will attempt here, but also how those active in or writing about health care in Southeast Asia shaped "the rural" in their assessments and how considerations of the rural landscape framed their thinking. As Marie Stenseke observes,

> [t]he landscape holds no values in itself, just those identified by people from different standpoints. People respond to landscapes according to their various mental maps and experiences, and do not value different landscape elements in the same way. Individual landscape valuation may just be a result of a visual impression, an intuitive emotion or something deeply rooted in the individual. . . . The individual relationship to a place varies, depending on how one has come to know a certain area, and how it corresponds to one's preferences.[2]

Western impressions and observations of the local environment, climate, and conditions often contributed to creating negative views of local medical and health practices. The major government health programs of the last century in rural Southeast Asia were mainly medical interventions by urban-based medical officials. In Southeast Asia's colonial period, these medical authorities were part of the colonial medical establishment, either Europeans or Indians, or indigenous doctors trained in Western medical schools and usually drawn from urban-based colonial elites. Later, in the early independence period, state medical programs were directed at rural areas by largely urban-based political elites, trained in Western schools. These programs were often implemented by doctors who had been in the colonial medical service since the 1930s and were established on the basis of those traditions and nationalism, the culture of national health planning that has largely persisted to the present.[3] The other major stream of major public health initiatives in Southeast Asia since the 1930s has been shaped by international health authorities, whether at the Rockefeller Foundation, the LNHO, the WHO, or in the other major NGOs, largely dominated by authorities external to the region. As a result, understandings of the rural at the heart of so many official health policies and programs have been heavily influenced by foreign understandings or external constructions.[4] This is not to say that philanthropic or international organizations were blind to the need to include local perspectives. Indeed, the Rockefeller Foundation went great lengths to do so. Nevertheless, the generalized institutional view developed in New York City remained as external to rural Southeast Asia as had colonial decision making in London, Paris, or The Hague had been in the colonial period. Identifying the agency of external authorities also helps to explain why perceptions of rural Southeast Asian health have changed over time in tandem with evolving or conflicting understandings of rural areas elsewhere, often in areas far distant from the region. I thus structure my discussion around the major understandings of "rural" Southeast Asia as held by the medical authorities who implemented health policies from the colonial period to the present.

Colonial Period and World War II

According to V. R. Savage, citing Manning Nash, nostalgic looks away from the city and to the countryside as the clean and healthy opposite of the city were underway since the eighteenth century in Europe, followed by America in the nineteenth, and has left its best-known evidence in the works produced by the Romantic movement.[5] It is difficult to discern, however, if the men who came as Indian Medical Service officers from England or as missionary doctors from the United States carried these ideas with them. If they did, they quickly abandoned them. During the colonial period, official medical reporting tended to use the term "rural" to excuse the limited colonial investment in indigenous health. Rural areas were areas far from the reach of medical authorities in major towns or civil stations, and areas lost to disease anyway. As Savage explains, it was true that Western impressions of and experiences in the Southeast Asian tropical environment led to both favorable and unfavorable views. However, due to the widely accepted and vehemently held miasma theory of the period, the "insalubrious and unwholesome tropical climate," dominated by moist climactic elements, was often viewed as a major cause of diseases.[6] Rural areas were also seen as places entirely under indigenous culture's grip and were thus out of reach to colonial medicine. Well into the first several decades of the twentieth century, until World War II, rural Southeast Asia continued to be seen as dangerous and off limits, but there was some effort into the 1920s to provide doctors at civil stations in towns who would then by tour or through native assistants vaccinate and collect statistics on births, deaths, and so on. But generally, colonial concern over health was limited to what was important for the maintenance of the colonial order, as shown in recent research on the selective nature of colonial interest in mental health.[7]

The most significant effort to mobilize indigenous doctors to treat rural Southeast Asians was the *dokters-djawa* in the Dutch East Indies who were the product of training begun from the 1850s. The *dokters-djawa* were drawn from indigenous Javanese elites and were at least supposed to be provided with extensive medical education and then sent to the villages. Nevertheless, as authorities on this medical group point out, about half of the *dokters-djawa* were not much more than vaccinators.[8] Burma similarly trained native assistants as vaccinators for village work, but set up a medical school in country only in the twentieth century, half a century after the Dutch in Indonesia. While the Dutch conception of the *dokters-djawa* was that they would compete with *dukun*, indigenous medical men on their home turf—in the rural areas, the British trained Burmese medical doctors in Western medicine to compete with indigenous medical men, *hse-hsayas*. As in the Dutch East Indies, failure to make significant inroads into the rural areas was blamed on the grip indigenous *hse-hsayas* or Burmese inoculators had on the village—making indigenous medical practitioners into colonial medical bogeymen. In 1916, the government began to seriously investigate the possibility of teaching indigenous doctors Western medicine to make up for staff shortages caused by World War I. However, in the end it was decided that although indigenous medical doctors did some good, their potential for doing bad far outweighed any advantage in mobilizing them in rural areas as official agents of colonial health policies. Despite this decision, some civil surgeons began to push Burmese medical authorities to do more to promote the use of Burmese *hse-sayas* with a limited amount of Western training to improve on their methods but leaving to them the essence and culture of their practices. Despite government approval in 1922 to open training institutes for Burmese *hse-hsayas*, by the end of the 1920s, the investigation to unify European and indigenous medicine in Burma was abandoned.[9]

Colonial regimes remained unable or unwilling to afford the costs of extending Westernized healthcare to rural populations. Generally, this provided space for an American philanthropic organization, the Rockefeller Foundation, to experiment with the improvement of rural health through improved sanitation and health education. In contrast to the colonial view, for whom the rural lay outside of the reach of the colonial state, the new international health organizations looked at rural Southeast Asia as part of a broader, transnational landscape neglected by prevailing state medical policies that favored urban populations. This condition was true of European countries as well, and Central and Eastern European countries were among the first targeted. But the situation was more severe in colonial possessions, where medical policies were designed to avoid major health expenditures as much as possible. International health organizations emphasized the teaching of rural populations to transform their own living environment. The emphasis on local conditions also meant greater attention to local nuances, rather than the standardized colonial policies that sometimes merely replicated policies developed in the metropole. Immediately after the Depression era, international organizations concerned with health such as the Rockefeller Foundation and the LNHO were advocating the necessity of "internationaliz[ing]" public health to fit variable local conditions by educating the rural population of the importance of hygiene and a good diet and leading them to gradually improve their own health conditions through programs such as rural reconstruction.[10]

Underlying the reorientation toward rural health promoted by some of the new international organizations was a different understanding of rural areas that saw rural health as central to the wellbeing of the nation. Anne Foster, for example, appropriately describes the Rockefeller doctors as secular missionaries. They, like the American Baptist missionaries that had come to Southeast Asia a century earlier to convert the population to Christianity, also came to the region "to spread American values."[11] Rockefeller doctors' views of rural health as crucial for the well-being of the nation drew in part upon the legacy of the Country Life Movement in the first few decades of the twentieth century in the United States. The Country Life Movement sought to develop a rural response to industrialization and urban development by modernizing the rural sector in America through "rural uplift," the application of new technologies and approaches to farming that would make rural life more efficient, and focused on the role of education for producing this change.[12] Although the spirit was clearly there, importantly and perhaps ironically, the Rockefeller doctors also shared with colonial regimes the desire to promote health in Southeast Asia at the least possible cost.

In the late 1920s and 1930s, the Rockefeller Foundation began a number of model health projects in rural Southeast Asia to test and teach the benefits of improved rural sanitation, water availability, midwifery, health education, and health data collection. At their model village of Hlegu in Burma, the Rockefeller Foundation began selecting certain diseases most likely to be demonstrable of their effective operations to serve as a convincing showcase.[13] But this remained a very local and small project. In the Philippines, the Rockefeller effort began in 1929 with a "demonstration unit for rural sanitation" at Calauan in Laguna Province, followed by a second at Navotas in Rizal Province in 1931.[14] In 1924, the Rockefeller Foundation began a hookworm control program in West Java.[15]

Expanding the Rockefeller projects in Java was difficult at first; Dutch officials resisted Rockefeller intervention in part because of their particular view of the unique village life of rural Java. As Gouda explains, the Dutch viewed rural Java as operating according to a special premodern logic that would not yield to the rational, scientific approaches of the Europeans; thus, villages could not be modernized in the way the Dutch suspected the Rockefeller Foundation wanted to improve them. It was thought that this effort to change how villages ran themselves might even prove dangerous.[16] Despite this resistance, Dr. John Lee Hydrick, who began his work on Java with the hookworm project in 1924, continued his work in the area until 1939. By 1933 he had selected sixty Javanese villages to serve as health models, although by the end of the 1930s the Dutch Public Health Service officially named the demonstration unit at Purwokerto as the center of rural hygiene for the entire colony.[17] This work left an important health legacy for central Java that remained unfelt elsewhere in the archipelago.[18] The core of the Rockefeller effort in Java was the training and utilization of health "technicians" (*mantris*) who were drawn from the same villages whose sanitary condition they would inspect and whose neighbors they would give rudimentary health education. Making use of such local talent who knew the vernacular languages, could make use of local networks, and could approach villagers from a position of superior status helped to guarantee their acceptance by villagers. A school to train these health *mantris* was established in 1936 in urban Banyumas, although Stein points out that the *mantris* never became full medical doctors per se, but remained merely technicians trained in the techniques of health propaganda and education. This was necessary given the nature of health provision to rural Indonesians in a colony that wanted to achieve improvements in health but at the lowest possible cost.[19] The health education technologies that were being used by Rockefeller were the same as those of other health bodies and would represent the beginning of a general approach to getting rural people to take care of their own health. The Rockefeller effort was joined in a few years by new international attention to rural health. In 1937, a conference that focused on rural hygiene was organized by the LNHO and held in Bandung, Indonesia. Several key issues raised in this conference related to the to the necessity of local participation in rural reconstruction and local support.

A major, region-wide interruption was brought by the Japanese occupation from late 1941 until the end of World War II in 1945, which either temporarily suspended the activities of colonial health agencies or ended them altogether (although many of the same indigenous staff would continue under Japanese tutelage and then reemerge in charge of health departments in newly independent states after the Japanese had left). Even where there was some continuity in personnel, public health services were severely curtailed, especially outside of the towns. Wartime destruction saw many outlying health stations simply erased, and widespread shortages made matters worse. Links with all sorts of international organizations and foundations that had undertaken health and fitness work in the region before the war—such as the League of Red Cross Societies, the Girl Guides, the Rockefeller Foundation, the League of Nations (from which Japan had withdrawn before the war), and others—were broken. In areas where Europeans were able to return, things were not picked up again immediately because European regimes focused on reestablishing rule rather than development, and some places ejected the Europeans again very quickly.

The reconstruction of rural health after World War II was uneven across Southeast Asia. After the independence of the Philippines in 1946, the U.S. Public Health Service invested very heavily in rebuilding the country's health infrastructure, rebuilding hospitals and rural health centers destroyed during the war.[20] In other colonies, by contrast, European medical workers came back to postwar Southeast Asia with a more racial view of health again. In these places, the Japanese occupation had a lasting impact on the equation of rural health with what was out of reach of central medical authorities and forgetting the lessons of the late 1930s. What was characterized by colonial health authorities as rural and unscientific medicine and related practices was redeployed on the other side of racial divisions by the returning Europeans. "Urban" and "rural," which had steadily become the chief colonial abstractions of medical space in Southeast Asia, were now overshadowed by a return to nineteenth-century categories of European and native health. Rural medicine in Burma, for example, now became firmly Burmese traditional medicine, a category that had begun to be used in certain contexts from the 1920s. When the Red Cross returned to Indonesia in 1945 its main concern was dealing with the malnutrition of the released populations from the POW camps. The Dutch were also unable to reassert control over the entirety of what had been the Dutch East Indies because of the civil war that followed the Japanese collapse. The report that was published was the result of work from 1945 to 1946 that focused on different groups—all defined by race (Chinese, Ambonese, Indo-Europeans, Europeans, Natives, etc.), without reference once to rural or urban origins. In this view, race rather than geography was the most important way of dividing people to understand the implications of the Japanese occupation.[21] Worse, during the Indonesian Revolution, the Dutch imposed a naval blockade that prevented the flow of medical supplies to rural Indonesians, leading life expectancy to drop from thirty-five to twenty-eight years by the end of the 1940s.[22]

The Javanese medical staff, trained in the Intensive Rural Hygiene approach in the Rockefeller villages, continued to conduct work in rural areas, although they were forced to shift locations to avoid fighting in the revolutionary war. The Hygiene Mantri School, reestablished in 1945 by health workers trained at the prewar Rockefeller unit, was moved to Magelang in 1947.[23]

The 1950s to Mid-1970s

The newly independent governments of Southeast Asia sought to improve national health as a conspicuous demonstration of their ability to match and exceed the achievements of the colonial period. But these new regimes lacked the resources that some of the colonial regimes had enjoyed, and as the new prime minister of independent Burma, U Nu, admitted, the country had to have a health plan that "was in consonance" with its ability to pay for it. The greatest and quickest gains could be achieved at the lowest cost in rural areas, where the colonial record had not been good at all. It could also be argued that this is where there was the greatest genuine need for health development and also where 85 percent of Burmese at independence still lived.[24] Whereas colonial regimes had treated rural areas as peculiarly indigenous cultural spaces, rural areas in independent Southeast Asia took on, in the postwar period, associations with underdevelopment.

In 1949, a year after Burmese independence, the Mass Education Council was created to train "educational workers" who would then be sent to the countryside to improve the rural economy, education, social welfare, and health.[25] For help and advice, the new government turned not to the British—who were unwelcome—but to the Americans, who emerged as the main developmental model and sources of technical assistance and aid money after the war (although they would see considerable competition as sources of development assistance and guidance from the Soviet Union and then the PRC as the Cold War emerged). In 1951, the Burmese Department of Social Services requested U.S. technical advisers to help with rural reconstruction. The United States sent twenty health specialists to Burma to conduct a health survey of the country and recommended development projects. In addition to defining villages and rural areas as separate development zones, these advisers found the entire country, including the major metropolitan areas, were in need of clean water and working sanitation systems. Nevertheless, the first project decided upon was the digging of new wells and the construction of latrines in rural areas of the country. Connected with this effort, the American specialists conducted health education in the rural areas until such time as indigenous health demonstrators could be trained. Interestingly, the only operating drilled well they found already in operation was a poorly maintained well at Hlegu, which was presumably that established by the Rockefeller project in the 1930s.[26] Several years later, Nu complemented this effort with the Welfare State Scheme for Health. This scheme was partly aimed at bringing national health back up to colonial standards (for urban areas) and extending modern health to rural areas (for the first time). In addition to training more doctors and health officers and building four hundred new rural health centers, this program also recommenced health propaganda through photographs, films, and lectures—but also Nu's pet project, the distribution of vitamin tablets.[27]

In Indonesia, Dr. R. Mochtar, who had been the colonial director of health propaganda in the 1930s, and in the 1950s headed the Division of General Hygiene, extended the rural hygiene approach. Under his leadership, hygiene *mantris* became hygiene educators and were assisted by village hygiene workers to guide rural sanitation projects. The educators and village workers numbered a total of seven hundred for the entire archipelago, as the postwar effort continued the colonial tradition of keeping costs to a minimum and rural health remained deprioritized. Throughout the Sukarno years, the real absence in rural areas were local health centers.[28] Instead, the Sukarno government also began to build maternal and child health centers in Indonesian villages with aid from UNICEF.[29]

These programs were encouraged by new international health bodies. In 1957, for example, the WHO SEA regional office sponsored a rural health conference in New Delhi, and reintroduced subjects discussed at 1937 conference. These included, for example, key issues such as the organization of the "multipurpose village worker, the formation of village committees to encourage the people to participate in health services and village improvement, the importance of health services development going hand in hand with other welfare and development programs."[30] Although Sunil Amrith argues that the WHO's techno-centric approach to diseases such as the indiscriminant application of DDT, antibiotics, etc., was unable to serve as a panacea because it did not resolve varying local socioeconomic problems, the WHO was successful in strengthening the national government's attention to the health needs of the rural areas.[31]

The major problem was that these states lacked the resources for a complete overhaul of rural health limitations. They thus focused instead on symbolic campaigns targeting particular diseases rather than general rural health problems. The Sukarno regime, for example, emphasized campaigns against smallpox, yaws, and malaria. Rural insurgencies throughout region also led to symbolic programs, in particular in the communist zones of Indochina, but the emphasis was still on urban indigenous populations. As a result, despite significant official hype about rural health projects, the 1960s actually saw a decline in rural health programs in many countries in the region. In some cases, rural political problems and hyperinflation brought the improvement of rural health to a standstill, such as in Indonesia from 1960 to 1967.[32] Some Southeast Asian countries even rejected foreign aid altogether as dangerous to the national project. In the case of Burma, its Burmese Way to Socialism Program, begun after the military take-over in 1962, "advocated Burmese control of the economy and self reliance."[33] This rejection of outside help would change in the mid-1970s.

The Mid-1970s to the Present

The mid-1970s brought renewed interest in the condition of rural health in Southeast Asia. This was partly because of the need to rebuild rural health in countries whose neglect had reached its limits, as in Burma, or in countries rebuilding after decades of war, such as Laos and Vietnam (in Cambodia, Khmer Rouge rule from 1975 to 1978 and the ensuing civil war afterward instead provoked dramatic rural health decline). Even before this, a change in U.S. foreign aid would help to promote rural health programs in other countries, when, from late 1973, USAID changed its aid structure to adopt new directions that focused on basic development assistance. In 1978 the WHO/UNICEF Regional Meeting on Primary Health Care in Alma-Ata set the goal of "Health for All People by the Year 2000."[34]

Research on the demand for health care in rural Java in the early 1970s under Suharto's New Order found that the government's focus on attempting to improve rural prosperity rather than health could be arguably justified by the fact that rural people approved of the prioritizing of higher rural incomes. In the 1970s in both Indonesia and Thailand, economic growth (as well as oil profits in the case of Indonesia) allowed the government to build more rural health centers in great numbers. Indonesia's construction of rural health facilities increased under Suharto, who had 2,300 health centers built in towns and villages from 1968 to 1970. In 1970, he began the Presidential Instruction program that made the development of rural physical and social infrastructure an important government goal and during the following decade built 2,000 health centers and 9,000 health subcenters, as well as local health posts and mobile health units.[35]

In both countries, however, political and institutional conflicts hindered the implementation of rural health programs. In Indonesia, for example, the Health Ministry could make health policies, but their successful implementation depended upon the Interior Ministry and the cooperation of local governments. There were also problems in translating rural health investment into improved rural health. Large numbers of health centers were built according to one formula or model with little attention to differences in local needs. Local governments tended to use local health centers, at least in Indonesia, to siphon off money for other investments. The main problem was that rural areas were unable to attract or retain staff, doctors, or nurses at rural health centers that had few amenities to offer young professionals. Such staff tended to concentrate in large cities.[36] As late as 1978, 50 percent of the health centers on Java, and 60 percent on the outer islands, had no physician on staff.[37]

In Thailand, one solution to the neglect of rural health provisions was the encouragement of self-reliance by the promotion of traditional medicine and village temple health centers. An NGO called the Traditional Medicine for Self-Curing Project was established in 1980; it promoted the use of traditional medicine to improve health, and its support included aid to the Foundation for the Revival and Promotion of Traditional Medicine, which established an Ayurveda college in the same year.[38] But the NGO also helped villagers collaborate with traditional health resources in rural areas. In one case reported by the *Bangkok Post*, this collaboration led to one village setting up in 1984 "their first local health centre and herbal garden in the temple compound" with the help of local "folk medicine men," the village temple, and government officials.[39] In Vietnam, from the 1960s to the 1980s, traditional medicine was the "crucial component of rural programs to promote public health" and became "a cultural symbol of the self sufficiency and age-old experiences of the Vietnamese people."[40] Citing Hoang Bao Chau, Wahlberg explains that after the temporal decline of traditional medical practices in Vietnam in the late 1980s, the government revived initiatives to educate local people about Vietnamese traditional medicine including "the 'Doctor at Home' and 'Drug at Home' programs" that promoted self-reliance in rural areas regarding common medical problems in the 1990s.[41]

New programs were embarked upon to rectify the problems of rural health. Thailand reacted to this problem from the late 1980s by aggressively recruiting more health staff to rural areas. In Indonesia, the government began two programs. The Village Health Development Program from 1978 represented the first nationwide rural primary healthcare initiative and included the recruitment training of members of the village as health care volunteers to maintain health centers and to improve the health environment of the village. The second program was the Village Midwife Program of 1989–96. The latter sought to alleviate rural health problems by placing a midwife, additionally trained in nutrition and immunization, in every village.[42] In the early 1970s, Burma began to open the door to outside development in reaction to the failure of the Burmese Way to Socialism policies; this increased from fifty million dollars a year in the early 1970s to four hundred million dollars a year in the late 1970s.[43]

The gravity of rural health planning and implementation has shifted since the mid-1990s in the region. In earlier decades, discussions about health in rural areas were directed from the political center. However, since the mid-1990s, there has been a change—NGOs have increasingly helped to fund local organizations in rural areas and mobilize local participation in them.

Imbalances in health care and problems have also shifted. Rigg warns us against viewing rural Southeast Asia as the clear opposite of urban due to the large and frequent movement of people from the countryside into the cities in contemporary Southeast Asia.[44] While attention to rural health has grown, problems related to urbanization and the rising costs of urban health care have led to poorer health conditions in growing urban slums. One of the ways to understand rural health may be better informed by reflecting on the health issues in urban areas in Southeast Asia. In a *Bangkok Post* article of October 15, 2010, Samlee Pilangbangchang, the regional director of WHO Southeast Asia, explained the urban health problem thus:

> In most countries of Southeast Asia, a well-structured rural health care infrastructure has been well developed, but the same degree of development does not apply to the public health system in urban areas, which therefore has many gaps and weaknesses.[45]

Urban health problems have worsened very quickly within the last twenty years or so, while rural health has steadily improved at first, slowly after the colonial period, but very quickly since the late 1980s. As a result, in 2010, the Ministries of Health in Southeast Asia adopted the Bangkok Declaration on Urbanization and Health, which highlighted the fact that the urban poor had the worst health situation in the region and that they suffered from the "Urban Equity Gap," which meant that they suffered from all the regular urban health problems yet could not afford health care.[46]

The Impact of Environmental Changes on Forest Peoples of Southeast Asia in the Twentieth Century
Alberto G. Gomes

We Have Eaten the Forest is a catchy title of a book about a forest people, the Montagnard (French for "People of the Mountains") in the Central Highlands of Vietnam by the late French anthropologist, Georges Condominas.[1] The title regrettably gives the impression that the mountain people have completely "consumed" the forest. In reality, the rapid and widespread depletion of the forests in the region is overwhelmingly a consequence of the expansion of commercial plantations, extractive industries, and large-scale settlement schemes almost exclusively for the benefit of corporations and non-forest peoples.[2]

Defined as "peoples who traditionally live in forests and depend on them primarily and directly for their livelihoods," Southeast Asia's forest peoples for centuries have engaged in hunting, gathering, forest-fallow swidden cultivation, and the collection and trading of non-timber forest products such as rattan, bamboo, wild fruit, and medicinal plants.[3,4] At the turn of the last century, there were several small bands of nomadic hunters and gatherers, such as the Negritos of the Philippines, Peninsular Malaysia and Southern Thailand, and the Penan of Borneo, inhabiting pockets of Southeast Asia's forested areas while dispersed across the region, but mostly in the interior and upland areas, were Tribal communities subsisting mainly on swidden cultivation (also referred to as shifting cultivation or pejoratively as "slash and burn" agriculture).[5,6] Typically, swidden farmers plant a range of cultigens in forest clearings and once the crops have been harvested, the farms are left to fallow and regenerate into forests, making it an ecologically efficient farming system well-suited for forest environments. Among people renowned for swiddening in Southeast Asia are the Dayaks of Borneo, the Orang Asli of Peninsula Malaysia, the Akha, Hmong, Lisu, Lahu, Karen and Khmu of Mainland Southeast Asia, and the Bataks and Tagbanua in the Philippines.[7] Today, there are very few communities in the region that depend on the forests for their livelihood as most have been resettled away from their forest homelands or the forests around their settlements have been completely destroyed.[8]

The sweeping political economic changes in the twentieth century in Southeast Asia have greatly altered both the region's forest landscape and the economic practices of forest communities.[9] Between 1900 and 1989, Southeast Asia's forested area shrunk from an estimated 250 million hectares to sixty million hectares and from the 1990s onwards, the annual deforestation rate hovered above one million hectares of forests.[10] While vast tracts of forests have been cleared for the sake of economic development, manifested as capitalist-oriented extractive industries (commercial logging and mining), agribusiness plantations (of rubber, oil palm, tea, and coffee), migratory land settlement, and large infrastructural projects (hydroelectric power installations and roads), thousands of hectares of forests, especially in Indo-China, have been denuded in counter-insurgency campaigns during the war in the 1960s and early 1970s.[11]

The twentieth century also witnessed the radical shift in the economies of forest peoples from subsistence-oriented forest dependence to market dependence.[12] This was due to the combined effects of deforestation and government-sponsored economic development programs. Both these processes led to the displacement of forest peoples and their inability to engage in their time-honored and ecologically sustainable subsistence forest activities. As forests are also integral to the social, spiritual, and historical lives of the forest communities, the loss of the forests has also had negative social and ontological implications for Southeast Asia's forest communities.[13] In a longitudinal study, spanning three decades, on the Menraq (also referred to as Semang or Negritos) of Malaysia who are descendants of hunter-gatherers who have inhabited Southeast Asia for about forty thousand years, I found that the government-sponsored development programs have paradoxically made matters worse for the people.[14] In 1972, the Malaysian government resettled the Menraq foragers away from their forest homelands into a patterned settlement where several market-focused economic projects, such as rubber and oil palm cultivation, were carried out.[15] Moving them out of their traditional territories and concentrating them in a smaller area had freed up forest land for exploitation by timber companies and for land settlement schemes for the dominant Malay population. With having lost access to, and control, of their traditional livelihood base and with their growing involvement in commodity production, the Menraq became increasingly dependent on market-oriented activities. Since they fetched low and fluctuating prices for their products, their incomes were meager and erratic. Their low incomes meant that they could afford to buy only poor quality food and with the disappearance of forests they could no longer rely on hunting and gathering for a balanced diet. As a consequence of deficient nutrition and diet and living in poor sanitary and crowded conditions, Menraq were extremely susceptible to health problems and diseases, leading to high levels of mortality.[16] I also found that increased commoditization as well as a drastic decline in their traditional economic activities had adverse social implications. Within the community, there was a shift from communal to private ownership of means of production and resources, a drop in sharing and generalized reciprocity, increase in accumulative tendencies, and concomitantly a rise in social differentiation in a society renowned for its egalitarianism. All this has severely disrupted intra-community social relations in these communities.[17]

The Menraq story of social, cultural, and economic transformations is common to almost all forest peoples in Southeast Asia and elsewhere.[18] With the disappearance of the forests in the region as a result of the advent and consolidation of modernity, especially capitalism, and the vicious cycle of the attendant environmental and political economic changes, the small-scale communities that once depended on these forests for their livelihood are struggling to survive as displaced, marginalized, and impoverished minorities. Their involvement with commodity production has induced the over-exploitation of the forests by the forest communities as they disregard their long-standing sustainable practices in their quest to increase their cash earnings. But the environmental catastrophe of deforestation in Southeast Asia is not by any stretch of imagination due to the region's forest peoples; the accusing finger should be pointed at the greed of corporations and governments driven by an obsession with economic growth at the expense of the natural environment and the livelihood of minorities like the forest peoples.

Notes

1. G. Condominas, *We have eaten the forest: the story of a Montagnard village in the central highlands of Vietnam* (London: Allen Lane, 1977).

2. M. Colchester and L. Lohmann eds., *The Struggle for land and the fate of the forests* (Penang, Malaysia: World Rainforest Movement, 1993); P. Hurst, *Rainforest politics: ecological destruction in South-East Asia* (London: Zed Books, 1990); T. P. Lye, W. de Jong, and A. Ken-ichi eds., *The political ecology of the tropical forests in Southeast Asia: historical perspectives* (Kyoto, Japan: Kyoto University Press, Melbourne: Trans Pacific Press; 2003); M. J. G. Parnwell and R. L. Bryant, eds., *Environmental change in Southeast Asia: people, politics and sustainable development* (London: Routledge, 1996); L. E. Sponsel, T. N. Headland, and R. C. Bailey eds., *Tropical deforestation: the human dimension* (New York: Columbia University Press, 1996).

3. S. Chao, "Forest peoples: numbers across the world," 2012, 4, available at http://www.forestpeoples.org/sites/fpp/files/publication/2012/05/forest-peoples-numbers-across-world-final_0.pdf.

4. F. L. Dunn, *Rain-forest collectors and traders: a study of resource utilization in modern and ancient Malaya* (Kuala Lumpur: Monographs of the Malaysian Branch, Royal Asiatic Society, No.5, 1975).

5. K. Endicott, *Batek Negrito religion: the world-view and rituals of a hunting and gathering people of Peninsular Malaysia* (Oxford: Clarendon Press, 1979); P. B. Griffin, A. Estioko-Griffin eds,. *The Agta of Northeastern Luzon: Recent studies* (Cebu City, The Philippines: San Carlos Publications, 1985).

6. J. B. Brosius, "Foraging in tropical rain forests: the case of the Penan of Sarawak, East Malaysia (Borneo)," *Human Ecology* 19 (1991): 123–50.

7. S. C. Chin, "Agriculture and resource utilization in a lowland rainforest Kenyah community," Special Monograph No. 4, *The Sarawak Museum Journal* 35, no. 56 (1985); H. Conklin, *Hanunoo agriculture: a report on an integral system of shifting cultivation in the Philippines* (Rome: FAO, 1957); M. Dove, *Swidden agriculture in Indonesia: the subsistence strategies of the Kalimantan Kantu'* (Berlin: Mouton Publishers, 1985); D. Freeman, *Iban agriculture: a report on the shifting agriculture of hill rice by the Iban of Sarawak* (London: Her Majesty's Stationery Office; 1955); D. Schmidt-Vogt, S. J. Leisz, O. Metz, A. Heinimann, T. Thiha, P. Messerli, et al., "An assessment of trends in the extent of swidden in Southeast Asia," *Human ecology* 37, no. 3 (2009): 269–280; J. E. Spencer, *Shifting cultivation in Southeastern Asia* (Berkeley: University of California Press, 1966).

8. H. Brookfield, L. Potter, Y. Byron, *In place of the forest: Environmental and socio-economic transformation in Borneo and the eastern Malay Peninsula* (Tokyo: United Nations University Press, 1995); J. P. Brosius, *After Duwagan: Deforestation, succession, and adaptation in Upland Luzon, Philippines.* Michigan Studies of South and Southeast Asia Number 2 (Ann Arbor: Center for South and Southeast Asian Studies, University of Michigan Press, 1990); E. Hong, *Natives of Sarawak: survival in Borneo's vanishing forests* (Penang: Institut Masyarakat, 1987); T. P. Lye, *Changing pathways: forest degradation and the Batek of Pahang, Malaysia* (Lanham, MD: Lexington Books, 2004).

9. V. T. King, *Anthropology and development in South-east Asia: theory and practice* (Oxford: Oxford University Press, 1999); V. T. King, W. D. Wilder, *The modern anthropology of South-east Asia* (London: Routledge, 2003); T. M. Li ed., *Transforming the Indonesian uplands: marginality, power, and production* (Amsterdam: Harwood Academic Publishers, 1999); J. Nevins and N. L. Peluso, *Taking Southeast Asia to market: commodities, nature, and people in the neoliberal age* (Cornell: Cornell University Press, 2008).

10. M. Poffenberger, "People in the forest: community forestry experiences from Southeast Asia," *Int. J. Environment and Sustainable Development* 5, no. 1 (2006): 57–69.

11. P. Hurst, *Rainforest politics: ecological destruction in South-East Asia* (London: Zed Books, 1990); S. Chao, "Forest peoples: numbers across the world," 2012, 4, available at http://www.forestpeoples.org/sites/fpp/files/publication/2012/05/forest-peoples-numbers-across-world-final_0.pdf; J. C. Scott, *The art of not being governed: an anarchist history of upland Southeast Asia* (New Haven: Yale University Press, 2009).

12. T. P. Lye, W. de Jong, A. Ken-ichi eds., *The political ecology of the tropical forests in Southeast Asia: historical perspectives* (Kyoto, Japan: Kyoto Univer-

sity Press, Melbourne: Trans Pacific Press, 2003); T. M. Li ed., *Transforming the Indonesian uplands: marginality, power, and production* (Amsterdam: Harwood Academic Publishers, 1999); J. Nevins and N. L. Peluso, *Taking Southeast Asia to market: commodities, nature, and people in the neoliberal age* (Cornell: Cornell University Press, 2008); R. A. Cramb, *Land and longhouse: agrarian transformation in the uplands of Sarawak* (Copenhagen: NIAS, 2007); R. A. Cramb, C. J. Pierce Colfer, W. Dressler, P. Laungaramsri, Q. T. Le, E. Mulyoutami et al., "Swidden transformations and rural livelihoods in Southeast Asia," *Human Ecology* 37, no. 3 (2009): 323–46; J. Fox, Y. Fujita, D. Ngidang, N. Peluso, L. Potter, N. Sakuntaladewi, et al., "Policies, political-economy, and swidden in Southeast Asia," *Human Ecology* 37 (2009): 305–22; P. Kunstadter, E. C. Chapman, and S. Sabhasri eds., *Farmers in the forest: economic development and marginal agriculture in Northern Thailand* (Honolulu: East-West Center, 1978); V. Lopez-Gonzaga, *Peasant in the hills: a study of the dynamics of social change among the Buhid swidden cultivators in the Philippines* (Diliman, Quezon City: University of the Philippines Press, 1983); O. Mertz, C. Padoch, J. Fox, R. A. Cramb, S. J. Leisz, T. L. Nguyen et al., "Swidden change in Southeast Asia: understanding causes and consequences," *Human Ecology* 37, no. 3 (2009): 259–64; C. Dallos, *From equality to inequality: social change among newly sedentary Lanoh hunter-gatherer traders of Peninsular Malaysia* (Toronto: University of Toronto Press, 2011); A. G. Gomes, *Looking for money: capitalism and modernity in an Orang Asli village* (Kuala Lumpur: Centre for Orang Asli Concerns, Melbourne: Trans Pacific Press, 2004); A. G. Gomes, *Modernity and Malaysia: settling the Menraq forest nomads* (London: Routledge, 2007); C. Nicholas, *The Orang Asli and the contest for resources: Indigenous politics, development and identity in Peninsular Malaysia* (Copenhagen: IWGIA Document No. 95, Subang Jaya, Malaysia: Centre for Orang Asli Concerns, 2000); R. K. Dentan, K. Endicott, B. Hooker, A. G. Gomes, *Malaysia and the "original people": a case study of the impact of development on Indigenous peoples* (New York: Allyn and Bacon, 1997); C. R. Duncan eds. *Civilizing the margins: Southeast Asian government policies for the development of minorities* (Singapore: National University of Singapore Press, 2008).

13. C. Dallos, *From equality to inequality: social change among newly sedentary Lanoh hunter-gatherer traders of Peninsular Malaysia* (Toronto: University of Toronto Press, 2011); A. G. Gomes, *Looking for money: capitalism and modernity in an Orang Asli village* (Kuala Lumpur: Centre for Orang Asli Concerns, Melbourne: Trans Pacific Press, 2004); A. G. Gomes, *Modernity and Malaysia: settling the Menraq forest nomads* (London: Routledge, 2007); C. Nicholas, *The Orang Asli and the contest for resources: Indigenous politics, development and identity in Peninsular Malaysia* (Copenhagen: IWGIA Document No. 95, Subang Jaya, Malaysia: Centre for Orang Asli Concerns, 2000).

14. A. G. Gomes, *Modernity and Malaysia: settling the Menraq forest nomads* (London: Routledge, 2007).

15. Ibid.

16. Ibid.

17. Ibid.

18. H. Brookfield, L. Potter, and Y. Byron, *In place of the forest: Environmental and socio-economic transformation in Borneo and the eastern Malay Penin-*

sula (Tokyo: United Nations University Press, 1995); J. P. Brosius, *After Duwagan: Deforestation, succession, and adaptation in Upland Luzon, Philippines.* Michigan Studies of South and Southeast Asia Number 2. (Ann Arbor: Center for South and Southeast Asian Studies, University of Michigan Press, 1990); E. Hong, *Natives of Sarawak: survival in Borneo's vanishing forests* (Penang: Institut Masyarakat, 1987); T. P. Lye, *Changing pathways: forest degradation and the Batek of Pahang, Malaysia* (Lanham, MD: Lexington Books, 2004); R. A. Cramb, *Land and longhouse: agrarian transformation in the uplands of Sarawak* (Copenhagen: NIAS, 2007); R. A. Cramb, C. J. Pierce Colfer, W. Dressler, P. Laungaramsri, Q. T. Le, E. Mulyoutami et al., "Swidden transformations and rural livelihoods in Southeast Asia," *Human Ecology* 37, no. 3 (2009): 323–46; J. Fox, Y. Fujita, D. Ngidang, N. Peluso, L. Potter, N. Sakuntaladewi, et al., "Policies, political-economy, and swidden in Southeast Asia," *Human Ecology* 37 (2009): 305–22; P. Kunstadter, E. C. Chapman, and S. Sabhasri eds., *Farmers in the forest: economic development and marginal agriculture in Northern Thailand* (Honolulu: East-West Center, 1978); V. Lopez-Gonzaga, *Peasant in the hills: a study of the dynamics of social change among the Buhid swidden cultivators in the Philippines* (Diliman, Quezon City: University of the Philippines Press, 1983); O. Mertz, C. Padoch, J. Fox, R. A. Cramb, S. J. Leisz, T. L. Nguyen et al., "Swidden change in Southeast Asia: understanding causes and consequences," *Human Ecology* 37, no. 3 (2009): 259–64; C. Dallos, *From equality to inequality: social change among newly sedentary Lanoh hunter-gatherer traders of Peninsular Malaysia* (Toronto: University of Toronto Press, 2011); A. G. Gomes, *Looking for money: capitalism and modernity in an Orang Asli village* (Kuala Lumpur: Centre for Orang Asli Concerns, Melbourne: Trans Pacific Press, 2004); A. G. Gomes, *Modernity and Malaysia: settling the Menraq forest nomads* (London: Routledge, 2007); C. Nicholas, *The Orang Asli and the contest for resources: Indigenous politics, development and identity in Peninsular Malaysia* (Copenhagen: IWGIA Document No. 95, Subang Jaya, Malaysia: Centre for Orang Asli Concerns, 2000); R. K. Dentan, K. Endicott, B. Hooker, and A. G. Gomes, *Malaysia and the "original people": a case study of the impact of development on Indigenous peoples* (New York: Allyn and Bacon, 1997); C. R. Duncan ed., *Civilizing the margins: Southeast Asian government policies for the development of minorities* (Singapore: National University of Singapore Press, 2008).

Conclusion

In this chapter, I have attempted to show that the history of rural health in modern Southeast Asia has been significantly affected by the availability of funds and views of the importance of rural areas to the state, whether it was in the hands of Europeans or indigenous rulers. As a result of the growth of the regional economy in the last few decades and because of the problems of urbanization, village health underwent a transformation. It went from the weaker health sector throughout much of the twentieth century to the stronger, in various ways, relative to the urban sector. During this period, however, terms did not remain constant and whether health conditions were based on rural or racial/ethnic grounds depended upon the agendas of those who controlled health policy. It is unclear how much new research from inside of rural Southeast Asia will change the way that we have looked the history of public health in the region. There is still much work to do. As Mark Harrison points out, aside from missionary medicine, the stories of "medical practice and health care in rural areas" is little known in South Asia.[47] I would suggest that this is even truer for Southeast Asia. But understanding how the history of public health has been influenced by external perception of rural landscape of the region is a necessary first step.

Notes

1. J. Rigg, *Southeast Asia: The Human Landscape of Modernization and Development,* 2nd ed. (London: Routledge, 2003).
2. M. Stenseke, "Whose Landscape Values? Central Goals Versus Local Perspectives in Planning and Management of the Rural Landscape," in *Claiming Rural Identities: Dynamics, Contexts, Policies,* ed. T. Haartsen, P. Groote, and Paulus P. P. Huigen (Assen, Netherlands: Uitgeverij Van Gorcum, 2000), 25–34.
3. T. G. McGee, *The Southeast Asian City: A Social Geography of the Primate Cities of Southeast Asia* (London: G. Bell and Sons, 1967).
4. A. Naono, "Inoculators, the Indigenous Obstacle to Vaccination in Colonial Burma," *Journal of Burma Studies* 14 (2010): 91–114.
5. V. R. Savage, *Western Impressions of Nature and Landscape in Southeast Asia* (Singapore: Singapore University Press, 1984), 23.
6. Savage, *Western Impressions.*
7. J. Saha, "Madness and the Making of a Colonial Order in Burma," *Modern Asian Studies* 47, no. 2 (2013): 406–35.
8. L. Hesselink, "The Unbearable Absence of Parasols: The Formidable Weight of a Colonial Java Status Symbol," *IIAS Newsletter* (Autumn 2007): 43.
9. Naono, "Inoculators," 91–114.
10. S. S. Amrith, *Decolonizing International Health: India and Southeast Asia, 1930–65* (London: Palgrave, 2006), 186.
11. A. L. Foster, *Projections of Power: The United States and Europe in Colonial Southeast Asia, 1919–1941* (Durham, NC: Duke University Press, 2010).
12. K. Jellison, *Entitled to Power: Farm Women and Technology, 1913–1963* (Chapel Hill: University of North Carolina Press, 1993).
13. J. R. Andrus, *Rural Reconstruction in Burma* (Bombay: Oxford University Press, 1936).
14. Warwick W. Anderson, *Colonial Pathologies: American Tropical Medicine, Race and Hygiene in the Philippines* (Durham, NC: Duke University Press, 2006), 199.
15. J. W. McGuire, *Wealth, Health, and Democracy in East Asia and Latin America* (Cambridge: Cambridge University Press, 2010).
16. F. Gouda, "Discipline versus Gentle Persuasion in Colonial Public Health: The Rockefeller Foundation's Intensive Rural Hygiene Work in the Netherlands East Indies, 1925–1940," *Rockefeller Archive Center Research Report* (2009), Rockefeller Archive Center website, www .rockarch.org/publications/resrep/gouda.pdf.

17. E. Stein, "Sanitary Makeshifts and the Perpetuation of Health Stratification in Indonesia," in *Anthropology and Public Health: Bridging Differences in Culture and Society,* ed. R. A. Hahn and M. C. Inbonn (Oxford: Oxford University Press, 2009), 541–65.

18. McGuire, *Wealth, Health, and Democracy.*

19. Stein, "Sanitary Makeshifts," 541–65.

20. Anderson, *Colonial Pathologies.*

21. Netherlands Red Cross Feeding team, *Report on Nutritional Survey in The Netherlands East Indies, Conducted during October 1945 till June 1946* (The Hague: Van Loon, 1948).

22. McGuire, *Wealth, Health, and Democracy.*

23. Stein, "Sanitary Makeshifts," 541–65.

24. R. Butwell, *U Nu of Burma* (Stanford, CA: Stanford University Press, 1963).

25. Butwell, *U Nu of Burma.*

26. C. J. Feldhake, "Well Drilling and Latrine Construction in Rural Burma," in *Public Health Reports* 69, no. 4 (April 1954): 391–97, esp. 392–93.

27. Butwell, *U Nu of Burma.*

28. Stein, "Sanitary Makeshifts," 541–65.

29. McGuire, *Wealth, Health, and Democracy.*

30. V. T. H. Gunaratne, *Voyage towards Health* (New Delhi: Tata McGraw-Hill, 1980), 23.

31. Amrith, *Decolonizing International Health.*

32. McGuire, *Wealth, Health, and Democracy.*

33. P. Strefford, "The Response of International Donors to Myanmar's Escalating Health Crisis," *Ritsumeikan Annual Review of International Studies* 5 (2006): 35–57, quotation on 38.

34. "Declaration of Alma Ata, 1978," World Health organization website, www.euro.who.int/__data/assets/pdf_file/0009/113877/E93944.pdf.

35. McGuire, *Wealth, Health, and Democracy.*

36. McGuire, *Wealth, Health, and Democracy.*

37. R. Sciortino, *CARE-takers of CURE; A Study of Health Centre Nurses in Rural Central Java* (Amsterdam: Jolly/Het Spinhuis Publishers, 1992).

38. P. T. Cohen, "Public Health in Thailand: Changing Medical Paradigms and Disease Patterns in Political and Economic Context," in *Public Health in Asia and the Pacific: Historical and Comparative Perspectives,* ed. Milton J. Lewis and Kerrie L. MacPherson (Abingdon, UK: Routledge, 2008), 106–21.

39. V. Chinvarakorn, "Business as Usual," *Bangkok Post,* August 19, 1998, www.oocities.org/rainforest/7813/0831_cop.htm.

40. A. Walhberg, "A Revolutionary Movement to Bring Traditional Medicine Back to the Grassroots Level: On the Biopolitization of Herbal Medicine in Vietnam," in *Global Movements, Local Concerns: Medicine and Health in Southeast Asia,* ed. L. Monnais and H. J. Cook (Singapore: NUS Press, 2012), 207–25, quotations on 216.

41. Walhberg, "A Revolutionary Movement," 207–25, quotation on 218.

42. McGuire, *Wealth, Health, and Democracy.*

43. Gunaratne, *Voyage Towards Health.*

44. Rigg, *Southeast Asia.*

45. Samlee Pilangbang, "'Health for All' Must Include Country's Urban Poor," *Bangkok Post,* October 15, 2010, www.thaiworld.org/en/thailand_monitor/answer.php?question_id=1013.

46. "Bangkok Declaration on Urbanization and Health," September 7, 2010, World Health Organization website, apps.searo.who.int/pds_docs/B4827.pdf.

47. M. Harrison, "Medicine and Colonialism in South Asia since 1500," in *The Oxford Handbook of the History of Medicine,* ed. Mark Jackson (Oxford: Oxford University Press, 2011): 285–301, quotation on 295.

7 Population Aging and the Family

The Southeast Asian Context

Theresa W. Devasahayam

POPULATION AGING IS one of the key demographic drivers of the rise in non-communicable chronic disease in Southeast Asia. The phenomenon of aging raises far-reaching questions about the locus of responsibility for elder care in the context of changing family structures and shifting public priorities. It is likely to present a formidable challenge to health policy in Southeast Asia in the foreseeable future, calling into question both the adequacy of public provision and its financial sustainability. This chapter follows from Peter Boomgaard's overview of Southeast Asia's demographic transition in the twentieth century, focusing on the past three decades. It shifts the terrain of this volume's discussion of health to the family, and it adopts a perspective informed by demography and sociology.

The phenomenon of population aging has been a cause of public concern for several reasons. From the perspective of the state, an aging population suggests pressures on government resources that, in turn, have called for swift and relevant policy responses in the areas of fiscal management, income support, the labor market, health care, housing, and social support services.[1] In Southeast Asia, the strategy of states has been to provide minimal or residual support to elder care largely with the aim of ensuring that families continue to undertake the role of primary caregiver to the elderly.[2] In light of this, we may ask how, then, have families been able to cope with the role of providing care to the elderly and whether population aging has posed unique challenges to these families.

That the family is far from being a static social institution is the point of departure of this chapter. Transformations in the family structure have been observed in countries across Southeast Asia, raising concerns on the impact this would have on the role of the family toward elder caregiving. Family structure is a composite term, taking into account the number, type, and location of kin who provide transfers of support through co-residence, financial provision, goods, and care. Focusing on the relationship between family support structures and aging, this chapter investigates older persons' concerns as a result of selected shifts in family structure. Studies conducted in a variety of social settings have suggested that the potential for vulnerability among older persons increases as a result of changes in the family structure. This chapter argues, however, that the situation for older persons in Southeast Asia is more varied and highly nuanced and dependent on context. To be more specific, old-age dependency and vulnerability need not necessarily be as pervasive as assumed, owing to shifts in family structure. In this regard, the literature on aging in the Southeast Asian region has proven to be useful in providing a glimpse into the lives, experiences, and conditions of the older population; the bulk of the literature consulted has been written by demographers, while other works were produced by scholars using qualitative methods. Based on the literature, it has been found that older persons are not entirely dependent on adult children for care and financial provision. Instead, for the most part, older persons have proven to be self-sufficient in regard to caring for themselves and, in fact, have been found to extend care toward others. Although this reflects the general situation, there are some pockets of older persons who may be more vulnerable than others—usually as a result of factors aside from being old, such as gender, deteriorating health, or poverty.

Transforming Southeast Asia: From the 1950s Onward

Since the 1950s to the 1960s, most countries in Southeast Asia have had a stable political leadership, albeit characterized by authoritarianism. President Suharto governed Indonesia for nearly thirty years, as it was the case with Lee Kuan Yew in Singapore. To an extent, a well-entrenched political leadership meant that the governments could implement longer-term economic strategies with little disruption.[3] Having successfully generated economic plans to stimulate economic growth, Indonesia, Malaysia, Singapore, and Thailand grew at a phenomenal rate of an average of over 5.5 percent annually in per capita terms between 1965 and 1990.[4] Initially poor, these countries became open to the global economy, generally taking advantage of new technologies, larger markets, and improved management techniques, as well as foreign direct investment. Such economies also tended to have fewer distortions and better resource allocation, and their firms were competitive in the world markets. There was also evidence of diversification in Indonesia and Malaysia, where a wide range of natural resources were exploited and manufactured exports were encouraged with the aim of responding to changing international circumstances. Moreover, as pointed out by Radelet, Sachs, and Lee, low levels of income in the 1960s provided the potential for rapid economic growth.[5] While macroeconomic management, especially in terms of government fiscal policy, should be credited with spurring economic growth, education also had its positive effects by raising the skills level of people.

While the region was seeing a growth in its economies, rapid urbanization was also taking place. In the region, the growth of cities led to the development of megacities with populations exceeding ten million. Examples of such megacities are Bangkok, Jakarta, and Manila. Some scholars have argued that globalization spurred the urbanization process as cities and regions became absorbed into "network landscapes" marked by "investment, production, and market opportunities" in "global 'space(s) of flows,'" particularly in the 1990s as urbanization became linked to globalization's economic activities.[6,7] In this case, structural transformation as a result of globalization has been an important factor in accelerating urbanization, with the city becoming the new economic space attracting capital flows.[8] In Southeast Asia, however, the urbanization process in the region was not confined to the inflow of global capital into a fixed built environment, but rather has been found to be occurring at multiple scales of analysis, including national political economies and cultures, national/regional interactions with hinterlands, and the differentially "'articulated' spaces of the city."[9] Because Cambodia, Laos, Myanmar, and Vietnam have been slower in embracing globalization, these countries have had low levels of urbanization. This is in contrast to the other countries in the region that saw sharp increases in the growth of the non-agricultural labor force, congregating mainly in the urban areas and, as a result, spurring further urbanization. In spite of variations in urbanization patterns across the region, cities have become magnets for rural people for generations. In Southeast Asia, the city represents the "center of new activities" adopted by the "new social class"; thus, for many, the city has come to symbolize the transition from the "traditional" to the "modern."[10,11]

In tandem with a boom in economic growth and urbanization after 1950, population rates in Southeast Asia were found to rise until the mid-1970s, when instead this growth in population was accompanied by declining mortality rates—especially in the cities—although it must be noted that the region as a whole records considerable variation in this regard.[12] Demographic figures from Southeast Asia attest to this dramatic population shift. In 1950–55, Indonesia's life expectancy at birth was thirty-eight years and in 1995, the figure jumped to sixty-three. In Vietnam, life expectancy figures were forty and sixty-eight respectively; while in the Philippines, they were forty-eight and sixty-seven; and in Thailand, fifty-one and sixty-seven.[13] The lowering of mortality and increase in fertility could be attributed to improved medical facilities. People in the cities no doubt have had easier access to better amenities and facilities. Thus, it comes as no surprise that people in the cities also tended to live longer.

Demographer Gavin Jones remarks that it was from the 1960s onward that "mortality continued to decline steadily, but fertility also declined, faster than any observer would have imagined in 1960," thereby contributing to a gradual drop in population growth.[14] In Malaysia, Singapore, and Thailand, development occurred at the same time fertility came down drastically.[15] Above all, the countries in the region were adamant about reducing population growth rates. In 1963, Vietnam became the first country in the region to adopt a specific policy to curb its population growth rates; it was followed by Singapore in 1965, Indonesia in 1968, and Thailand and the Philippines in 1970 and 1971, respectively. In Thailand, the fertility rate dropped from 5.0 in the early 1970s to 1.8 children in the early 2000s.[16] Having seen the implications of shrinking fertility rates, in later years Thailand implemented modifications to its population policy in order to prevent further fertility decline.[17] Singapore also implemented incentives to raise fertility rates, but these efforts have proven to be unsuccessful. By way of contrast, the drop in fertility rate was not as drastic in Indonesia and the Philippines. Considered an intermediate case, Indonesia experienced a moderate decline from the end of the 1970s before leveling off at 2.4 children per woman in the early 2000s. Demographic surveys of the Philippines indicate that the drop in fertility rates showed a marginal decline compared with other countries in the region, resulting in a fertility rate of 3.5 children per woman in 2000–5, compared with 7.3 children in the 1950s.[18]

In the following sections, I provide an assessment of the relationship of these broader economic and demographic changes to population aging in the context of Southeast Asia. Specifically, one may ask whether these shifts in family structure as a result of economic and demographic changes in the region have affected old-age care and, if so, in what ways.

The Extended Family in Southeast Asia: Is It Disappearing?

Sociologists have argued that as societies become more industrialized and urbanized, families become increasingly isolated.[19] The characteristic of being more nuclear enables the family to be more mobile, so as to secure jobs when suitable opportunities arise. While this theoretical assertion has received its share of criticisms, nonetheless the question of whether families have become increasingly nuclear as a result of industrialization and urbanization has also been raised in the Southeast Asian context. If, indeed, the family has become more nuclear, what effect, then, has this had on older persons in terms of living arrangements as well as the care they receive? Demographers have emphasized that the probability of living with a child increases with the number of living children.[20] In other words, the odds of living alone reduce significantly as a result of a very large household. Conversely, if family size shrinks, the probability of living with a child decreases and the odds of living alone increases.

At the outset, it must be noted that Southeast Asian kinship systems have been bilateral, which renders equal importance to the paternal and maternal kin on either side of the kinship lineage. The exception, however, is that of Vietnam, where there is greater preference for patrilineal kin, especially in the north.[21]

What this suggests is that in most parts of Southeast Asia, a newly married couple does not prioritize either kin group in terms of place of residence. Instead the norm is for a couple to set up a household independently, making it almost nuclear in its structure—although in the first few years of marriage, living with the bride's kin is not uncommon. This residential pattern is found among the Malays in Malaysia, in Indonesia, and in the Philippines.[22] In the case of the Javanese nuclear family, Jay and Geertz mention that although children leave the parental home sometime after marriage, they maintain regular and close contact with their parents while each household functions as a separate and self-sufficient unit.[23,24] Nonetheless, it is not uncommon for parents and children to engage in various forms of social exchange, such as giving gifts of money and food and paying frequent visits. Jones, citing Castillo, makes this statement about family structure in the Philippines, which she describes as "residentially nuclear but functionally extended."[25,26] In this sense, it can be said that family structures in Southeast Asia have not changed as they have in the Western Hemisphere, where the nuclear family is regarded as a more recent social phenomenon.

Although households are largely nuclear in Southeast Asia, there is a tendency for older parents to reside close to adult children.[27] Because of falling fertility rates, however, this has led to households shrinking in size and fewer children living near their aged parents, even as they move out of the household with the intention of setting up their own household. This suggests that there is a reduction in potential carers for elderly parents, as well as an increase in solitary living among the elderly, which has become a cause for concern among policy makers.[28,29] According to data from the National Statistical Office, Thailand, the average household size in Thailand was 3.9 in 2000, compared with 5.6 in 1960.[30] The same trend was found in Malaysia, where the average household size in 2010 was 4.31, dropping from 5.22 in 1980.[31] Although this concern may not apply to the current cohort of elderly in Indonesia, for example, whose fertility may not have dropped as drastically as compared to that of their own children, having fewer grandchildren is considered a liability since the elderly have fewer grandchildren to depend on, thereby suggesting that grandchildren also play a role in elder caregiving.[32]

But on a more positive note, research in Southeast Asia has suggested that the effect of smaller family sizes on co-residence with children in later life has only had a minimal impact.[33] For example in Singapore, rates of co-residence continue to be high, although this may be in part because of the urban nature of Singapore as well as the high cost of living, which makes it difficult for young adults to live independently from their parents.[34] In a study by Zimmer and Korinek, a difference was made between proximate residence and co-residence.[35] The authors assert that while there would be further declines in proximate residence should there be further changes in family size—which would be inevitable for the forthcoming generations of elderly—the study confirmed that co-residence rates continue to be high, and that proximate residence is even more pervasive than assumed. Moreover, if co-residence was not found, it was more likely that older adults decided to live independently from their children out of individual choice, suggesting that "provid[ing] support and care according to traditional approaches are evolving, and so too are residential preferences."[36]

Nevertheless, changes in family size and residence patterns are critical issues to be examined, since adult children play a significant role in supporting elderly parents. Their role is significant in a number of ways: adult children undertake the health-care costs, housing, and other day-to-day living expenses of their aging parents.[37] Aside from these economic needs, adult children also provide for the social needs of their aged parents such as family care, housekeeping, social support, and personal care. In Vietnam, it was found that the marital status of an older parent determined the kind of support received; for example, non-married parents were found to receive money and durables from sons, while married parents received food and clothing from sons—with the exception of non-married mothers in the north, who were also likely to receive food or clothes from their sons.[38] In the Philippines, Thailand, and Singapore, it was found that between 88 percent and 91 percent of the elderly receive financial support from family members.[39]

In fact, in urban and rural Southeast Asia, there continues to be a strong sense of responsibility toward parents.[40] Here, it was found that "intra-familial bonds are increasingly expressed in terms of care and support rather than obedience and obligation."[41] Surveys conducted in Malaysia and Singapore revealed that generally even the youth held a strong sense of filial duty.[42] That adult children saw it as their duty to support needy parents or parents-in-law was found in another context. In a study conducted in Sungei Petani, Kedah, West Malaysia, in 2008, 65.6 percent of 186 co-residing children maintained that caring for their aging parent was their responsibility.[43] It was also found that having a "close relationship . . . facilitate[d] and enable[d] care and support to be more completely and readily transferred."[44]

Because the role of adult children is critical to the well-being of the elderly, there have been fears of families breaking down and not fulfilling this role—especially with the rise of modernization and Western values such as individualism.[45] While by and large the younger generation provides care for their elderly parents out of their own volition, there have been aberrations in this pattern. Such is the case of Singapore, where there have been a number of instances of parental neglect. In response, the state took deliberate steps to enforce the Maintenance of Parents Act in 1996 in order to ensure a safety net for all aging individuals. Essentially the law uses "the rhetoric of filial piety to emphasize the principle of familism. . . . [In doing so] the bill clearly places financial risks and responsibilities not on the community but solely on the individual, i.e., the older person first and then his or her adult children."[46] Under this law, any elderly person who is unable to maintain him- or herself adequately may claim maintenance from children who are capable of supporting him or her but are not doing so by approaching the tribunal. Since the act came into force, there were 1,411 applications for maintenance; of this number, 1,047 maintenance orders were made.[47] Since then, there has been an increase in the number of applications filed from the usual annual rate of 100. Most applicants tended to be fathers of Chinese descent, and were single parents who were either divorced or widowed.

While there is evidence to show that older persons depend on the care and assistance provided by their children or other close kin, this relationship is far from being one-sided. Instead, intergenerational flows and reciprocal caregiving aptly describes the relationship across the generations—a pattern found to be on the increase in the region. In spite of families shrinking, there is evidence to show that many families, whether they are aging parents or dependent or independent adult children, are committed to caring for and supporting their kin both in expressed attitudes and behavior. In this sense, "parent-care and childcare have become more equal and the resource flows more balanced" and, as such, "there has been a shift away from the dominance of the older generation and the precedence accorded to resource flows towards parents."[48] In this regard, the expanding role of the elderly within the family has to be acknowledged.[49]

In Indonesia, parents see it as their responsibility to care for their children from birth until adulthood. It was found that for mothers to be able to provide financial support to their children was important to their life satisfaction; at the same time, they did not expect that their children would reciprocate.[50] That mothers derived greatest satisfaction in response to the appreciation they received from daughters was most evident in the urban areas. Kreager and Schröder-Butterfill explain that in some family networks in Java, "parents provide far-reaching support to some children, while receiving assistance from others."[51] In fact, these authors found that Javanese villagers emphasize their "life-long responsibility" toward their children and maintain that "'parents can never be heartless' towards their children in need."[52] While aging parents were found to be taking on responsibility for school- or university-age children or grandchildren through downward transfers from parent to child, older women provided childcare support to grandchildren in exchange for material support from their children. In this case, the position of the elderly is not necessarily one of dependence but rather authority. Among those who are struggling to get by or are even poor, however, this decision to render help to their children may, in turn, be a source of vulnerability.

The caregiving role of older people toward their own children has been evident in the context of health. In Thailand, persons infected with HIV relied on parental assistance, especially in the months leading up to their deaths.[53] Mothers, more than fathers, undertook the role of primary caregiver, even though both parents might still be living. Older women rendered assistance to the adult children by preparing food, doing laundry, and assisting in eating, dressing, bathing, and using the toilet. It has been suggested that while providing this kind of care is regarded as onerous and painful, these women have been found to believe that they are able to improve their *karma* and release *dukkha* (attachment), because as women they have fewer opportunities to release *dukkha* than do men, who may join the monkhood.[54] Moreover, parents usually shouldered the expenses incurred as a result of providing care to their children with AIDS, including undertaking the costs related to the funeral. In the event the deceased had children, grandparents also undertook the responsibility to provide care and support for these children if the deceased did not have a spouse.

The World of Women: The Choice between Working and Caregiving

In Southeast Asia, women's lives have undergone massive changes as a result of vibrant economic growth. The rising demand for women's labor in the electronics, textile, clerical, service, teaching, and nursing sectors in response to labor shortages in these industries has meant that vast numbers of women have moved from the rural areas to the more urbanized areas.[55] In 1990, women's share of the adult labor force in Southeast Asia was 59 percent, whereas in 2010 it was 57 percent, indicating that women's engagement in the labor force has been relatively consistent.[56] But taking into account all stages of the life cycle, women's labor force participation in the region has been far lower than men's. For example, in 2010, women's labor force participation rate of 57 percent stood in sharp contrast to men's labor participation rate, which was recorded to be 83 percent. Nonetheless, there has been a surge in the numbers of women receiving tertiary-level education simultaneously, which has enabled greater proportions of women to take on higher-status and higher-paid jobs in the workforce. In this case, increasing levels of education among women as a result of greater educational opportunities has enhanced women's bargaining power in the labor market.

Although the labor sector has changed, resulting in the recruitment of large numbers of women into the workforce, the organization of care in the household has not changed from previous times. Cultural norms continue to posit women's primary role as caregivers in the family in spite of their being employed.[57] Walker's notion of how women's caregiving role at the individual level may be traditionally explained in terms of their stronger emotional ties to family members compared to those of men is also applicable to the Southeast Asian context.[58] Moreover, there is the presumed notion that women are naturally suited to the caregiving role. In this case, women's caregiving role is bound up with their capacity to be more sacrificial and giving—qualities central to the identity of a "good woman."

In spite of these persistent cultural norms linking women to the caregiving role, the path working women from the more affluent families in Southeast Asia have had to tread in fulfilling their career objectives has been much easier than that of their sisters in the Western Hemisphere. Among them, balancing familial commitments and work demands has been made possible because of the option of employing women from the poorer countries in the region or from the rural areas to whom they can transfer their own domestic responsibilities, including their role of elder caregiver.[59] In Singapore, for example, increasingly families are employing live-in domestic workers (or maids) specifically to provide care for elderly parents.[60] These women come mainly from Indonesia, the Philippines, Myanmar, and Sri Lanka. The recent arrivals in particular would have received skills training required specifically for providing care to the elderly in their own countries before departing for Singapore. Although households with higher income levels are more likely to employ foreign domestic workers, a study found that the presence of individuals with higher levels of education and those belonging to the Chinese ethnic group increased the likelihood that the elderly person residing in that household would receive the aid of a domestic worker.[61] The same study found that older persons in households with more male or female adult children are less likely to employ a domestic worker, while those with fewer male or female adult children were more likely to do so, implying that domestic workers substitute for the care provided by adult children. Moreover, while the likelihood of employing a domestic worker increases in households with co-resident grandchildren or great-grandchildren, in households where the elderly person had a co-resident spouse, the likelihood of employing a domestic worker is far less. It was also suggested in this study that foreign domestic workers employed to provide care to an elderly person were more likely to assist the elderly with dressing, bathing, and toileting or performing housework; other principal caregivers were mainly found to take on the tasks of feeding the elderly, administering medication and/or injections, exercising or walking the elderly person, shopping, and preparing the meals.[62] In another study, it was found that unmarried working women in particular could not have engaged in wage work without the help of a domestic worker.[63] But having a domestic worker does not completely relieve them of their caregiver role, since these women usually end up having to supervise the domestic worker. Because the involvement of daughters or daughters-in-law in care provision to the elderly on a day-to-day basis is seen as a woman's prerogative and not a man's, the effort and time a daughter or daughter-in-law puts into caregiving is much greater than a son's.

While cultural norms associating women with the caregiver role continue to be strong in Southeast Asia, there have been observable changes in women's responses to these persistent cultural expectations of their roles in the family, especially in regard to attitudes toward marriage and fertility. For example, there has been a marked shift toward a delay in marriage throughout Southeast Asia, suggesting that marriage is losing its appeal. If women are not delaying marriage, they are certainly resisting it—as may be deduced from the rising numbers of unmarried women, significant proportions of whom are highly educated. In Indonesia, these women now make up 2 percent, while in Singapore they constitute 13 percent; in Thailand, the figure for unmarried women jumped from 3 percent in 1960 to 8 percent in 2000.[64] Increasing levels of education has been identified as one factor for this demographic trend among women; the lack of government policies to help women balance their work demands and family commitments may be identified as another. In Southeast Asia, countries demonstrating the trend toward delayed marriage include Malaysia, Myanmar, the Philippines, Thailand, Singapore, and, to a lesser extent, Indonesia—a trend found to be more pronounced in the urban areas than the rural areas.[65]

These shifts in attitudes towards women's role in the family raise questions as to how women view their elder caregiving role and the extent to which this may pose a threat to the care and support received by elderly persons.[66] Southeast Asian countries continue to demonstrate a strong sense of filial piety and obligation toward older kin. Evidence from Myanmar reveals that rejection of marriage has been beneficial to older persons. Usually it is the eldest daughter who denies herself of marriage in order to take on the task of primary elder caregiver to aging parents.[67] In Singapore, elder care policy emphasizes a "crowding in" approach, in which the family is regarded as the primary site of elder caregiving. National public housing policy through the Housing Development Board encourages children to provide care for their aging parents by providing subsidies to children, irrespective of gender, who choose to live close to their parents after marriage.[68] A woman who provides care for her elderly parent(s) or parent(s)-in-law also has the option of claiming a tax relief in her yearly income tax returns.[69]

Migrating for Work: Implications for the Elderly

Population aging is "emerging in the context of globalization."[70] What this means is that countries are aging while simultaneously becoming absorbed into a global economy marked by transnational flows of human and economic capital. From the 1980s onward, migrating for work across national borders has taken off in leaps and bounds in Southeast Asia. Although initially labor migration in the region was dominated by men, since the late 1980s, growing numbers of women have been migrating in search of wage work, their numbers overtaking that of men in some countries, such as the Philippines and Indonesia.[71,72] There has been substantial research undertaken on the "care crisis," particularly the impacts on children resulting from the absentee mother in the family.[73] Much less, however, has been documented on how migrant women (as well as men) affect the care she or they would provide for an aging parent. The question then arises as to the extent to which the migration of younger people from the rural to the urban areas raises the proportion of rural older people left without family support since "labour migration, predominantly of younger people, exacerbates age-structure imbalances in rural areas . . . by removing young adults at the very time that the older population is increasing."[74,75]

In Southeast Asia, the Philippines is the largest labor-exporting country, resulting in high numbers of older parents having to cope with residing alone.[78] Such is also the case in Thailand, as recorded by different researchers, where adult children were found to continue to maintain close contact with parents in spite of living apart from them.[79] Evidence from Thailand demonstrates that rural-urban migration is most common among young adults, leading to a decline in co-residence. From 1985 to 2003, significant numbers of young adults left the countryside to find jobs outside agriculture, given that the country's urban economy is one of the fastest-growing in the world.[80] In 1985, 78 percent of the young rural workforce employed in agriculture comprised males in the age group 15–39; in 2003, the numbers dropped to 59 percent. Among females, there was a larger drop in proportion of those employed in agriculture; in 1985, 80 percent of the rural workforce comprised females, whereas in 2003, it was only 53 percent. Such a trend has also led to rapid aging among the agricultural workforce.

Studies demonstrate that labor migration invariably alters the living arrangements of older people. In research conducted in Thailand, although it was found that the preference among older people would be to live with family members, circumstances were such that family members had to migrate to other places in order to find wage work, leaving the older person to reside alone. It was found that an incremental increase in one labor migrant from the household "doubles the odds" that the older person will end up living alone.[76] Older people living alone were vulnerable in another respect. As the results of this study showed, older people who live alone are more likely to possess fewer assets than those who live with others. However, they were better off because of the financial support they received through remittances. In fact, a related study found that remittances had the effect of reducing the levels of intra-rural household income inequality, beyond helping the older person.[77]

According to the existing literature, migrant children were found to provide for their aging parents, aside from sending home remittances and goods as well as maintaining daily contact. Although older persons may benefit from the remittances and goods sent home by their migrant children, the disadvantage is that if they decide to take on wage work away from their natal families, migrant adult children are not available to help the elderly on a daily basis.[81] This is most pronounced when adult daughters migrate for wage work, since daughters would help out more in the household than sons.

In migrant communities in Java, it was found that greater numbers of older women tended to rely on remittances of adult migrant children compared with older men. Because remittance amounts were usually less than work income, older women were at an economic disadvantage compared with older men because the latter had access to work income, and if they were not working they would be receiving pensions and investment income. For this reason, older women tended to be better off living with spouses than living alone.[82] In another study conducted in Java and Sumatra of Indonesia, the role of networks was found to ensure the security of the older person. Even small amounts of remittances were found to go a long way in maintaining family solidarity and the social status of the elderly, but mostly in conjunction with support provided by local family members. But among the very poor elderly, there were those who were subject to low levels of support and, in turn, were forced to rely on charity. In this case, what created vulnerability was not crises as such but status and network differences over the life course. For this reason, higher-status families did better as they were able to take advantage of migration opportunities.[83] That dependence was not shunned but rather a point of honor was a differentiating factor among the elderly in Indonesia. Unlike in Java, the elderly in Minangkabau tended to take pride in their dependence on their children, although they were relatively solvent because of their agricultural income. The younger generation, in turn, felt compelled to give their parents money even though the latter did not require it. For this reason, Minangkabau migrants tended to send remittances back to their families more frequently and in larger amounts compared with migrants from Java.[84]

Concluding Remarks

What, then, can we conclude about the traditional support system provided by families for older adults in this time of immense changes? Research in the region has affirmed that families continue to play a prominent role in care provision towards the elderly. In spite of demographic changes having resulted in smaller families, the family continues to be the primary site of old-age care. But older persons are never only receiving care. The literature is replete with examples of older persons who have been found to extend care to others residing in the same household. In this regard, intragenerational ties continue to be strong, with both the elderly and adult children reinforcing intra-familial obligations.

While the familial role in caregiving continues to be strong, state intervention in bolstering the family in this regards cannot be ignored. Governments are aware that declining family size, the growing numbers of women joining the workforce, and the geographic mobility of family members have the potential to reduce the number of potential caregivers within the family and the options of old-age care. Because of these trends, the state has taken proactive measures to ensure in different ways that the family has the capacity to cope with the problems associated with caring for the elderly. For example, governments have established supplementary services such as daycare centers to help lighten the burden of the family.[85] Tax incentives and subsidies have also been enforced to encourage families to care for the elderly. Although these structural interventions may have strengthened the role of the family, it is "unlikely that [such efforts] alone could have encouraged the renegotiation of such a robust and resilient reciprocal inter-generational contract if it was not also based on mutual need and dependence."[86] Thus, as Croll compellingly argues, "it is the familial contract and familial exclusion rather than a social contract and social exclusion that are more pertinent to individual well-being."[87]

While "aging in place" has numerous benefits for older persons, it must be noted that overreliance on the family may be a double-edged sword for some groups of elderly. Elderly women constitute a case in point, since they tend to rely on family support more than elderly men because of having had fewer savings as a result of not having engaged in wage work or not having worked as long as men.[88] This suggests that elderly women would feel the negative impacts much more than elderly men should there be significant shifts in the family structure. To this end, targeted programs directed at older women become imperative, especially in cases where the family is unable to exercise its familial role in elder care. As such, states cannot take it for granted that since family ties continue to be strong in the region, they need play only a minimal role in supporting the elderly. Although this may be the current trend, it is uncertain for how long the family would be able to live up to the expectations of its role in old-age care given the demographic, social, and economic transformations taking hold in the region. Should there be a time the family is not able to execute its role in elder care, the state would have to step in and play a greater role than it had before.

Notes

1. A. Börsch-Supan, "Global Ageing: What Is at Stake?" *Ageing Horizons* 4 (2006): 3–5; A. C. D'Addio, M. Keese, and E. Whitehouse, "Population Ageing and Labour Markets," *Oxford Review of Economic Policy* 26 (2010): 613–35; J. M. Wiener and J. Tilly, "Population Ageing in the United States of America: Implications for Public Programmes," *International Journal of Epidemiology* 31 (2002): 776–81; S. Hillcoat-Nalletamby, J. Ogg, S. Renaut, and C. Bonvalet, "Ageing Populations and Housing Needs: Comparing Strategic Policy Discourses in France and England," *Social Policy and Administration* 44 (2010): 808–26.

2. A. Chan, "Aging in Southeast and East Asia: Issues and Policy Directions," *Journal of Cross-Cultural Gerontology* 20 (2005): 269–84.

3. D. L. Lindauer and M. Roemer, "Legacies and Opportunities," in *Asia and Africa: Legacies and Opportunities in Development*, ed. D. L. Lindauer and M. Roemer (San Francisco: Institute for Contemporary Studies, 1994), 1–24.

4. S. Radelet, J. Sachs, and J-W. Lee, *Economic Growth in Asia*, HIID Development Discussion Paper No. 609 (Cambridge, MA: Harvard Institute for International Development, 1997), www.cid.harvard.edu/hiid/609.pdf.

5. Radelet, Sachs, and Lee, *Economic Growth in Asia*.

6. P. F. Kelly and T. G. McGee, "Changing Spaces: Southeast Asian Urbanization in an Era of Volatile Globalization," in *Southeast Asia Transformed: A Geography of Change*, ed. Lin Sien Chia (Singapore: Institute of Southeast Asian Studies, 2003), 257–85, quotation on 268.

7. Kelly and McGee, "Changing Spaces," 258.

8. D. Forbes, "Metropolis and Megaurban Region in Pacific Asia," *Tijdschrift voor Economische en Sociale Geografie* 88 (1997): 457–68; P. F. Kelly, "Globalization, Power and the Politics of Scale in the Philippines," *Geoforum* 28 (1997): 151–71.

9. Kelly and McGee, "Changing Spaces," 258.

10. A. E. Goodman, "The Political Implications of Urban Development in Southeast Asia: The 'Fragment' Hypothesis," *Economic Development and Cultural Change* 20 (1971): 117–30.

11. V. T. King, *The Sociology of Southeast Asia: Transformations in a Developing Region* (Copenhagen: Nordic Institute of Asian Studies, Honolulu: University of Hawai'i Press, 2008).

12. I. Attané, and M. Barbieri, "The Demography of East and Southeast Asia from the 1950s to the 2000s: A Summary of Changes and a Statistical Assessment," *Population* (English edition) 64 (2009): 9–146.

13. United Nations, *World Population Prospects: The 2006 Revision* (New York: Population Division of the Department of Economic and Social Affairs of the United Nations Secretariat), esa.un.org/unpp, as cited in Attané and Barbieri, "The Demography of East and Southeast Asia," 135.

14. G. W. Jones, "Population and the Family in Southeast Asia," *Journal of Southeast Asian Studies* 26 (1995): 184–95, quotation on 184.

15. Jones, "Population and the Family in Southeast Asia."

16. Attané and Barbieri, "The Demography of East and Southeast Asia"; Jones, "Population and the Family in Southeast Asia."

17. Jones, "Population and the Family in Southeast Asia."

18. Attané and Barbieri, "The Demography of East and Southeast Asia."

19. T. Parsons, "The American Family: Its Relations to Personality and to the Social Structure," in *Family, Socialization and Interaction Process,* ed. T. Parsons and R. F. Bales (London: Routledge and Kegan Paul, 1956), 3–33.

20. M. Qin, S. Punpuing, P. Guest, and P. Prasartkul, "Labour Migration and Change in Older People's Living Arrangements: The Case of Kanchanaburi Demographic Surveillance System (KDSS), Thailand," *Population, Space and Place* 14 (2008): 419–32.

21. D. Belanger, "Regional Differences in Household Composition and Family Formation Patterns in Vietnam," *Journal of Comparative Family Studies* 31 (2000): 171–89.

22. Jones, "Population and the Family in Southeast Asia," 184–95.

23. H. Geertz, *The Javanese Family: A Study of Kinship and Socialization* (New York: The Free Press of Glencoe, 1961).

24. R. R. Jay, *Javanese Villagers: Social Relations in Rural Modjokuto* (Cambridge, MA: MIT Press, 1969).

25. Jones, "Population and the Family in Southeast Asia," 189.

26. G. T. Castillo, *Beyond Manila: Philippine Rural Problems in Perspective* (Ottawa: International Development Research Centre, 1979), 116, as cited in Jones, "Population and the Family in Southeast Asia," 189.

27. A. I. Hermalin, "Theoretical Perspectives, Measurement Issues, and Related Research," in *The Well-Being of the Elderly in Asia: A Four-Country Comparative Study,* ed. A. I. Hermalin (Ann Arbor: The University of Michigan Press, 2002), 101–41.

28. K. O. Mason, "Family Change and Support of the Elderly in Asia: What Do We Know?" *Asia-Pacific Population Journal* 7 (1992): 13–32.

29. K. Glaser, E. M. Agree, E. Costenbader, A. Camargo, B. Trench, J. Natividad, and Y.-L. Chuang, "Fertility Decline, Family Structure, and Support for Older Persons in Latin America and Asia," *Journal of Aging and Health* 18 (2006): 259–91.

30. National Statistical Office: The 2000 Population and Housing Census (Thailand: National Statistical Office, Ministry of Information and Communication Technology), web.nso.go.th/en/census/poph/prelim_e.htm.

31. Table 3: Average Household Size by State, 1980–2010, Department of Statistics Malaysia website, www.statistics.gov.my/portal/images/stories/files/LatestReleases/banci/jadual3.pdf.

32. L. Rudkin, "Gender Differences in Economic Well-Being among the Elderly of Java," *Demography* 30 (1993): 209–26.

33. J. Knodel, N. Chayovan, and S. Siriboon, "The Impact of Fertility Decline on Familial Support for the Elderly: An Illustration from Thailand," *Population and Development Review* 18 (1992): 79–103.

34. Z. Zimmer and K. Korinek, "Does Family Size Predict Whether an Older Adult Lives with or Proximate to an Adult Child in the Asia-Pacific Region?" *Asian Population Studies* 4 (2008): 135–59.

35. Zimmer and Korinek, "Does Family Size Predict?"

36. Zimmer and Korinek, "Does Family Size Predict?" 154.

37. L. G. Martin, "Living Arrangements of the Elderly in Fiji, Korea, Malaysia, and the Philippines," *Demography* 26 (1989): 627–43; J. Knodel and N. Chayovan, "Family Support and Living Arrangements of Thai Elderly," *Asia-Pacific Population Journal* 12 (1997) 12: 51–68; Hermalin, *The Well-Being of the Elderly in Asia.*

38. J. Friedman, J. Knodel, T. C. Bui, and S. A. Truong, "Gender Dimensions of Support for Elderly in Vietnam," *Research on Aging* 25 (2003): 587–630.

39. A. Chan, "Formal and Informal Intergenerational Support Transfers in South-Eastern Asia," United Nations Expert Group Meeting on Social and Economic Implications of Changing Population Age Structures, Population Division Department of Economic and Social Affairs, Mexico City, Mexico, August 31–September 2, 2005, www.un.org/esa/population/meetings/Proceedings_EGM_Mex_2005/chan.pdf; E. M. Agree, A. E. Biddlecom, M.-C. Chang, and A. E. Perez, "Transfers from Older Parents to Their Adult Children in Taiwan and the Philippines," *Journal of Cross-Cultural Gerontology* 17 (2002): 269–94; G. R. Andrews and M. M. Hennink, "The Circumstances and Contributions of Older Persons in Three Asian Countries: Preliminary Results of a Cross-National Study," *Asia-Pacific Population Journal* 7 (1992): 127–46; Knodel and Chayovan, "Family Support and Living Arrangements of Thai Elderly," 51–68.

40. E. J. Croll, "The Intergenerational Contract in the Changing Asian Family," *Oxford Development Studies* 34 (2006): 473–91.

41. Croll, "The Intergenerational Contract in the Changing Asian Family," 483; E. C. Y. Kuo, "Confucianism and the Chinese Family in Singapore: Continuities and Changes," in *Confucianism and the Family,* ed. W. H. Slote and G. A. DeVos (Albany: State University of New York Press, 1998), 231–48; Chan, "Aging in Southeast and East Asia."

42. Kuo, "Confucianism and the Chinese Family in Singapore."

43. R. A. Aziz and F. Yusooff, "Intergenerational Relationships and Communication Among the Rural Aged in Malaysia," *Asian Social Science* 8 (2012): 184–95.

44. Aziz and Yusooff, "Intergenerational Relationships and Communication," 191.

45. Croll, "The Intergenerational Contract in the Changing Asian Family."

46. P. A. Rozario and S-L. Hong, "Doing It 'Right' by Your Parents in Singapore: A Political Economy Examination of the Maintenance of Parents Act of 1995," *Critical Social Policy* 31 (2011): 618, 616.

47. P. L. Lim, "Maintenance of Parents Act," *Singapore Infopedia,* 2009, http://eresources.nlb.gov.sg/infopedia/articles/SIP_1614_2009=11=30.html.

48. Croll, "The Intergenerational Contract in the Changing Asian Family," 484.

49. K. A. Roberto and J. Stroes, "Grandchildren and Grandparents: Roles, Influences, and Relationships," in *The Ties of Later Life,* ed. J. Hendricks (New York: Baywood, 1995), 141–53.

50. B. Schwarz, I. Albert, G. Trommsdorff, G. Zheng, S. Shi, and P. R. Nelwan, "Intergenerational Support and Life Satisfaction: A Comparison of Chinese, Indonesian, and German Elderly Mothers," *Journal of Cross-Cultural Psychology* 41 (2010): 706–22.

51. P. Kreager and E. Schröder-Butterfill, "Indonesia against the Trend? Ageing and Inter-generational Wealth Flows in Two Indonesian Communities," *Demographic Research* 19 (2008): 1791.

52. Kreager and Schröder-Butterfill, "Indonesia against the Trend?" 1790.

53. J. Knodel and C. Saengtienchai, "Older-Aged Parents: The Final Safety Net for Adult Sons and Daughters with AIDS in Thailand," *Journal of Family Issues* 26 (2005): 665–98.

54. A. Sankar, M. Luborsky, T. Rwabuhemba, and P. Songwathana, "Comparative Perspectives on Living with HIV/AIDS in Late Life," *Research on Aging* 20 (1998): 885–911.

55. S. B. Westley and A. Mason, "Women Are Key Players in the Economies of East and Southeast Asia," *Asia-Pacific Population and Policy* 44 (1998): 1–4; B. P. Resurreccion, "Gender Trends in Migration and Employment in Southeast Asia," in *Gender Trends in Southeast Asia: Women Now, Women in the Future*, ed. T. W. Devasahayam (Singapore: Institute of Southeast Asian Studies, 2009), 31–52.

56. Department of Economic and Social Affairs, *The World's Women 2010: Trends and Statistics* (New York: United Nations, 2010), United Nations Statistics Division website, unstats. un.org/unsd/demographic/products/Worldswomen/WW_full report_BW.pdf.

57. T. W. Devasahayam and B. S. A. Yeoh, eds., *Working and Mothering in Asia: Images, Ideologies and Identities* (Singapore and Copenhagen, Denmark: National University of Singapore Press and Nordic Institute of Asian Studies, 2007).

58. A. J. Walker, "Conceptual Perspectives on Gender and Family Caregiving," in *Gender, Families, and Elder Care*, ed. J. W. Dwyer and R. T. Coward (Newbury Park, CA: Sage, 1992), 34–46.

59. A. Brooks and T. Devasahayam, *Gender, Emotions and Labour Markets: Asian and Western Perspectives* (London: Routledge, 2011); P. A. Rozario and A. L. Rosetti, "'Many Helping Hands': A Review and Analysis of Long-Term Care Policies, Programs, and Practices in Singapore," *Journal of Gerontological Social Work* 55 (2012): 641–58.

60. L. M. Verbrugge and A. Chan, "Giving Help in Return: Family Reciprocity by Older Singaporeans," *Ageing & Society* 28 (2008): 5–34.

61. T. S. Sobieszczyk, *Domestic Servants Assisting the Elderly in Singapore: Current Situation and Future Research Recommendations*, Comparative Study of the Elderly in Asia, Research Report No. 02-59 (Ann Arbor: University of Michigan Population Studies Center, 2002), University of Michigan Population Studies Center, Institute for Social Research website, www.psc.isr.umich.edu/pubs/pdf/eao2-59.pdf.

62. Sobieszczyk, *Domestic Servants Assisting the Elderly in Singapore*.

63. T. W. Devasahayam, *Organisations That Care: The Necessity for an Eldercare Leave Scheme for Caregivers of the Elderly in Singapore*, Asian MetaCentre Research Paper Series no. 10, Asian MetaCentre website, January 2003, www.populationasia.org/Publications/Research-Paper/AMCRP10.pdf.

64. Attané and Barbieri, "The Demography of East and Southeast Asia."

65. G. W. Jones, "Women, Marriage and Family in Southeast Asia," in *Gender Trends in Southeast Asia: Women Now, Women in the Future*, ed. T. W. Devasahayam (Singapore: Institute of Southeast Asian Studies, 2009), 12–30.

66. V. Desai and M. Tye, "Critically Understanding Asian Perspectives on Ageing," *Third World Quarterly* 30 (2009): 1007–25.

67. Jones, "Women, Marriage and Family in Southeast Asia."

68. V. Chew, "Housing and Development Board (HDB)," Singapore Infopedia, 2009, http://eresources.nlb.gov.sg/infopedia/articles/SIP_1589_2009=10=26.html; A. Chan, A. E. Biddlecom, M. B. Ofstedal, and A. I. Hermalin, *The Relationship between Formal and Familial Support of the Elderly in Singapore and Taiwan,* Asian Metacentre Research Paper Series no. 9, Asian MetaCentre website, January 2003, www.populationasia.org/Publications/RP/AMCRP9.pdf.

69. P. A. Rozario and A. L. Rosetti, "'Many Helping Hands': A Review and Analysis of Long-Term Care Policies, Programs, and Practices in Singapore," *Journal of Gerontological Social Work* 55 (2012): 641–58.

70. S. Harper, "Addressing the Implications of Global Ageing," *Journal of Population Research* 23 (2006): 205–23, quotation on 208.

71. J. W. Huguet, "International Migration and Development: Opportunities and Challenges for Poverty Reduction," in *Fifth Asian and Pacific Population Conference,* Asian Population Studies Series 158 (New York: United Nations, 2003), 117–36.

72. A. Brooks and T. Devasahayam, *Gender, Emotions and Labour Markets.*

73. R. Salazar Parrañes, *Children of Global Migration: Transnational Families and Gendered Woes* (Stanford, CA: Stanford University Press, 2005); G. Battistella and M. C. G. Conaco, "The Impact of Labour Migration on the Children Left Behind: A Study of Elementary School Children in the Philippines," *Sojourn: Journal of Social Issues in Southeast Asia* 13 (1998): 220–41.

74. P. Kraeger, "Migration, Social Structure and Old-Age Support Networks: A Comparison of Three Indonesian Communities," *Ageing & Society* 26 (2006): 37–60, quotation on 37.

75. Qin et al., "Labour Migration and Change in Older People's Living Arrangements."

76. Qin et al., "Labour Migration and Change in Older People's Living Arrangements," 429.

77. P. Guest, "Assessing the Consequences of Internal Migration: Methodological Issues and a Case Study on Thailand Based on Longitudinal Household Survey Data," in *Migration, Urbanization, and Development: New Directions and Issues,* ed. R. E. Bilsborrow (New York: United Nations Population Fund and Kluwer Academic Publishers, 1998), 275–318.

78. G. T. Cruz, A. M. C. Lavares, M. P. N. Marquez, J. N. Natividad and Y. Saito, "Gender and Economic Well-Being among Older Filipinos," in *Gender and Ageing: Southeast Asian Perspectives,* ed. T. W. Devasahayam (Singapore: Institute of Southeast Asian Studies, 2014), 288–314.

79. J. Knodel and N. Chayovan, "Gender and Ageing in Thailand: A Situation Analysis of Older Women and Men," in *Gender and Ageing: Southeast Asian Perspectives,* ed. T. W. Devasahayam (Singapore: Institute of Southeast Asian Studies, 2014), 33–67.

80. J. Bryant and R. Gray, *Rural Population Ageing and Farm Structure in Thailand,* Food and Agriculture Organization website, September 2005, www.fao.org/sd/dim_pe3/docs/pe3_051001d1_en.pdf.

81. L. Rudkin, "Gender Differences in Economic Well-Being among the Elderly of Java," *Demography* 30 (1993): 209–26.

82. Rudkin, "Gender Differences in Economic Well-Being among the Elderly of Java."

83. Kraeger, "Migration, Social Structure and Old-Age Support Networks," 37–60.

84. Kreager and Schröder-Butterfill, "Indonesia against the Trend?" 1781–1810.

85. Croll, "The Intergenerational Contract in the Changing Asian Family."

86. Croll, "The Intergenerational Contract in the Changing Asian Family," 487.

87. E. J. Croll, "The Intergenerational Contract in the Changing Asian Family," 473.

88. T. W. Devasahayam, "Growing Old in Southeast Asia: What Do We Know about Gender?" in *Gender and Ageing: Southeast Asian Perspectives,* ed. T. W. Devasahayam (Singapore: Institute of Southeast Asian Studies, 2014), 1–32.

8 Epidemic Disease in Modern and Contemporary Southeast Asia

Mary Wilson

Epidemics can cross borders and encircle the globe. Dynamic and dramatic events, they can seem unpredictable and capricious. They can spread rapidly or slowly and can be caused by old, familiar pathogens, like the bacillus that causes tuberculosis, or by never previously recognized ones, like the SARS coronavirus. They can be introduced from another region or can originate locally and disseminate. They can spread directly from one person to another or can require an intermediary, such as a food or water vehicle, a mosquito or flea vector, or exposure to a contaminated environment. They can kill, sometimes rapidly, or cause only minor symptoms in the majority of cases. Animals are also vulnerable—in some instances to pathogens that are the same as or similar to those that infect humans. Outbreaks of disease in animals, called epizootics, can also have serious indirect consequences for human life and well-being. Epidemics are often highly visible, especially if they cause death, disability, or disfigurement—and especially if the cause is unknown or not well understood. They engender fear and precipitate irrational behavior. Economic consequences often extend well beyond those directly affected. This chapter will discuss epidemics in Southeast Asia and some of the forces that have changed the nature, size, sources, characteristics, and drivers of epidemics over the past 100 to 150 years in this region. Although non-infectious diseases, such as beriberi in the past and obesity today, can also occur in epidemic form, most of the examples in this chapter will be infectious diseases. Because it has been discussed in Kirsty Walker's chapter, pandemic influenza of 1918–19 will not be included in this chapter.

In addition to demographic, psychological, and economic impacts, epidemics can also affect governance domestically and internationally.[1] Epidemics can lead to a shift in power to the state in an attempt to control spread and limit impact. States can suppress reports of disease and deaths. By their policies and provision of resources, they can also generate or exacerbate conflicts between ethnic groups, geographic regions, and social classes. Attempts to find and explain the origins and drivers of epidemics can lead to scapegoating and assigning blame, often targeting minorities and impoverished populations.

Several key themes thread through this chapter:

- The spectrum of causes and patterns of spread of epidemic diseases in Southeast Asia have been shaped by the geography, ecology, and demography of the region. The rapid increase in urbanization and growth of large cities has altered the landscape of more recent epidemics.
- Infections causing epidemics can come from within the region or can be introduced from the outside. The high level of connectedness and population mobility in recent decades is associated with an increased probability of spread of epidemics within, into, and out of Southeast Asia.
- Epidemics can be characterized as fast or slow. Both have affected Southeast Asia. Epidemic diseases—especially fast ones with rapid onset and spread, such as cholera—are disruptive, receive intense attention, and can have a profound economic impact, but may account for a small proportion of overall deaths.
- In recent decades, Southeast Asia has experienced a transition in the burden of disease from being predominantly infectious diseases to an increasing burden of chronic diseases, such as diabetes and heart disease, now responsible for 60 percent of deaths in the region.[2]

Southeast Asia: The Geography

The region of Southeast Asia is highly diverse in culture, traditions, language, economic resources, and natural resources. Most of it lies in tropical and subtropical zones, characterized by rich biodiversity. It is hot and humid much of the year and has abundant rainfall. The countries are found between the latitudes of 30°N and 10°S. It has been described as the part of Asia that spills into the sea, and water is a constant presence in daily life and an important mode of transport and trade.[3] Many of the major cities developed on rivers or in marshy coastal areas. Water is essential for human survival—but also can provide ideal breeding sites for mosquitoes. Large concentrations of the population were often in port cities, which were vulnerable to introductions of infections that arrived by ship—diseases carried by the human travelers (e.g., smallpox, typhus, cholera) or in stowaways, such as rats that could carry fleas and the plague bacillus. Advances in the development of steamships and their increasing deployment in the second half of the nineteenth century dramatically increased the speed and volume of travel and trade.[4] Steamships appeared in Philippine waters in the mid-1880s and drew the islands closer together. By 1890 the mail steamer could make the trip from Manila to Iloilo (a distance of 564 km) in less than thirty-six hours.[5]

At the end of the nineteenth century and beginning of the twentieth century many of the classic epidemic diseases still periodically caused outbreaks. In the Philippines, for example, the five leading causes of death in 1902–3 were malaria, cholera, tuberculosis, diarrheal diseases, and smallpox (although precise numbers are recorded, reporting was incomplete and diagnostic capabilities limited).[6] Epidemic diseases can be dramatic and highly visible, but analysis of data from Java (Indonesia) over a sixty-year period from 1820 to 1880 suggested that excess mortality due to epidemics (especially cholera, smallpox, typhoid fever, and malaria) and other disasters, such as famine, was only about 10 percent of the total mortality.[7]

Vulnerabilities to Epidemics

Although pathogenic microbes may be necessary for an epidemic, many socio-economic, ecoclimatic, demographic, and political factors work synergistically to set the stage for an epidemic event and may influence its size and consequences. Several of these will be explored in the section that follows.

Among the many factors that make a population or region vulnerable to epidemics of infectious diseases are ecoclimatic conditions. In general, areas that are closer to the equator have greater biodiversity, which decreases as distances from the equator increase. Known as the species latitudinal gradient, it also applies to parasites and microbes that are pathogenic for humans.[8] Ecoclimatic factors influence the survival and propagation of many pathogens, vectors (such as mosquitoes), and intermediate hosts (such as rats)—and the ease or difficulty in controlling their spread. Biologists have also identified twenty-five areas globally called biodiversity hotspots, or areas that are especially rich in endemic species, and ones that are also threatened by human activities.[9] Notably, the Philippines and Indo-Burma are among these hotspots. Human population density is a significant predictor of emerging infectious disease events.[10] Wildlife species richness is also a predictor for emergence of human infections with animal origin, the zoonoses.[11] Although many parts of Southeast Asia are sparsely populated, the region includes many densely populated urban areas, and the region has an abundance of diverse wildlife.[12]

Famines alone can cause deaths, but undernutrition and malnutrition (including micronutrient deficiencies) make humans more susceptible to many infectious diseases, including epidemic diseases, such as tuberculosis, measles, and cholera. Many massive epidemics with high death rates have occurred in populations weakened by lack of food. Often famine occurs in the setting of other disasters—such as war and conflict and extreme events, such as floods—that can displace populations and disrupt access to food. The confluence of many factors working synergistically can favor appearance of epidemic disease and its spread. Healthy, well-nourished populations are more resistant to many infections.

The density of population can influence the probability of spread of infections that pass from person to person. The size of the population also matters. To be maintained in a population, smallpox, for example, requires a population size of at least one hundred thousand to two hundred thousand.[13] Smallpox could not become endemic in the small, dispersed populations that were found in many parts of Southeast Asia, but these areas were vulnerable to periodic introductions. Mortality could be high in unvaccinated populations, averaging 30 percent in some outbreaks.

Cultural beliefs and traditions can facilitate spread of infection, epidemic or otherwise. In the Philippines, for example, the tradition that friends and relatives visit and draw near the sick and dying—even when they had a contagious infection like smallpox—would facilitate spread to others, especially in an era before most were vaccinated.[14] Likewise, the bathing of and close contact with a body after death could fuel the spread of epidemic diseases, such as cholera.

War and conflicts historically and in the twentieth century were associated with epidemic disease in Southeast Asia and elsewhere. Victims include civilians as well as those fighting. The multiple disruptions that accompany conflicts include malnutrition, starvation, displacement of populations and crowding together in temporary shelters, loss of clean water and sanitation, and increased exposure to vectors—all of which increase the risk of epidemics and their spread.

The scale of human migration within Asia since the mid-nineteenth century has been greater than at any other time and place in history.[15] To this we superimpose vast movements of populations into and out of Asia to other parts of the world. Singapore, in particular, has become a major hub for international travel, with international passenger numbers climbing from about 2.2 million per month in 2000 to peaks of almost 4 million monthly a decade later.[16]

Today the burden from communicable diseases is highly variable by country within Southeast Asia; Cambodia and Myanmar (Burma) have the highest burden as reflected in disability-adjusted life years (DALYs), and Singapore the lowest.[17] Cambodia, the Philippines, and Indonesia have the highest burdens of tuberculosis in the region; Thailand, Cambodia, and Burma bear the greatest burden from HIV/AIDS. In Burma, the cumulative probability of malaria death in individuals aged five years or older is 51.8 per 1,000 population, by far the highest in the region.[18] In the region, communicable diseases contribute approximately 42 percent of DALYs, which is slightly more than the 40 percent in the world as a whole.[19]

Epidemics can be characterized as fast or slow. Cholera and influenza are fast epidemics. Exposed individuals can become ill within hours of exposure. Infected individuals can spread infection before they know they are infected or during asymptomatic infection. When combined with rapid, long-distance transport, these infections, carried by humans, can be introduced and spread in new areas. Influenza can infect all—rich and poor, old and young—whereas cholera thrives only where sanitation is poor and clean water not available. HIV/ AIDS has caused a slow epidemic. Because of the long period required before most infected individuals develop characteristic signs of infection, it became entrenched in many populations in many countries before it was recognized, characterized, and its several mechanisms of spread identified.

What is notable is that many of the factors that favor the propagation of an epidemic are associated with poverty and lack of education about simple protective measures. In most instances, the poorest and least advantaged suffer the greatest burden from infections, including during epidemics. Historical examples illustrate the multiplicity of factors that can participate synergistically in overlapping epidemics and in those involving animals and noninfectious diseases.

Rinderpest

Rinderpest is an infection of bovines that in May 2011 was declared by the World Health Organization (WHO) to have been globally eradicated.[20] Until recent decades it caused massive die-offs in cattle. Caused by an RNA virus, a morbillivirus in the same genus as the measles virus, it can wipe out a herd of cattle within days. There is no treatment for it. Although it does not directly infect humans, it can destroy human livelihood and access to food. In the 1960s a tissue culture vaccine was developed, and mass vaccination campaigns were started shortly thereafter. Wide use of the vaccine facilitated disease control and, ultimately, led to its eradication. The history of rinderpest outbreaks in the Philippines illustrates the interrelatedness of multiple events and importance of animal disease in human health and survival.

Rinderpest was first introduced into the Philippines in 1887, and is thought to have reached the Philippines from Indochina with animals imported for breeding.[21] Local cattle and domestic buffalo were susceptible and died rapidly. Mortality reached 90 percent in some bovine populations. These draft animals allowed Filipinos to work the land. With the loss of the animals, rice harvests declined and production dropped precipitously. Agricultural production collapsed. This aggravated malnutrition. With the death of the animals, the local mosquitoes turned to humans for blood meals.[22] Malaria was already present, but the increased biting of humans was associated with massive outbreaks in malaria in humans. A major epidemic of cholera in 1889 hit a population already weakened by malnutrition.

Similar events were observed in other areas. A large malaria epidemic in West Java in 1880 occurred in an area experiencing a severe attack of rinderpest. One of the mosquito vectors in that region, *Anopheles maculatus,* apparently prefers cattle blood to that of humans, but may have turned to human blood following the death of many of the domestic buffaloes.[23]

Beriberi

Multiple interacting events contributed to the epidemics of beriberi, a noninfectious disease, in the Philippines. Caused by a deficiency of thiamine, beriberi can lead to disability and death. In 1902 and 1903, more than ten thousand deaths—thought to be an undercount—were attributed to beriberi, making it the sixth leading cause of death after malaria, cholera, tuberculosis, diarrheal disease, and smallpox.[24] Although the disease is easily prevented by eating foods containing thiamine, the cause was not generally understood at that time and speculation about its cause included a bacillus, a nonbacterial toxin, as well as dietary deficiency.[25] The stage for large outbreaks had been set over several decades. Because of better ships and port services, agriculture in the Philippines had shifted from rice to other exportable crops, such as sugar, hemp, and tobacco. By 1902, the Philippines no longer grew sufficient rice for its population and was importing >300 million kilos of rice annually.[26] The highly milled imported rice was deficient in thiamine—in contrast to the locally grown rice, which was only partially milled. Those who ate only milled rice, not supplemented by fish and other foods, could develop symptoms of beriberi within three months of subsisting only on rice. Other factors contributed to the large outbreaks of beriberi among the Filipinos: movement to towns and cities, hence the loss of locally grown foods to supplement the rice diet, and relentless poverty among many who could not afford other foods. The cholera epidemic polluted the waters and made people fearful of eating fish—so the poorest subsisted on milled rice alone and were those affected by beriberi.[27]

Dengue Infections

In considering a variety of epidemics from infectious diseases in Southeast Asia, it is useful to examine the origin or source of the pathogen, factors that have enabled the dispersal within the region, the geographic reach, and the consequence or impact of the epidemic on health. In some instances, it is relevant to also examine the economic impact. Table 8.1 summarizes these factors for five infections, and these are described more fully in the text that follows.

Dengue is among the most dramatic examples of an infection that has had broad impact in Southeast Asia.[28] Epidemics continue to occur regularly throughout the region and show no evidence of abating. Caused by an RNA virus, dengue infections range from mild or asymptomatic to hemorrhagic fever with shock and death.[29] Children in many parts of Asia are the most severely affected. The dengue virus is transmitted by mosquitoes, most commonly *Aedes aegypti*. Four serotypes of the virus exist globally—and all four circulate in Southeast Asia. Infection with one serotype provides transient immunity against all four virus types, but lifelong immunity against only the infecting serotype. Subsequent infection with a different serotype is associated with a greater likeli-

Table 8.1. Examples of epidemic infections: Drivers and consequences

Infection/agent	Origin/source	Enablers; drivers of dispersal	Geographic reach	Consequences; impact
Dengue virus	Human-to-human; transmitted by mosquitoes; originally from non-human primates	Urbanization; population mobility; poor vector control	Widespread in Southeast Asia, especially urban areas; tropics/subtropics globally; expanding reach and severity of epidemics	High morbidity; deaths from severe dengue; economic consequences from lost productivity and health care
Chikungunya virus	Originally primate-to-human in Africa; transmitted by mosquito	Population mobility; urbanization; widespread infestation by competent mosquitoes; mutation of virus to enable more efficient transmission	Widespread outbreaks in countries of Southeast Asia; co-circulation with dengue virus and co-infection in some instances; Asia, Africa; recent transmission in the Americas	Low mortality but persistent, disabling joint pain is common
SARS coronavirus	Reservoir host: bats; transmitted to humans from civets, then person-to-person spread; initial cases in China in 2002	Travel of infected persons; spread in hospitals, airplanes, housing	Spread to at least 30 countries and regions before virus was contained in 2003; health care workers and their contacts were most affected	>8000 probable SARS cases resulted in 916 deaths. Spread of virus was contained through use of isolation and quarantine; major disruption of global travel in 2003
H5N1 influenza virus	Avian host (chickens, ducks, other) Limited person-to-person spread. First recognized in 1997	Large poultry populations; mixing of different avian species; poultry trade; migration of birds	Primarily Asia with limited, sporadic spread in avian species in Europe and Africa; human cases in Asia, Africa	Millions of poultry culled to prevent spread; reported human cases 650; deaths 386 (as of January 2014)
HIV/AIDS	Primates in Africa	Human contact with primates; perhaps via hunting, preparing bushmeat; travel; medical care; sex; IV drug use	Global spread over several decades	Estimated 1.6 million died from AIDS (2012); Estimated 36 million deaths since start of epidemic; 35 million persons currently living with HIV/AIDS (2012)

Sources: World Health Organization, "Summary Table of SARS Cases by Country, 1 November 2002–7 August 2003," August 15, 2003, World Health Organization website, www.who.int/csr/sars/country/2003_08_15/en; World Health Organization, "Cumulative Number of Confirmed Human Cases for Avian Influenza A(H5N1) Reported to WHO, 2003–2014," World Health Organization website, www.who.int/influenza/human_animal_interface/EN_GI P_20140124CumulativeNumberH5N1cases.pdf; "2103 Global Fact Sheet," UNAIDS website, www.unaids.org/en/media/unaids/contentassets/documents/ epidemiology/2013/gr2013/20130923_FactSheet_Global_en.pdf.

hood of severe disease and death. This means that an individual can have dengue up to four times—and later infections may be more severe than the first. Since World War II, epidemics in Southeast Asia have become more widespread and severe.[30] The first known outbreaks of hemorrhagic dengue in the world occurred in the Philippines in 1953–54 with another appearing two years later. Thailand had sporadic cases of hemorrhagic disease in the 1950s but had its first epidemic of hemorrhagic disease in 1958. Epidemics have seasonality and a cyclical pattern, with more severe epidemics occurring about every three years. Even Singapore, with its excellent surveillance and vector control programs, has been unable to prevent outbreaks.

Although the original hosts for the dengue virus were nonhuman primates, the virus has now become well adapted to humans, and the virus is perpetuated almost exclusively in a human–mosquito–human cycle. It can also be passed from one generation to another in the mosquito. The virus is well adapted to an urban mosquito that is well adapted to contemporary urban life.[31] The mosquito is abundant in urban tropical and subtropical areas globally. *Aedes aegypti* is an efficient vector that is hard to avoid. It prefers to take blood meals from humans (rather than animals), enters houses, and bites during the daytime. It can breed in small pools of water that can be found in discarded plastic cups and cans, gutters, used tires, flowerpots, and decorative fountains. Its life cycle is influenced by temperature and rainfall, but the mosquito eggs are resistant to desiccation, so the virus can survive dry and cool seasons.

Among the factors fueling the increase in dengue cases are increasing urbanization, especially in tropical and subtropical areas, and increased population mobility.[32,33] Humans who are infected, whether they know it or not, can easily carry the virus in their blood from one place to another. If suitable mosquitoes are present in the new location and bite an infected person, the mosquito can subsequently transmit infection to one or more other humans halfway around the world. Today most of the global population growth is occurring in low-latitude areas, like Southeast Asia, and in urban areas. In Southeast Asia, currently almost half of people live in urban areas, and this is projected to grow to >70 percent by 2050.[34] Many live in periurban slum areas without reliable water supplies. This leads them to store water in containers that provide good breeding sites for the vector mosquitoes. More humans are living in transmission zones—and more humans have already had at least one episode of dengue, which may put them at higher risk for severe disease. More urban areas have reached a population size, somewhere between 150 thousand and 1 million, that is large enough to allow the ongoing circulation of dengue viruses. Besides urbanization and travel, other factors that have contributed to the spread of dengue are poor vector control and poor surveillance programs in many areas. In tropical areas that lack adequate health facilities, the specific cause of a fever—whether malaria, dengue, or something else—often is never identified.

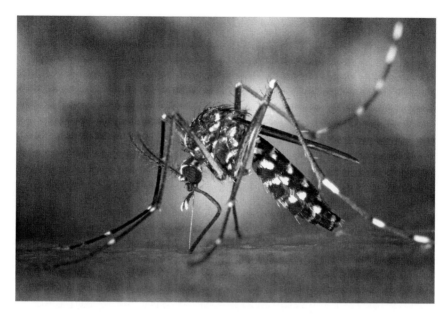

Figure 8.1. *Aedes albopictus.* Photo from the U.S. Centers for Disease Control and Prevention, Atlanta, GA.

To complicate the situation other mosquitoes can also transmit dengue, and one in particular, *Aedes albopictus,* is becoming more widespread.[35] It can be transported in used tires, bamboo, and other materials that are moved by ship from one continent to another. As a vector it is not as efficient as *Aedes aegypti,* but it lives in a broader habitat and can be found in forested areas as well as in cities and has been implicated in some outbreaks.

Currently there is no licensed vaccine to protect people against dengue, although hundreds of millions of dollars have been spent trying to develop one that can prevent infections by all four serotypes. Protective efficacy of a quadrivalent vaccine in a trial carried out in Thailand and published in 2012 showed reasonable protection against three dengue serotypes, but no significant protection against the fourth.[36] Many other vaccine studies are in progress. Although there is no specific drug treatment for dengue, expert management by knowledgeable clinicians can reduce mortality in severe dengue from >10 percent to <1 percent.[37] Even though most people infected with dengue virus survive, the large number of hospitalizations for dengue-related illnesses drains resources in endemic areas.

Studies have assessed the cost of dengue. A study in Malaysia estimated the economic burden of dengue illness to be US$56 million per year. This did not include the costs associated with dengue prevention and control, dengue surveillance, and late sequelae of dengue.[38] In Vietnam, in families with a confirmed dengue infection, 47.2 percent had to borrow money for medical care and after six months >70 percent had not started or had only made partial repayment.[39]

Chikungunya

Another virus that is spread by similar mosquito vectors is chikungunya virus. It was first identified in Tanzania in the 1950s and subsequently spread to Asia. Infection also causes fever and rash that may resemble dengue, but chikungunya infections often are associated with severe and disabling joint pain, to the point that patients find it difficult to walk. Joint symptoms can be persistent, lasting months or longer. Although it is rarely fatal, infection can sweep through a susceptible population causing short-term incapacity in a large percentage of the population. Infections can also be spread via blood transfusions and tissue transplantation.[40]

Epidemics are known to have occurred in Southeast Asia since 1954, when an outbreak was reported in the Philippines. Outbreaks also occurred in 1956 and 1968. Sporadic outbreaks occurred in the 1970s; in the 1980s it spread to Indonesia. It was first recorded in Malaysia in 1998 and in Singapore in 2006.[41] Although the origin of the virus was Africa, it has repeatedly been introduced into Asia.[42]

Cases have increased in many areas in the past decade. A genetic mutation in the viral gene encoding the envelope protein of the virus appears to enhance the replication efficiency of the virus in *Aedes albopictus,* a mosquito vector that is widespread in Asia (Asian tiger mosquito).[43,44] The mutation has been present in >90 percent of viral sequences in some recent outbreaks, suggesting that this mutation confers enhanced survival benefit for the virus. Mosquitoes are more easily infected (a lower level of virus in human blood is required), and the mutation also allows the virus to disseminate more rapidly into the mosquito salivary glands, both of which facilitate the cycle of infection. The mutation is thought to be one of the drivers of recent widespread outbreaks. As is the true of dengue, however, travel, urbanization in the tropics, and poor vector control have contributed to its spread. Chikungunya virus arrived in Southeast Asia from Africa; today, with the high volume of travel from and through Southeast Asia, the virus can also be carried from Southeast Asia to other regions of the world with competent mosquito vectors and climates that are warm enough to support the transmission cycle.

Influenza A (H5N1)

Influenza is caused by an RNA virus that is highly mutable. Although influenza viruses have a wide host range—humans and many other mammals including swine, bats, and marine animals—all influenza viruses have come from aquatic birds. In 1997 an influenza virus, H5N1, was first identified in humans in Hong Kong. The same virus was found to be circulating in the live bird markets and in other avian species. It rapidly killed flocks of domestic poultry. Because six of the eighteen humans in Hong Kong infected with the virus in 1997 died, a decision was made to cull the poultry populations in Hong Kong in an attempt to eliminate the reservoir for this virus. Human cases temporarily ceased but the virus was never eliminated from its avian reservoir. The virus reappeared in humans in 2003 and 2004 in China, Vietnam, and Thailand. Domestic poultry are highly susceptible to the virus and die rapidly if infected, but other avian species, such as ducks and wild aquatic birds, can carry the virus without showing symptoms. They can excrete the virus in their feces and contaminate the environment. The virus can be moved from place to place—sometimes over long distances—by migratory birds and in poultry moved from one market to another.[45] In Indonesia, where infections have been reported every year since 2005, pigs have also been documented to carry the virus—without showing symptoms of infection. During three rainy seasons between 2005 and 2009, more than 7 percent of nasal (snout) cultures obtained from pigs (702 specimens) were positive for H5N1. On phylogenetic analysis the viruses were found to be closely related to ones isolated from poultry located near the pigs.[46] Pigs are believed to be possible mixing vessels because they can be infected with both avian and human influenza viruses. Infections of pigs could allow the virus to acquire mutations that could potentially increase its ability to infect humans to spread among them.

As of January 24, 2014, of 650 reported cases, 386 have been fatal—a mortality of almost 60 percent. Human infections have been reported in Southeast Asia since 2003, and Indonesia currently leads the world in the number of reported cases (195) and deaths (163).[47] Other Southeast Asian countries that have reported human cases and deaths include Cambodia, Laos, Burma, Thailand, and Vietnam. Although the human death toll has been low relative to other influenza epidemics, the toll on the poultry industry has been extensive. Millions of chickens have been culled in the multiple attempts to prevent spread of the virus. Residents have suffered economically and have lost an important source of protein. And the virus is now entrenched in avian populations in Southeast Asia and beyond—and it continues to evolve.

Most human cases have followed direct or indirect contact with infected live or dead poultry. So far, the virus has not become readily transmissible from person to person, although recent research suggests that a few mutations in the virus could potentially make the virus transmit more easily between humans. Seasonal influenza causes fast epidemics because it is easily transmissible from person to person. H5N1 in humans has had a stuttering course—and is not likely to disappear from its avian hosts.

The ecological setting in Southeast Asia makes it favorable for the evolution of new strains of influenza viruses. Large, densely populated cities are linked to rural populations locally as well as to global populations via air and ocean travel.

Many residents, especially in rural areas and small towns, have animals—including chicken, ducks, and other avian species—and live in close proximity to them. Studies have found an association between the presence of influenza H5N1 and the abundance of free-ranging ducks and with rice farming intensity and human population.[48] There is also evidence that global influenza A epidemics caused by H3N2—at least during the period from 2002 to 2007—were seeded annually by viruses that first appeared in East and Southeast Asia.[49] In tropical areas influenza does not show the strong seasonality observed in temperate regions, and transmission can occur throughout the year.

Tens of millions of poultry have died or been culled in attempt to control spread.[50] In Vietnam in 2003–4 policies put in place because of the H5N1 outbreak led to the culling of 45 million birds at an estimated cost of almost US$118 million.[51] Poultry meat exports were banned after outbreaks in Thailand, causing a precipitous drop in exports, an important contributor to the national economy.

SARS Coronavirus

In 2003, the world was alerted to the appearance and spread of a respiratory disease that was severe, often fatal, and appeared to spread from person to person. Before the causative virus was identified, the disease was named severe acute respiratory syndrome, or SARS. This was the first pandemic of the twenty-first century. International collaboration among scientists, many of whom had worked together in an influenza network, led to the rapid identification and sequencing of an RNA virus, a novel coronavirus, named the SARS-coronavirus or SARS-CoV.[52] Early studies showed that that SARS-CoV was necessary and sufficient to cause illness. Infection spread rapidly from an infected individual in Hong Kong to people who traveled to multiple other cities, including Beijing, Singapore, and Toronto. The virus spread from person to person during symptomatic infection and internationally via airplanes. In retrospect, the first cases had occurred in southern China in Guangdong Province in November 2002. Before the outbreak was halted by use of isolation and quarantine, 8,422 cases and 916 deaths in thirty countries had been identified.[53] Much of the transmission occurred in hospitals and involved hospital workers and their family members. The last reported case of SARS-CoV was in 2004 in a laboratory worker in China. Surveillance since then has not identified continued circulation of this specific virus, although a different coronavirus that causes sporadic severe respiratory infection was identified in late 2012.[54]

The early identification of the agent causing SARS was useful, but the biological characteristics of the virus made it feasible to stop the spread. The virus caused fever and symptoms in virtually every person who was infected, and infected individuals did not transmit the virus until after they became symptomatic. In contrast to HIV/AIDS, an infection in which individuals can carry and transmit the virus for years before they are aware that they are infected, SARS caused acute visible illness.[55] Patients either died or cleared the virus. Even though no specific antiviral treatment was available, it was possible to halt the spread by strictly isolating those who were infected and to closely monitor those who might have been exposed to identify any early evidence of infection.

At the time, the SARS pandemic generated widespread fear that extended beyond the countries directly affected and had a profound effect on global travel. The specter of a pandemic that might rival the 1918–19 influenza pandemic was raised early in its course. It was notable that the virus was dispersed by humans traveling by plane to and from some of the most developed cities in the world— Hong Kong, Toronto, and Singapore. The economic impact was disproportionate to the number of cases and deaths that it ultimately caused. In Southeast Asia, there were 331 reported probable cases and 44 deaths in Singapore, Vietnam, Thailand, Malaysia, and Indonesia. Passenger travel into Hong Kong, Singapore, Bangkok, Taipei, and Beijing—all major travel hubs—plummeted. The largest numbers of cases were in China (5,327), Hong Kong (1,755) Taiwan (665), Canada (251) Singapore (238), Vietnam (63) and the United States (33).[56] The estimated cost to East and Southeast Asia was US$18 billion.[57] Other studies suggest the global macroeconomic impact of SARS was in the range of US$30–100 billion, spread across many sectors, but mainly in travel and tourism.[58,59,60]

One exceptional cluster of 321 SARS cases occurred at the housing complex, the Amoy Gardens, in Hong Kong. This densely populated complex consists of nineteen high-rise apartment blocks, each with thirty-three floors and eight units per floor. A study of the building design, ventilation, and airflow patterns; computational fluid dynamics simulations; meteorological data; spatial and temporal analysis; and mapping and genetic sequence analysis led investigators to conclude that airborne spread of the virus could explain this large outbreak.[61] The pattern of spread was consistent with virus-laden aerosols (from an index case with high concentrations of virus in urine and feces excreted into a toilet) being carried by a rising plume of warm air in the air shaft between buildings. The investigators postulated that air entered apartments through open windows. Nonfunctional seals of floor drain traps allowed aerosols from drainage pipes to reach the air shaft. This event also has implications for potential unusual routes of spread of epidemics in urban areas and in the built environment at present and in the future.

Investigations started during the SARS outbreak found evidence that palm civets (*Paguma larvata*) farmed for food and sold at wet markets in southern China were infected with a coronavirus similar to the virus infecting humans. Although civets may have been the proximate source for human infection, results from other studies suggest that bats are the natural reservoir host for the virus. Apparently healthy horseshoe bats trapped in their local habitat from four different locations in China, including Guangdong, were found to be infected with a SARS-like coronavirus.[62] Antibody prevalence ranged from 38 percent to 71 percent, suggesting infection in bats is common. It is postulated that the palm civets became infected with the SARS-like coronavirus by having contact with bats. In Asia, bats have also been shown to be the reservoir host for another virus, the Nipah virus, which can infect pigs and can cause fatal encephalitis in humans.[63] These are examples of spillover events from viruses in wild animal populations that reach humans—and sometimes can spread easily and widely within the human population. The population growth and development of new areas, encroachment on areas with abundant wildlife, and hunting and farming of wild animals for food have all played a role in the entry of animal viruses and bacteria into the human population—these zoonoses that can propagate in humans and cause epidemics.

As a consequence of the emergence of SARS, the International Health Regulations, which govern international health regimes and specify what diseases must be reported to the WHO, were finally revised and adopted by the World Health Assembly in May 2005 and went into force globally in June 2007.[64]

Many infections with epidemic potential have emerged from Southeast Asia or southern Asia. In addition to the SARS-CoV and influenza H5N1 viruses, Nipah virus was first recognized in Southeast Asia (Malaysia), the hemorrhagic form of dengue was first reported in Southeast Asia and new strains of dengue viruses continue to emerge and spread to other continents, and the variant of *Vibrio cholerae* o1 El tor first appeared in Indonesia in 1961.[65]

One infection that was introduced from the outside is HIV/AIDS. Because its spread can be relatively silent early in the epidemic, it became widespread in Southeast Asia, especially Thailand, early in the pandemic. HIV/AIDS epidemics unfold slowly but have a lifetime of consequences for those who are infected. In the region, the greatest burden from HIV/AIDS as measured in DALYs is borne by Thailand, Cambodia, and Burma.[66]

Drug Resistance

Especially noteworthy in a review of epidemics in Southeast Asia is growing resistance of pathogens to antimicrobials—including some of those that caused epidemics in the nineteenth and early twentieth century—malaria, tuberculosis, cholera, and typhoid fever. Antimicrobial resistance could threaten some of the impressive gains that have been made in the control of infectious diseases in Southeast Asia over the last century.

Although cholera no longer causes the waves of epidemics that occurred in the nineteenth and early twentieth century in Southeast Asia, infection still periodically occurs. The recent report of *Vibrio cholerae* from India that harbors two beta-lactamase genes, including NDM-1, making it resistant to commonly

The Eradication of Smallpox in Indonesia
Vivek Neelakantan

South Asia (India, Afghanistan, Pakistan, and Nepal), the Indonesian archipelago, Brazil, and the Horn of Africa were the only smallpox-endemic regions of the world in 1967 when the World Health Organization (WHO) executed the Intensified Smallpox Eradication Program (INSEP). Although smallpox eradication in postcolonial South Asia has been well documented in contemporary historiography, a parallel historiography assessing the smallpox eradication campaign as it unfolded in post-independence Indonesia is lacking. A part of this problem relates to the compartmentalisation of Indonesian history into distinct periods such as the Dutch period, the period of Japanese occupation, the Indonesian Revolution, the Sukarno Era, the Suharto Era, and the Reformasi Era. Smallpox was decimated in the Indies archipelago at the turn of World War II (1939) and made a comeback during the revolutionary period (1947)—a period of political transition—that fits untidily into the colonial or the postcolonial state, or both, which is problematic. In this article, I argue that the Indonesian smallpox eradication campaign (1947–74) serves as a crucible to examine the shift in strategy—from mass vaccination to surveillance and containment—within the policy circles of the WHO that ultimately contributed to the worldwide eradication of smallpox in 1980.

Since the introduction of vaccination on the island of Java in 1804, the colonial state in the Dutch East Indies (today known as Indonesia) successfully tackled smallpox through a series of mass vaccination campaigns consisting of the dual system—that is, primary vaccination, which immunized as many infants as possible—and revaccination of the entire population once every seven years. Consequently, the transmission of smallpox was reduced to near-zero levels by 1939–40. However during World War II (1942–45) due to the slackening of primary vaccination and revaccination, the immunity of the Indonesian population to smallpox weakened.

Waves of smallpox outbreaks began to affect Sumatra beginning October 1947. The Dutch medical resident in Riaow, Van Waardenburg, had reported that the first case of smallpox in post–World War II Indonesia occurred in an unvaccinated Chinese child in the island of Koendoer on the Riaow archipelago; the child's father sailed frequently across the Straits of Malacca to the island of Batu Pahat in Ma-

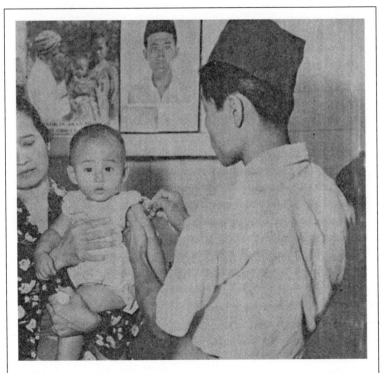

Figure 8.2. "Do not fear vaccinating your infant against smallpox." *Lukisan Mingguan,* 1949. Photo taken at Batavia during the 1949 smallpox epidemic. Image courtesy Perpustakaan Nasional Image Collection, Jakarta.

lacca, which was smallpox endemic in 1947. In October and November 1947, smallpox outbreaks were reported amidst the Orang Mantang community (sea nomads native to the Straits of Malacca) who would evade vaccination in the past owing to their antagonism to Western medicine. Of the 89 reported smallpox cases from Kundur in 1947, 81 cases happened to be from the Orang Mantang community. The inter-island coastal traffic between Sumatra and Java acted as conduits for transmitting smallpox from endemic areas in Sumatra to Java, which was smallpox free in 1948. In December 1948, smallpox was imported into Batavia (now known as Jakarta). By June 1949, Batavia recorded a smallpox epidemic, with 4,841 reported cases (fig. 8.2). During the Batavia epidemic (1949) the separation of smallpox patients from their families and subsequent transportation to the quarantine station on the island of Kramat Djati proved too radical, leading to patient unrest.

In the 1950s, Indonesia did not have a national smallpox eradi-cation program. Mass-vaccination campaigns involving the earlier colonial dual system of separating vaccination of infants from revac-cination of the older population continued. The Pasteur Institute at Bandung manufactured Otten's vaccine (a dried vaccine sourced from buffalo lymph), which was used in mass vaccinations. The Pasteur In-stitute at Bandung and the Department of Health at the central level rarely achieved a consensus on questions such as the potency of the vaccine or standardization of the vaccination technique.

In 1958, the Soviet Union proposed the global eradication of small-pox at the Eleventh World Health Assembly. The Global Strategy for the Eradication of Smallpox aimed to eradicate the disease from endemic areas of the world through a program of mass vaccination involving at least 80 percent of the population of the affected countries. In 1963, Indonesia launched a five-year program to combat smallpox, under the overall control of the malaria eradication program (implemented first as a pilot project in West Java, then in the provinces of South Suma-tra, West Sumatra, and East Java). Implementing Indonesia's five-year program proved to be a thorny issue, as the central government was in charge of epidemic control, whereas the provincial governments were in charge of administering routine vaccinations. Achieving coor-dination between epidemic control and the administration of routine vaccinations proved to be almost impossible in the 1950s. The World Health Organization's Regional Office for Southeast Asia (SEARO) criticized Indonesia's policy of diverting malaria eradication person-nel and infrastructure to smallpox eradication as being premature, as the nation had not yet eradicated malaria.

The Nineteenth World Health Assembly formulated the basic strategy of the INSEP in 1966. The two components of the INSEP were mass vaccination, involving vaccination of at least 80 percent of the population; surveillance, detecting smallpox cases and containment of outbreaks as they occurred. Indonesia initially introduced the INSEP on the islands of Java and Bali in 1968 which later included Sumatra, Sulawesi, and Kalimantan in 1969.

In West Java, backlog fighting (mass vaccination of infants, mi-grants) had covered 25 percent of the population in 1969 but had failed to interrupt the transmission of the pox. Nurses and vaccinators would not report smallpox outbreaks to the regency health officials as they were not given specific instructions as to how to do so. It was custom-ary in West Java to carry sick children to visit relatives. Isolation of the sick patient at home and vaccinating the immediate contacts in order to contain an outbreak proved unworkable.

North Sumatra was smallpox endemic when the INSEP was launched in the province in 1969. Plantations employed up to 40 percent of North Sumatra's workforce. There was little coordination between plantation hospitals and the regency health services in the implementation of the INSEP. Smallpox surveillance in North Sumatra was not effective in detecting cases because surveillance activities were carried on during the day, when the majority of villagers were at work on the plantation. As a result there was a huge backlog of unvaccinated individuals. Plantation hospitals lacked coordination with the regency health services in North Sumatra. In the plantation hospital at Simelungun, it was observed that children with symptoms of chickenpox were misdiagnosed with smallpox and isolated in a smallpox ward where they were infected with the smallpox virus. They began to initiate new smallpox outbreaks soon after their discharge. Case notifications from village heads to the regency health services were incomplete as the disease was not suspected.

When the INSEP began in Indonesia in 1968, 17,380 cases of smallpox were officially recorded. In 1970, Indonesia recorded 10,081 cases—33 percent of the world's total cases of smallpox. In 1972, Indonesia recorded its last case of smallpox. The WHO-sponsored *Smallpox and its Eradication* states that smallpox transmission in Indonesia was interrupted in 1972, three years after the INSEP was introduced due to shift in eradication strategy from mass vaccination to surveillance and containment.[1] However, the reported success of the surveillance-based component of the INSEP in Indonesia was more apparent than real. Surveillance in the initial stages of the campaign was weak, since chickenpox cases were misreported as smallpox. An unnamed vaccinator in Bandung would successfully use color photographs of smallpox cases published in a WHO teaching folder to obtain numerous case notifications with remarkable success. The WHO staff adapted this field experience by printing smallpox recognition cards, which were used successfully for case detection in smallpox-endemic South Asia.

With smaller number of smallpox outbreaks since 1971, the vaccinators discontinued routine vaccination to look for cases. Every case of smallpox was considered by the health authorities to be a national emergency. The Department of Health announced a reward of five thousand rupiahs to anyone who reported a suspected case that was confirmed in the laboratory for smallpox. Despite all efforts, no smallpox case has been discovered in Indonesia since 1972. Indonesia was declared free of the pox, thus providing hope for the SEARO that smallpox eradication was attainable.

Smallpox was virtually eliminated in the Dutch East Indies by 1939–40 due to successful primary vaccination of infants and revaccination of the population every seven years. But during World War II, the immunity of the population to smallpox declined as routine vaccinations were disrupted. From 1947 to 1968, Indonesia did not have a coordinated plan to eradicate smallpox. The Indonesian chapter of the INSEP (1968–72) proved to be the crucible in which ideas related to mass vaccination and surveillance formulated at the WHO headquarters in Geneva were evaluated and adapted based on their applicability to local geographic and cultural factors. The success of the INSEP in Indonesia was based on a strategic shift from mass vaccination involving the total population to using smallpox recognition cards for case detection.

Note

1. F. Fenner, D.A. Henderson, I. Arita, Z. Jezek, and I. D. Ladnyi, *Smallpox and Its Eradication* (Geneva: WHO, 1988), 627–57.

used antibiotics, is ominous.[67] This is a reminder that a pathogen causing an old disease still has new tricks—and can still surprise.

Extensively drug resistant tuberculosis has been reported in Indonesia, Burma, and Thailand; figures published in 2008 showed that 3 percent of new cases and 18 percent of retreatment cases had multidrug-resistant tuberculosis—figures that are undoubtedly higher now.[68] Chloroquine-resistant malaria first became established in Southeast Asia, and resistance to mefloquine has been present for many years, especially in western Cambodia and along the Thai-Burma border.[69] More recently *Plasmodium falciparum* parasites resistant to artemisinin, an essential part of malaria treatment programs globally, appeared in Cambodia and appear to be spreading.[70] Drug-resistant forms can hobble treatment and thwart control programs.

Southeast Asia today has largely controlled the epidemic diseases that plagued the region a century ago. However, population size, density, mobility, and connectedness combined with pockets of poverty and large periurban slums, ecoclimatic factors, the diversity and proximity of wildlife populations, and the susceptibility of the region to disasters (especially earthquakes, floods, and tsunamis) create an environment in which epidemics can still appear—even under times of political stability. The region is heterogeneous and vulnerable—but more highly networked and able to provide surveillance for, and response to, outbreaks than in past decades.

Notes

1. A. T. Price-Smith, "Theory and Exegesis: On Health and the Body Politic," in *Contagion and Chaos: Disease, Ecology, and National Security in the Era of Globalization* (Cambridge, MA: MIT Press, 2009), 11–32.

2. A. Dans, N. Ng, C. Verghese, E. S. Tai, R. Firestone, and R. Bonita, "The Rise of Chronic Non-communicable Diseases in Southeast Asia: Time for Action," *Lancet* 377 (2011): 680–89.

3. K. W. Taylor, "Diseases and Disease Ecology of the Modern Period in Southeast Asia," in *The Cambridge World History of Human Disease*, ed. K. F. Kiple (Cambridge: Cambridge University Press, 1993), 440–47.

4. A. Cliff and P. Haggett, "Time, Travel and Infection," *British Medical Journal* 69 (2004): 87–99.

5. K. De Bevoise, *Agents of Apocalypse. Epidemic Disease in the Colonial Philippines* (Princeton, NJ: Princeton University Press, 1995), 38–40.

6. De Bevoise, *Agents of Apocalypse*, 135.

7. P. Boomgaard, "Morbidity and Mortality in Java, 1820–1880," in *Death and Disease in Southeast Asia: Explorations in Social, Medical and Demographic History*, ed. Norman G. Owen (Oxford: Oxford University Press, 1987), 48–69.

8. V. Guernier, M. E. Hockberg, and J-F. Guegan, "Ecology Drives the Worldwide Distribution of Human Diseases," *Public Library of Science Biology* 2, no. 6 (2004): 740–46.

9. R. P. Cincotta, J. Wisnewski, and R. Engelman, "Human Population in the Biodiversity Hotspots," *Nature* 404 (2000): 990–92.

10. K. E. Jones, N. G. Patel, M. A. Levy, A. Storeygard, D. Balk, J. L. Gittleman, and P. Daszak, "Global Trends in Emerging Infectious Diseases," *Nature* 451 (2008): 990–94.

11. Jones et al., "Global Trends in Emerging Infectious Diseases."

12. Even within a city, geography can matter. In Batavia (now Jakarta) in the early twentieth century, the three main ethnic groups, the Indonesians, Chinese, and Europeans, lived in different sections of the city. The oldest part of the city was built on lower ground, frequently flooded, and was heavily infested with anopheline mosquitoes, which can transmit malaria. During a cholera epidemic of 1910–11, the death rates were 73 per 1,000 inhabitants in the upper town and 148 per 1,000 in the lower town. In one crowded older subdistrict of the lower town, mortality reached 394.7 per 1,000 residents during the cholera epidemic of 1911–12. S. Abeyasekere, "Death and Disease in Nineteenth Century Batavia," in *Death and Disease in Southeast Asia: Explorations in Social, Medical and Demographic History*, ed. Norman G. Owen (Oxford: Oxford University Press, 1987), 194–95.

13. De Bevoise, *Agents of Apocalypse*, 97.

14. De Bevoise, *Agents of Apocalypse*, 101.

15. S. S. Amrith, *Migration and Diaspora in Modern Asia* (Cambridge: Cambridge University Press, 2011), 2–3.

16. K. Khan, "Bio.Diaspora," www.biodiaspora.com.

17. R. J. Coker, B. M. Hunter, J. W. Rudge, M. Liverani, and P. Hanvoravongchai, "Emerging Infectious Diseases in Southeast Asia: Regional Challenges to Control," *Lancet* 377 (2011): 599–609.

18. C. Murray, L. C. Rosenfeld, S. S. Lim, K. G. Andrews, K. J. Foreman, D. Haring, N. Fullman, M. Naghavi, R. Lozano, and A. D. Lopez, "Global Malaria Mortality between 1980 and 2010: A Systematic Analysis," *Lancet* 379 (2012): 413–31.

19. I. Gupta and P. Guin, "Communicable Diseases in the South-East Asia Region of the World Health Organization: Towards a More Effective Response," *Bulletin of the World Health Organization* 88 (2010): 199–205.

20. J. C. Mariner, J. A. House, C. A. Mebus, A. E. Sollod, D. Chibeu, B. A. Jones, P. L. Roeder, B. Admassu, and G. G. M. van 't Klooster, "Rinderpest Eradication: Appropriate Technology and Social Interventions," *Science* 337 (2012): 309–12.

21. De Bevoise, *Agents of Apocalypse*, 158–59.

22. De Bevoise, *Agents of Apocalypse*, 148.

23. Boomgaard, "Morbidity and Mortality in Java," 57.

24. De Bevoise, *Agents of Apocalypse*, 135.

25. De Bevoise, *Agents of Apocalypse*, 118.

26. De Bevoise, *Agents of Apocalypse*, 122–24.

27. De Bevoise, *Agents of Apocalypse*, 129–30.

28. E-E., Ooi and D. J. Gubler, "Dengue in Southeast Asia: Epidemiological Characteristics and Strategic Challenges in Disease Prevention," *Cadernos de Saude Publica* 25 (2008) suppl 1: S115–S124.

29. C. P. Simmons, J. J. Farrar, N. v. V. Chau, and B. Wills, "Dengue," *New England Journal of Medicine* 366, no. 15 (2012): 1423–32.

30. D. J. Gubler, "Epidemic Dengue/Dengue Hemorrhagic Fever as a Public health, Social and Economic Problem in the 21st Century," *TRENDS in Microbiology* 10, no. 2 (2002): 100–103.

31. D. J. Gubler, "Cities Spawn Epidemic Dengue Viruses," *Nature Medicine* 10 (2004): 129–30.

32. Gubler, "Cities Spawn Epidemic Dengue Viruses."

33. M. E. Wilson, "Global Travel and Emerging Infections," in *Infectious Disease Movement in a Borderless World: Microbial Threats Forum, Institute of Medicine, Workshop Summary* (Washington, DC: The National Academies Press, 2010): 90–104; 126–29.

34. Coker et al., "Emerging Infectious Diseases in Southeast Asia."

35. R. N. Charrel, X. de Lamballerie, and D. Raoult, "Chikungunya Outbreaks—The Globalization of Vectorborne Diseases," *New England Journal of Medicine* 356 (2007): 769–71.

36. A. Sabchareon, D. Wallace, C. Sirivichayakul, K. Limkittikul, P. Hanthavnich, S. Suvannadabba, V. Jiwariyavej, W. Dulyachai, K. Pengsaa, et al., "Protective Efficacy of the Recombainant, Live-Attenuated, CYD Tetravalent Dengue Vaccine in Thai Schoolchildren: A Randomised, Controlled Phase 2b Trial," *Lancet* 380 (2012): 1559–67.

37. Simmons et al., "Dengue," 1423–32.

38. D. S. Shepard, E. A. Undurraga, R. S. Lees, Y. Halasa, L. C. S. Llama, and C. W. Ng, "Use of Multiple Data Sources to Estimate the Economic Cost of Dengue Illness in Malaysia," *American Journal of Tropical Medicine and Hygiene* 87, no. 5 (2012): 796–805.

39. P. T. Tam, N. T. Dat, L. M. Huu, X. C. P. THi, H. M. Duc, T. C. Tu, S. Kutcher, P. A. Ryan, B. H. Kay, "High Household Economic Burden Caused by Hospitalization of Patients with Severe Dengue Fever Cases in Can Tho Province, Vietnam," *American Journal of Tropical Medicine and Hygiene* 87, no. 3 (2012): 544–58.

40. T. Couderc, F. Gangneux, F. Chrieien, V. Caro, T. L. Luong, B. Duclous, H. Tolou, M. Lecuit, and M. Grandadam, "Chikungunya Virus infection of Corneal Grafts," *Journal of Infectious Diseases* 206 (2012): 851–59.

41. F. J. Burt, M. S. Rolph, N. E. Rulli, S. Mahalingam, and M. T. Heise, "Chikungunya: A Re-emerging Virus," *Lancet* 379 (2012): 662–71.

42. Y. S. Leo, A. L. Chow, L. K. Tan, D. C. Lye, L. Lin, and L. C. Ng, "Chikungunya Outbreak, Singapore, 2008," *Emerging Infectious Diseases* 15 (2009): 836–37.

43. K. A. Tsetsarkin, D. L. Vanlandingham, C. E. McGee, and S. Higgs, "A Single Mutation in Chikungunya Virus Affects Vector Specificity and Epidemic Potential," *Public Library of Science Pathology* 3, no. 12 (2007): e201.

44. K. A. Tsetsarkin, R. Chen, G. Leal, et al., "Chikungunya Virus Emergence is Constrained in Asia by Lineage-Specific Adaptive Landscapes," *Proceedings of the National Academy of Sciences USA* 108 (2011): 7872–77.

45. J. Keawcharoen, D. van Reiel, G. van Amerongen, et al., "Wild Ducks as Long-Distance Vectors of Highly Pathogenic Avian influenza (H5N1)," *Emerging Infectious Diseases* 14, no. 4 (2008): 600–607.

46. C. A. Nidom, R. Takano, S. Yamade, Y. Sakai-Tagawa, S. Daulay, D. Aswadi, T. Suzuki, et al., "Influenza A (H5N1) Viruses from Pigs, Indonesia," *Emerging Infectious Diseases* 16, no. 10 (2010): 1515–23.

47. World Health Organization, "Cumulative Number of Confirmed Human Cases for Avian Influenza A(H5N1) Reported to WHO, 2003–2014," World Health Organization website, www.who.int/influenza/human_animal_interface/EN_GIP_20140124CumulativeNumberH5 N1cases.pdf.

48. M. Gilbert, X. Xiao, U. R. Pfeiffer, et al., "Mapping H5N1 Highly Pathogenic Avian Influenza Risk in Southeast Asia," *Proceedings of the National Academy of Sciences* 105, no. 2 (2008): 4769–74.

49. C. A. Russell, T. C. Jones, I. G. Barr, et al., "The Global Circulation of Seasonal Influenza A (H3N2) Viruses," *Science* 320 (2008): 340–46.

50. F. A. Taha, *How Highly Pathogenic Avian Influenza (H5N1) Has Affected World Poultry-Meat Trade* (Washington, DC: United States Department of Agriculture, 2007).

51. J. Rushton, R. Viscarra, E. Guernebleich, and A. McLeod, "Impact of Avian Influenza Outbreaks in the Poultry Sectors of Five South East Asian Countries (Cambodia, Indonesia, Lao PDR, Thailand, Vietnam) Outbreak Costs, Responses and Potential Long Term Control," *Proceedings of the Nutrition Society* 61 (2005): 491–541.

52. J. S. M. Peiris, K. Y. Yuen, A. D. M. E. Osterhaus, and K. Stohr, "The Severe Acute Respiratory Syndrome," *New England Journal of Medicine* 349 (2003): 2431–41.

53. World Health Organization, "Summary Table of SARS Cases by Country, 1 November 2002–7 August 2003," August 15, 2003, World Health Organization website, www.who.int/csr /sars/country/2003_08_15/en.

54. S. Van Boheemen, M. de Graaf, L. Lauber, et al., "Genomic Characterization of a Newly Discovered Coronavirus Associated with Acute Respiratory Distress Syndrome in Humans," *mBiosphere* 3, no. 6 (2012): e00473–12; available at *mBio* website, www.mbio.asm.org.

55. C. Fraser, S. Riley, R. M. Anderson, and N. M. Ferguson, "Factors That Make an Infectious Disease Outbreak Controllable," *Proceedings of the National Academy of Sciences* 101 (2004): 6146–151.

56. World Health Organization, "Summary Table of SARS Cases by Country."

57. Emma Xiaoqin Fan, "SARS: Economic Impacts and Implications," in *Asian Development Outlook 2003 Update* (Manila: Asian Development Bank, 2003), Asian Development Bank website, www.adb.org/publications/sars-economic-impacts-and-implications.

58. J. W. Lee and W. McKibbin, "Globalization and Disease: The Case of SARS," *Asian Economic Papers* 3, no. 1 (Winter 2004): 113–31.

59. S. Hanna and Y. Huang, "The Impact of SARS on Asian Economies," *Asian Economic Papers* 3, no. 1 (Winter 2004): 102–12.

60. R. D. Smith, "Responding to Global Infectious Disease Outbreaks: Lessons from SARS on the Role of Risk Perception, Communication and Management," *Social Science and Medicine* 63 (2006): 3113–23.

61. I. T. S. Yu, Y. Li, T. W. Wong, W. Tam, A. T. Chan, J. H. W. Lee, D. Y. C. Leung, and T. Ho, "Evidence of Airborne Transmission of the Severe Acute Respiratory Syndrome Virus," *New England Journal of Medicine* 350 (2004): 1731–39.

62. W. Li, Z. Shi, M. Yu, et al., "Bats are Natural Reservoirs of SARS-like Coronaviruses," *Science* 310 (2005): 676–69.

63. K. B. Chua, K. J., Goh, K. T. Wong, et al., "Fatal Encephalitis due to Nipah Virus among Pig Farmers in Malaysia," *Lancet* 354 (1999): 1257–59.

64. A. T. Price-Smith, "Epidemic of Fear: SARS and the Political Economy of Contagion in the Pacific Rim," in *Contagion and Chaos: Disease, Ecology, and National Security in the Era of Globalization* (Cambridge, MA: The MIT Press, 2009), 139–57.

65. Chua et al., "Fatal Encephalitis due to Nipah Virus."

66. Coker et al., "Emerging Infectious Diseases in Southeast Asia."

67. J. Mandal, V. Sangeetha, V. Ganesan, et al., "Third-Generation Cephalosporin-Resistant *Vibrio cholerae,* India," *Emerging Infectious Diseases* 18, no. 8 (2012): 1326–28.

68. N. Nair, F. Wares, and S. Sahu, "Tuberculosis in the WHO South-East Asia Region," *Bulletin of the World Health Organization* 88 (2010): 164–65.

69. A. P. Phyo, S. Nkhoma, K. Stepniewska, et al., "Emergence of Artemisinin-Resistant Malaria on the Western Border of Thailand: A Longitudinal Study," *Lancet* 379 (2012): 1960.

70. A. M. Dondorp, F. Nosten, P. Yi, et al., "Artemisinin Resistance in Plasmodium Falciparum Malaria," *New England Journal of Medicine* 361 (2009): 455–67.

PART IV

THE POLITICS OF HEALTH

9 The Internationalization of Health in Southeast Asia

Sunil S. Amrith

SCHOLARS OF SOUTHEAST Asia have been more self-conscious than most about the arbitrary boundaries of the region they study. "Southeast Asia" as a term and a concept did not come into widespread use until World War II, when the Allies' South East Asia Command was established to mirror the geography of Japanese military conquest. In the second half of the twentieth century, the region's boundaries were defined politically: above all, by the membership of the Association of Southeast Asian Nations (ASEAN), established in 1967. At the same time, the area studies tradition institutionalized the study of Southeast Asia as distinct from South Asia and East Asia.[1] In the field of health, too, the emergence of Southeast Asia as a region of knowledge and intervention is closely connected with the development of transnational and international institutions in the twentieth century. However, a recent collection of essays by public health specialists has argued that Southeast Asia's identity as a region in global health remains ambiguous, its unity obscured by "UN agency groupings of the region that do not take into account historical and geopolitical ties."[2]

This chapter goes back before World War II to examine two stages in the emergence of Southeast Asia as a region in the field of health. The first came in the second half of the nineteenth century, arising from the (predominantly British) imperial tradition of tropical medicine and tropical geography, applied to the specific problem of governing migration. The second key period, from the 1910s to the 1930s, witnessed the development and spread of international networks concerned with health in Asia. The health of Southeast Asia has always been understood relationally. It was not until the 1940s that policy makers began to treat Southeast Asia as a distinctive grouping; in the field of health this division between South and Southeast Asia was never as firmly enforced as in some other policy areas.

Climate, Mobility, and Region

The earliest European travel accounts of Southeast Asia are filled with descriptions of its tropical environment. Southeast Asia's lucrative spices, its forest products, its *materia medica,* and its landscapes captured the attention of European naturalists and artists and investors. The "tropical Edens" of Southeast Asia furnished the imagination of European writers: distant, exotic, and threatening.[3] Even after most of the Indian subcontinent had come under European control, Southeast Asia presented an untamed frontier for exploration and exploitation. Southeast Asia represented the furthest reaches of the tropics, or the tropics in their essence. Their understandings of both nature and culture predisposed Europeans to treat Southeast Asia as a natural extension of India: this is reflected in the geographical terms used at the time—the Indian Archipelago; Further India; or, simply, the East Indies. In the second half of the nineteenth century, a revolution in mobility and an aggressive expansion of European colonial conquest raised new kinds of distinctions between South and Southeast Asia.

By the 1870s, the British Empire had established primacy in the eastern Indian Ocean: with the exception of Siam, the whole arc of coasts around the Bay of Bengal, from Ceylon to Malaya, was under formal or informal British control. As such, it was often in British imperial debates—as they traversed networks of administrators, scientists, doctors, and lawyers—that new distinctions between South and Southeast Asia emerged. As European and Chinese investors moved into the forest frontiers of Southeast Asia, new scientific knowledge was needed to turn nature to profit; as new colonial administrations sifted administrative structures and legal codes, the applicability of Indian precedents came under review. Above all, the magnitude of migration between India, China, and Southeast Asia posed new epidemiological challenges.[4]

In the century between 1840 and 1940, close to twenty million Chinese and nearly thirty million Indians journeyed across the Bay of Bengal and the South China Sea to the frontier regions of Southeast Asia.[5] This movement altered the very landscape, the ecology, and the disease environment of Southeast Asia. It provoked discussion about what might make Southeast Asia distinctive—and it was in this period that the idea emerged that the extent of its population mobility was what made Southeast Asia unique. As Eric Tagliacozzo's chapter also shows, international and imperial concern focused on the threat posed by the scale and velocity of mobility from and within the region—including the mobility of Southeast Asian pilgrims to Mecca.

To colonial geographers, the differences in climate between India and the tropical plantation colonies made migration seem a natural redistribution of population to where the soil was most fertile. Southeast Asia appeared, in this view, healthier than India; its tropical climate was beneficent, its inhabitants freed from the tyranny of a fickle monsoon. "A glance at the map . . . will show that the colonies importing Indian labour are in the belt of the tropics," colonial administrator and linguist George Grierson argued, and those colonies possessed "an equable climate, free from sudden or extreme variations, and an amazing fertility." Grierson's historical account of the need for Indian labor in tropical colonies combined culture and climate. "When an Indian cooly is transported to a tropical colony," Grierson concluded, "he finds himself in a place quite beyond his experience. He finds a soil capable of yielding good crops with hardly any cultivation." What Grierson neglected to note was that—in contrast to the situation facing the white settlers of the New World—the obstacles in the way of Indian emigrants' acquiring land of their own were almost insurmountable, as the products of the "good soil" went straight to the planters.[6]

This perspective failed to explain the shockingly high mortality experienced by Indian emigrants to Malaya, particularly in the 1870s and 1880s. The quest to understand that mortality, and the need to justify the continued export and import of Indian labor, led to a more searching debate on the epidemiological frontiers that migrant workers had crossed as they crossed the Bay of Bengal. In the environmentalist view, still common in the late nineteenth century, the soil of the Malayan jungle harbored miasma harmful to Indian recruits. Bacteriology taught that the local ecology was home to pathogens to which migrant workers had little natural resistance. Dysentery, diarrhea, and "fevers" were a constant presence. Labor recruiters boasted of Malaya's "healthful climate," but the death rates on the plantations were higher than in almost any other part of the British Empire. Malaria posed the greatest risk of all. Malaria was hyperendemic in the Malayan jungle, unlike in southern India; Tamil migrant workers had little natural immunity to it. The ecological rupture caused by land clearance might even have worsened the problem. Only in the 1910s—with the abolition of indentured labor, with the gradual improvement of sanitation, and, perhaps, with growing immunity among workers now more used to Malayan conditions—did death rates decline. As late as the 1920s, a Malayan medical officer lamented that "the wastage was too rapid; it was not worthwhile to bring coolies over from India, however strictly they were bound to fulfil their term of contract if, in fact, they died before the term was up."[7]

To justify the high rates of mortality among indentured laborers, planters argued that recruits had arrived from India in poor health to begin with: they came from an unhealthy land frequented by famine; they lacked the resilience to adapt to Malaya's climate. In this view, Tamil estate workers were responsible for their own suffering: "the filthy habits of the natives as regards conservancy are too well known to require explanation," a Malayan magistrate wrote in defense of the planters. By contrast, Indian officials argued that "ill usage" and poor conditions turned healthy emigrants into "sickly" returnees. A Nagapatnam port surgeon put it starkly in 1880: "For the authorities on the other side of the water to pretend that the sickly, starved, ill-used looking wretches who return to this port from Penang . . . owe their present appearance to the weakly state in which they were when they emigrated," he wrote, was "a contention far worse than ridiculous." Malnutrition was an insidious cause of debility. A Tamil worker, rescued from the notorious Malakoff Estate in Province Wellesley, suffered from what the examining medical officer called "a degree of emaciation unsurpassed in my experience." If the Malayan government argued that Indian emigrants should be grateful for the escape that Malaya offered them from famine, a port surgeon in India had quite a different view: he saw workers returning from Malaya "in a worse state than the famine-stricken and diseased creatures I have seen in the hospitals of famine camps."[8]

By the turn of the twentieth century, health inequalities between India and Southeast Asia became a political issue. Within the British Empire the causes of ill health among migrant laborers was a matter of conflict between the Indian and Malayan colonial governments. It also became a matter of much wider public discussion. Indian journalists and nationalist politicians highlighted health inequalities as one of the indicators of the exploitation of Indians overseas. Colonial officials produced a ranked list of Malayan plantations, ranked by their mortality and morbidity rates; policy interventions followed, restricting the supply of migrant workers to estates that fared poorly. Humanitarian concern combined with the fear of political protest to bring about an improvement in estate and general health facilities in Malaya. The archives are full of telegrams and petitions by Tamil migrant workers appealing to various levels of government with their grievances, many of which were concerned with health and living conditions.[9]

Debates surrounding migration sharpened the epidemiological distinctions between South and Southeast Asia: they did so by affirming a whole series of dichotomies—between tropical and seasonal climates; between levels of infection and resistance; and, most fundamentally, between healthy and unhealthy lands. For reasons of economic self-interest as much as humanitarian concern, the colonial state and employers in Malaya expanded their provision of medical facilities. The Institute for Medical Research, established in Kuala Lumpur in 1901, studied local health conditions in depth—focusing on malaria and beriberi, and no longer dependent on knowledge and expertise from India.

Far beyond British Malaya, European colonies in Southeast Asia emerged as sites of experiment and innovation. One major influence, as Warwick Anderson has shown, was the American colonial administration in the Philippines, which projected an image of itself as self-consciously progressive—a different kind of empire, founded on education and hygiene and relentless improvement. In the Netherlands East Indies, too, the Ethical Policy brought questions of welfare to the forefront of debate. The Burma-based British scholar and administrator J. S.

Furnivall pioneered the comparative study of colonial administrations across Southeast Asia. Above all what these territories had in common was their diversity. The idea emerged that the management of ethnic and cultural diversity was the fundamental challenge for health and social policy in a part of the world shaped by migration—this idea has had a long life.[10]

Southeast Asia and International Health Networks, 1914–1930

By the 1910s, these discussions had an international and a comparative dimension, thanks to the interest taken in them by the Rockefeller Foundation; in the 1920s and 1930s, the League of Nations and the International Labour Organization, too, expanded their activities to Southeast Asia. An overlapping set of networks and institutions wove together fragmented local experiments in sanitation across South and Southeast Asia into a more unified set of ideas and practices. These initiatives were imbued with a stronger faith in intervention that most colonial administrations could muster: that contrast in approach would be a point of tension between imperial and international health throughout the 1920s and 1930s.

The internationalization of health in Asia after World War I can be traced back to the nineteenth century. As Eric Tagliacozzo's chapter in this volume shows, the mid-nineteenth century saw the development of international institutions to coordinate information regarding the spread of epidemics, quarantine regulations, and medical surveillance. The International Sanitary Conferences, which began in 1851, were concerned centrally with Asia as the "source" of contagion.[11] Within Asia, the American administration in the Philippines inaugurated the Far Eastern Association of Tropical Medicine in 1904—this became a forum for coordination between colonial regimes across East and Southeast Asia.[12]

The second lineage of international health in Southeast Asia lies in the growth of international humanitarianism. Although the rise of international humanitarianism is often associated with the development of the Red Cross movement, Henrietta Harrison has shown recently that religious networks—such as the Catholic Church's Holy Childhood Association—were often those with the widest reach, and the greatest ability to raise funds; China featured prominently in this international humanitarian imagination.[13] The reach of international humanitarian organizations spread to Southeast Asia at the turn of the twentieth century. The Thai branch of the Red Cross Society was founded as the Red Unalom Society in 1893, and was incorporated into the International League of Red Cross Societies in 1921.[14]

It was a new kind of American philanthropy, however, that transformed the scale and the intensity of interregional connections in the shaping of health and welfare in Asia.[15] Unshackled by the opportunities presented by World War I to intervene first in Europe, and subsequently across the globe, the new American philanthropy—epitomized by the expanding work of the Rockefeller Foundation—took techniques pioneered in the American South to Asia and Latin America.

No network had the reach of the Rockefeller Foundation's by the 1920s. The foundation was established in 1913, but had first intervened in public health activities through the work of the Rockefeller Sanitary Commission for the Eradication of Hookworm Disease in the southern United States. With the opening of the Panama Canal in 1914, General William Gorgas, surgeon general of the U.S. Army, urged the Rockefeller Foundation to support efforts to eradicate yellow fever.[16] The same year, 1914, saw the foundation of the China Medical Board, the foundation's first foray into Asia, and one of its most significant interventions in the field of health. The China Medical Board focused its attention on medical education. In 1917 the board established the Peking Union Medical College (designed to be the "Johns Hopkins of China"), taking over the premises from an American missionary hospital.[17] Following relief efforts during World War I, the Foundation expanded its health work farther overseas, initiating a tuberculosis control and education project in France in 1917.[18] Despite the U.S. government's walking away from the League of Nations, the Rockefeller Foundation took an early interest in the league's Health Organization: between 30 and 40 percent of its health budget came from the Rockefeller Foundation.[19] The foundation's health division went on to launch research-driven public health campaigns in Europe, Latin America, South Asia, and China—targeting yellow fever, malaria, and tuberculosis, as well as developing medical education.[20]

By funding study tours, consultancies, and scholarships, the Rockefeller Foundation and the League of Nations Health Organization fostered new kinds of connection in the field of public health. These connections were embodied in personal journeys, now, as much as in the reading of comparative statistics or law. The journeys of doctors and consultants brought together disparate sites of experiment in rural locales across Asia, linking them in turn to places and institutions in eastern Europe and America. While colonial public health efforts touched a very small proportion of colonized populations, the international purview of rural public health brought together a diverse range of interventions on the fringes of colonial policy. As Atsuko Naono's chapter in this volume shows, the internationalization of public health formed part of a broader consideration of rural poverty, which emerged with particular force as a problem in the light of the agrarian decline and agricultural depression. "Rural hygiene," as it was known, built upon new scientific knowledge, including the knowledge of nutrition, and advances in sanitary engineering. A socioeconomic focus, as opposed to climatic determinism ("tropics"), led to a wider set of comparisons and connections—across Southeast Asia, between Southeast Asia and South Asia, and between Asia and Eastern Europe.

The lands of Eastern Europe were locus of the Rockefeller Foundation's activities in the 1920s, and this had a significant impact on subsequent interventions in Asia. The foundation had established schools of public health in Warsaw, Zagreb, Budapest, Prague, and Bucharest by 1930. The Rockefeller approach to Eastern Europe came out of its experience in the American South, which had convinced them that only the state, supported by philanthropic funds, could effect a transformation of public health in so-called backward agricultural areas. The American approach gained a number of admirers throughout Europe, including the French social medic Jacques Parisot, and the Croat Andrija Stampar.[21] At the Zagreb School of Public Health, Stampar pioneered an approach to rural medicine based on mass education, agricultural extension projects and the techniques of the cooperative movement.[22] His vision of public health, shaped by his nationalism and his commitment to social medicine, complemented the educative social medicine of the Rockefeller Foundation.[23]

In 1933 Stampar accepted an invitation by the League of Nations to travel to nationalist China as a consultant on rural public health.[24] After three years traveling through China, Stampar was convinced that "successful health work is not possible where the standard of living falls below the level of tolerable existence." The best health policy, he argued, would be to "raise the standard of living of the people and to increase their resources." Education would be central to this project. Stampar pointed out that "unless the farmer can read pamphlets, and is given a rudimentary scientific attitude, it is very difficult to reach him by propaganda." Even more important was "the removal of social grievances, such as the sense of exploitation by the landlord."[25] Ultimately, public health was dependent upon the "co-operation of the people, and this will only be given by a population which is reasonably optimistic about the future, and which is willing to give at least qualified acceptance [to] the social order."[26] Stampar was not alone in his global travels: the Rockefeller Foundation and the League of Nations also enabled visits to China by the Polish doctor Ludwig Rajchmann and the American Selskar Gunn.[27]

By the early 1930s, the Asian arena was central to debates about agrarian poverty in the world. India became an important node in the transnational networks of expertise concerning public health, and particularly rural health. As Subir Sinha has shown, from the late nineteenth century the problem of "the Indian village" was constituted through the convergence of diverse transnational networks of expertise—encompassing American missionaries and scholars, colonial officials, and Indian social reformers of all kinds. Attempts to address the problems of rural India led to the deployment and translation of a range of techniques from around the world: cooperative societies, agricultural extension projects, and new methods of animal husbandry.[28] From Bombay to Bengal, local and philanthropic initiatives in public health proliferated.[29]

The networks of international public health—the patchwork of private, philanthropic and inter-governmental initiatives—spread throughout Southeast Asia in the 1920s and 1930s. The Rockefeller Foundation's activities in Southeast Asia were directed by its Far Eastern Directorate, headed by Victor G. Heiser, a veteran health official who had served the American administration in the Philippines.[30] Training centers and demonstration projects across the region formed part of a global web of others: sharing information, generating data, and comparing results. The foundation's global campaign to eradicate hookworm left an imprint on health systems across Southeast Asia; as in Latin America, the hookworm campaign often paved the way for more intensive interventions in rural health, and in the training of health workers.

Under American colonial rule, the Philippines was an early, and obvious, target for the foundation's health work. The Rockefeller hookworm eradication campaign began there in 1913; by the early 1920s, the foundation was involved in funding the training of female public health nurses to replace male sanitary inspectors as part of a broader campaign to carry the civilizing gospel of hygiene to the indigenous population through its enlightened women. The Laguna Health Unit—established in 1929 as a collaboration between the foundation and the provincial government of Laguna—sought to demonstrate the effectiveness of this new approach to rural hygiene.[31]

As Atsuko Naono's chapter also shows, the Rockefeller Foundation was equally involved in Dutch colonial Indonesia. There, too, the hookworm eradication campaign gave way to a more ambitious attempt to reshape rural health. Led by John L. Hydrick, who spent the years between 1924 and 1939 in Indonesia, the foundation focused on rural hygiene and health education. The Dutch colonial government was skeptical of—and even hostile to—their early initiatives, but eventually accepted the foundation's advice. The centerpiece of Hydrick's work was the Poerwokerto health demonstration unit in Banyunas, Java. Hydrick pioneered the use of health education films and emphasized the role of hygiene *mantris*—locally trained indigenous health workers: the Dutch government had used them from the nineteenth century. Hydrick wove his experiences into a manifesto for the new gospel of rural hygiene, published in 1936 in Dutch and English (the English title was *Intensive Rural Hygiene Work in Netherlands India*), and soon translated into French. The aim was to "awaken in the people a permanent interest in hygiene and to stimulate them to adopt habits and to carry out measures which will help them secure health and remain healthy." One colonial health minister wrote of Hydrick's miraculous techniques that they were "so planned that they quietly and gradually penetrate and become a part of normal village life."[32]

The rationale for deploying the subtle power of persuasion to shape individual and communal conduct lay in the very weakness of the colonial state in large parts of rural Java. "There would be no objection whatever to the use of coercion," Hydrick declared, "if its use could secure permanent results." Yet that would require "a large personnel to enforce all the rules and regulations and this makes it far too expensive." He concluded that "if it were possible to secure results at a reasonable cost by coercion then conditions in all countries would be much better than they actually now are."[33]

The successful hygiene *mantri* had to meet rigorous criteria. He was to be "polite and modest and no circumstances will excuse rudeness or misuse of authority," but he could not be "too shy," as this would "not inspire confidence." The list of virtues continues:

> He must possess an inexhaustible patience, because he will be obliged to talk daily to many people about things which they do not understand. A monotonous voice practically disqualifies an applicant. . . . [E]fforts for improvement of his technic [*sic*] must never cease. . . . The manner in which the mantri approaches the house and calls to the people to see if anyone is at home; the way in which he enters the house and finally gets all the members of the family together; his method of leading the conversation; where he sits; his manner of talking; his skill in keeping the interest of all members of the family; his patience; his answers to questions which are asked; his ability to make people talk, etc., are all points of the technic for which a long and thorough training is necessary.[34]

The hygiene *mantri* was at once distinctively Indonesian, and part of a global movement of health workers and assistants charged with the promotion of rural health—from Zagreb to Sriniketan to Poerwokerto. As Eric Stein has argued—based on fieldwork in Java, and interviews with elderly local people who had memories of the rural hygiene experiments of the 1930s—the Foundation used laughter and entertainment as a way to permeate the domestic sphere. Health education films, he argues—following Bruno Latour—were a "theatre of proof," through which the epistemological claims of modern medicine were instilled in local people.[35]

In un-colonized Siam (Thailand), the relationship between international health institutions and a modernizing state reached even further, as Stefan Hell's important work shows. The Siamese government drew on the expertise and the advice of the League of Nations Health Organization in its own efforts to improve the nation's health. Siamese medical officials participated in the Far Eastern Association of Tropical Medicine; the Rockefeller campaign against hookworm was active in the country between 1917 and 1928. But the closest relationship, Hell shows, was between the Siamese state and the League of Nations. Siamese officials were influential in the establishment of the league's Far Eastern Bureau in 1925; they received League of Nations commissions of enquiry on leprosy, malaria, cholera, and rural health. Hell argues that the Siamese government used these commissions to "present itself as modern and civilized" both domestically and in the international arena.

The work of the League of Nations Malaria Commission was particularly important to Siam. In 1931, a malarial survey of Siam was conducted by Ludwig Anigstein—a Polish malariologist who then worked at the Institute for Medical Research in Kuala Lumpur, and who was a member of the commission. His tour of Siam culminated in a report that recommended a wide-ranging malaria control program that focused on its root causes: poverty and environmental degradation, particularly in Siam's dry north.[36] The Depression ended any hopes of state financing for such an ambitious scheme—this was, of course, a common theme—but Hell argues, nevertheless, that the league was very important to the development of modern public health in Siam. Perhaps more than anywhere else in Southeast Asia, interactions with the league had direct results in terms of policy, including the national nutrition policy of 1938, and the establishment of an autonomous Ministry of Public Health two years later.[37]

Rural Health and the Problems of Development

The logic of the experiment characterized the connected health projects and demonstrations established in India, China, and Southeast Asia in the 1920s. The word conveyed a sense of self-realization by modern men: scientific exploration confined neither to the laboratory nor to Europe, producing incremental innovations that would result in social transformation. But the focus on experiment also conveyed a sense of limited scale, and of uncertain results.

In the context of the Depression, Asia's role within international health networks evolved. Suddenly, the problems of the periphery impinged upon those of the center: the problems of undernutrition in distant colonies no longer seemed too distant from the crises of subsistence in deprived urban and rural corners of Europe. There was a leap in scale when it came to thinking about problems of health—especially rural health—within Asia. Efforts to draw a wider picture of distress, and to generalize the lessons of localized experiments, came together in 1937 at the League of Nations conference on rural hygiene in Bandung. At the same time, the thin walls separating international health experts from the clamor of popular politics began to collapse. Technical debates on health became more entangled with moral and political debates about power.

French historian Lion Murard has argued that the enthusiasm for participatory rural hygiene—"[g]radualist, indigenous development"—was widespread in the 1930s: the League of Nations was a major conduit for the transmission of these ideas. Beginning with a conference on rural hygiene in Europe in 1931—the brainchild of Ludwik Rajchman—the League expanded its discussions beyond Europe with a Pan-African Health Conference, held in Johannesburg in 1935, and a conference on rural health convened in Bandung, Indonesia in 1937. Two further meetings were planned, but never took place: one on rural health in the Americas (scheduled to meet in Mexico in 1938), and the other an ill-fated European Conference on Rural Life, scheduled for the summer of 1939. In this context, the Bandung meeting of 1937 placed Asia's fragmented experiments in rural health in relation to one another, and also in a wider global context.[38]

It was with rural health particularly in mind that a group of three League of Nations consultants set out on a journey across the continent in 1936. The team consisted of A. S. Haynes, formerly colonial secretary of the Federated Malay States; C. D. De Langen, formerly dean of the Batavia Faculty of Medicine, and E. J. Pampana, a Venezuelan malariologist who was Secretary of the League of Nations Malaria Commission.[39] Between April and August 1936, the three men toured India, Burma, Siam, Malaya, Indochina, the Philippines, the Netherlands East Indies, and Ceylon.[40] They sought to identify the different approaches to public health that were on display for their consideration across imperial frontiers; and they sought a language with which to discuss these changes. Writing from the *SS Maloja,* traversing the Red Sea, Haynes wrote to the private secretary of the viceroy of India, thanking him for receiving the commission, and summarizing his impressions of his visit:

> The countries we have visited are almost entirely agricultural. . . . [I]n each country, "rural reconstruction" is prominent in the papers, and is on everyone's lips. It is perhaps somewhat strange that this should occur simultaneously in all the countries concerned and that it should be so recent and so comparatively sudden. But it is indisputable that a reorientation of governmental policies is taking place and that the needs of the distant and inarticulate peasant are being weighed in the council chambers . . . where his voice has been little heard.

The letter concludes with Haynes expressing excitement about the upcoming League of Nations conference on rural hygiene in Bandung: "there has been no such meeting of Eastern Nations before."[41]

The August 1937 League of Nations conference on rural hygiene in the Far East met in the modernist Dutch colonial city of Bandung. Its geographical delimitation—the "Far East"—was expansive, and it had deep institutional roots: both the Rockefeller Foundation's Far Eastern Directorate and the Far Eastern Association of Tropical Medicine had used the term. However, the meaning of the term "Far East" had undergone a subtle shift, at least partly as a result of the many interventions and experiments that international institutions had launched in Southeast Asia. In 1925, the League of Nations had chosen Singapore as the headquarters of its Far Eastern Bureau. The bureau's chief responsibility was the collection and dissemination of epidemiological surveillance. On a map charting the transmission of data between stations, Singapore sits at the heart of a web that reaches from India to China to the southern Indian Ocean. In this definition of the Far East, Southeast Asia was no longer peripheral—no longer an extension either of India or of China—but now central.[42]

The Bandung conference included representatives from across South and Southeast Asia. It was at once interimperial and international, and it went further than its predecessors (including the Far Eastern Association of Tropical Medicine) in the scope of its discussions and the range of its participants.[43] The conference was attended by representatives from each of the British territories in Asia, including separate representation of individual provinces in British India, and the Indian princely states; French Indochina; Japan (despite its withdrawal from the league after the Manchurian invasion, and, indeed, after the outbreak of the Second Sino-Japanese War); the Netherlands Indies; the Philippines; China; and Siam.[44] The meeting gave much scope, too, to a range of experts not directly linked to colonial or national states.

The discussions at the Bandung conference emphasized that the fundamental problem was poverty. In this connection, the new nutritional thought was never far from the forefront of discussion. In particular, the Bandung conference focused on the problem of rice "throughout the east." The discussants emphasized "the fact that the degree of milling to which rice is subjected is of vital importance in connection with the problem of nutrition throughout the East." They deplored "the tendency of urban and rural populations in the East to consume highly-milled rice." More strongly still, the conference resolution "recommends that Governments should make a thorough investigation of the nutritional, commercial, economic and psychological aspects of the problem, attention being given to the *possibility of checking the spread of mechanical rice mills in rural areas* . . . with a view to conserving the healthy habit of consuming home-pounded rice."[45] Influenced by the South Indian research of W. R. Aykroyd and his colleagues, the League of Nations saw that restraining the advance of mechanization might be necessary to conserve healthy habits.

As important as nutrition was the problem of malaria, and here, too, the potential tension between health and colonial development was all too evident. Going back to the 1920s, the League of Nations Malaria Commission had long taken a social approach to the problem, arguing that a focus on the problems of poverty and the environment, rather than a focus on the vector of transmission, was the most sensible approach to the problem of malaria in Eastern Europe.[46] The 1937 conference's consideration of the problem of malaria illustrates the concern of this new international public health with the relationship between health, poverty, and agricultural development. Some of the blame for the devastation caused by malaria lay squarely upon the effects of colonial capitalism on rural areas in Asia. The 1937 conference issued a resolution declaring that "the amount of *engineer-made malaria* . . . is appalling." Participants in the conference highlighted the problem of "malaria due to improper siting and housing; indiscriminate aggregation of labourers; uncontrolled jungle clearing . . . obstruction of natural drainage by road, railway and canal embankments with culverts too few and too high; impounding of water without regard to leakages, seepages and raised water-table levels; irrigation without drainage."[47] Despite this growing recognition of common factors underlying the causes and consequences of malaria, the league's experts stated emphatically that "the problems which it raises cannot be dealt with—or settled—without intimate knowledge of local conditions. Any attempt to proceed on standardized lines would be disastrous."[48]

The conclusion of the commission's discussion of malaria encapsulates the growth of international social medicine in Asia:

> It must be admitted that, except for a few quinine tablets distributed here and there, the health conditions of, say, a peasant living with his family in a hut in the middle of a marshy plain . . . have received very little attention. . . . Malaria is a health and social problem; it must be attacked simultaneously from both these angles. While, on the one hand, marked economic progress may depend on the success of anti-malarial measures, these, on the other hand, will be facilitated by an adequate diet, healthier dwellings, more widespread education—in a word, by rural reconstruction.[49]

This was the perspective of concerned scientists, disillusioned with the neglect of their findings in the operation of the colonial state and economy. More expansively, the views expressed on malaria and nutrition alike at the Bandung conference reflected the aspirations of those who saw in rural public health a panacea to "extremism," and even a path to national consciousness.[50] Murard's conclusion is apt: "the health demonstrations of the 1930s were outcroppings in a flattened landscape. The links among the outcroppings—which spanned large distances—gave a sense of (scale and) unity to reform-minded healers. But diversity, not unity, was the hallmark of the age."[51]

Colonial states were not immune to these international discussions of nutrition and health. The government of the Dutch East Indies was the most advanced in this, making a display of their commitment to widening and implementing the kinds of reforms the Rockefeller Foundation's J. L. Hydrick had advocated.[52] British colonial governments, too, indicated their increasing interest in public health. The "model colony" of Ceylon saw an expansion of maternal and child welfare services.[53] Reflecting the influence of rural hygiene and nutritional thinking on colonial officials, one 1935 report on public health in India argued,

> No preventive campaign against malaria, against tuberculosis or against leprosy, no maternity relief or child welfare activities, are likely to achieve any great success unless those responsible recognize the vital importance of this factor of defective nutrition and from the very start give it their most seri-

ous consideration. . . . The first essentials for the prevention of disease are a higher standard of health, a better physique, and a greater power of resistance to infection.[54]

Yet such views coexisted with a deepening colonial pessimism about their ability to affect the conditions of health in tropical Asia. As David Arnold has argued, colonial officials faced a "growing awareness of the complex and vulnerable nature of the Indian environment and the cultural and political difficulties involved in trying to effect any change."[55]

Referring explicitly to the findings of the League of Nations, British health officials conceded that "adequate diet, healthier dwellings, more widespread education are all needed if anti-malarial measures are to be fully effective."[56] Yet those were hardly realistic aspirations for a colonial state running on a tight budget. Instead, British colonial authorities argued that "it would be difficult to over-estimate the importance from an economic aspect of a successful campaign against the disease."[57] If rural reconstruction was too expensive, at least "the provision of anti-malarial drugs could be given an important place amongst the essential social services directed towards building up of national health and efficiency."[58] The logic was clear: if a cost-effective intervention against malaria could be found, "there could hardly be a more important contribution in present circumstances to the prosperity and well-being of tropical countries than an effective attack upon the disease."[59] The gulf between the aspirations for a transformation of health and welfare in rural Asia, and the capacity to bring it about, would make itself felt repeatedly in the decades to come.

Conclusion: Regions and the Limits of Internationalism

International health initiatives in Southeast Asia in the 1920s and 1930s were characterized by their pluralism and by their small scale. To a far greater extent than their postwar successors, the projects of the 1930s paid attention to variations in local conditions; they emphasized the importance of locality; they took an interest in "culture," however narrowly defined. The scales of comparison they deployed are, to our eyes, unfamiliar ones: by the 1930s, a focus on rural life meant that the most obvious parallels and models for South and Southeast Asia often came from Eastern Europe. The small-scale demonstration project was their quintessential mode of operation. To many observers, these stood removed from what we might call policy, or the aspiration to govern.[60]

The limitation of their ambitions was a reflection of weakness. International initiatives were dependent on fluctuating philanthropic funding; they failed to attract the interest—and very often they attracted the hostility—of colonial states until well into the 1930s. Their interventions were too limited, too piecemeal to satisfy the ambitions of a new political generation who imagined a far more sweeping social, economic, and political transformation in Asia. As I have argued elsewhere, the modernizing left of the Indian National Congress party drew inspiration and statistical ammunition from the work of international bodies, but they envisaged a far greater role for the state and a larger scale of operations.[61] Similarly, throughout Southeast Asia, a new political leadership confronted colonialism more directly in the 1930s: among their criticisms of colonial rule was the colonial governments' failure to embrace more ambitious programs of development.

Partha Chatterjee writes of the "normative acceptance over a wide spectrum of political opinion of the nation-state as the universally normal, legitimate form of the modern state" throughout the 1920s and 1930s.[62] In this context, the fact that the League's health work continued to be an interimperial as much as an international organization limited its reach. The postwar WHO learned this lesson well: from the outset, it was a more statist organization that achieved its goals by working with its member governments and by utilizing the power of the modern state to enact standardized mass campaigns that covered as much of each country as possible. International health campaigns drew on both the language and the technologies of nationalist mobilization to sustain mass vaccination and disease eradication campaigns. It is perhaps unsurprising that the most lasting legacy of the interwar experiments in health can be found in the work of individuals who went on to exercise state power: for instance in the work of Dr. Raden Mochtar, who worked on Rockefeller projects in Java in the 1930s, and went on to play a leading role in the Indonesian Department of Health in the 1950s.[63]

This chapter has shown that Southeast Asia emerged as a meaningful region within the networks of global health in the 1920s and 1930s, but never in a self-contained or limited way. Rather, it was Southeast Asia's role as a crossroads of migration and ethnic diversity that seemed to be its primary characteristic. At the time of its foundation in 1948, the WHO opted—for both geopolitical and practical reasons—to include India (and even Afghanistan) within its Southeast Asian Regional Office, headquartered in Delhi.[64] In some ways this works against the unity of Southeast Asia as a health region: in the WHO's conception, Indonesia, Thailand, and Myanmar are part of Southeast Asia, along with India; whereas Malaysia, the Philippines, and Hong Kong are in the Western Pacific. In other ways, however, intentionally or not, these groupings gesture toward historical and geographical ties that precede nation-states: they are neither more nor less arbitrary than Southeast Asia itself. The history of these other geographies is worth reexamining at a moment when the interregional ties that bind Southeast Asia to South Asia and to East Asia are of growing economic, political, and epidemiological importance in the twenty-first century.

Notes

1. Paul H. Kratoska, Remco Raben, and Henk Schulte Nordhold, "Locating Southeast Asia," in *Locating Southeast Asia: Geographies of Knowing and Politics of Space*, ed. Paul H. Kratoska, Remco Raben, and Henk Schulte Nordhold (Singapore: NUS Press, 2005), 1–19.

2. Cecilia S. Acuin, Geok Lin Khor, Tippawan Liabsuetrakul, et al., "Maternal, Neonatal, and Child Health in Southeast Asia: Towards Greater Regional Collaboration," *Lancet*, 377 (2011): 516–25, quotation on 517. See also Jose Acuin, Rebecca Firestone, Thein Thein Htay, Geok Lin Khor, Hasbullah Thabrany, Vonthanak Saphonn, and Suwit Wibulpolprasert, "Southeast Asia: An Emerging Focus for Global Health," *Lancet* 377 (2011): 534–35.

3. Richard Grove, *Green Imperialism: Colonial Expansion, Tropical Island Edens and the Origins of Environmentalism, 1600–1860* (Cambridge: Cambridge University Press, 1995); Jeyamalar Kathirithamby-Wells, *Nature and Nation: Forests and Development in Peninsular Malaysia* (Copenhagen: NIAS Press, 2005).

4. For a more detailed discussion of these themes, see Sunil S. Amrith, *Crossing the Bay of Bengal: The Furies of Nature and the Fortunes of Migrants* (Cambridge, MA: Harvard University Press, 2013), chaps. 3 and 4.

5. Adam McKeown, "Global Migration, 1846–1940," *Journal of World History* 15, no. 2 (2004): 155–89.

6. George Grierson, *Report on Colonial Emigration from the Bengal Presidency* (Calcutta: Government Printer, 1883), 35.

7. Amrith, *Crossing the Bay of Bengal*, 128.

8. Sources cited in Amrith, *Crossing the Bay of Bengal*, 128–30.

9. Sunil S. Amrith, "Indians Overseas? Governing Tamil Migration to Malaya, 1870–1941," *Past and Present* 208 (August 2010): 231–61.

10. Warwick Anderson, *Colonial Pathologies: American Tropical Medicine, Race, and Hygiene in the Philippines* (Durham, NC: Duke University Press, 2006); Peter Boomgaard, "The Welfare Services in Indonesia, 1900–1942," *Itinerario* 1 (1986): 57–82.

11. Neville Goodman, *International Health Organizations and their Work* (London: Blakiston, 1952).

12. Karine Delaye, "Colonial Co-operation and Regional Construction: Anglo-French Medical and Sanitary Relations in Southeast Asia," *Asia Europe Journal* 3 (2004): 461–471.

13. John F. Hutchinson, *Champions of Charity: War and the Rise of the Red Cross* (Boulder, CO: Westview Press, 1996); Henrietta Harrison, "'Penny for the Little Chinese': The French Holy Childhood Association in China, 1843–1951," *American Historical Review* 113, no. 1 (2008): 72–92.

14. Stefan Hell, *Siam and the League of Nations: Modernisation, Sovereignty and Multilateral Diplomacy, 1920–1940* (Bangkok: River Books, 2010), 128.

15. Paul Weindling, "American Foundations and the Internationalizing of Health," in *Shifting Boundaries of Public Health: Europe in the Twentieth Century*, ed. Susan Gross Solomon, Lion Murard, and Patrick Zylberman (Rochester, NY: University of Rochester Press, 2008), 63–86.

16. On the history of the Rockefeller Foundation's International Health Division, see J. Farley, *To Cast Out Disease: A History of the International Health Division of the Rockefeller Foundation (1913–1951)* (Oxford: Oxford University Press, 2004).

17. Farley, *To Cast Out Disease*; Mary Brown Bullock, *The Oil Prince's Legacy: Rockefeller Philanthropy in China* (Stanford, CA: Stanford University Press, 2011).

18. Lion Murard and Patrick Zylberman, "L'autre guerre (1914–1918): La santé publique en France sous l'oeil de l'Amérique," *Révue historique* 276 (1986): 367–98.

19. J. Farley, "The International Health Division of the Rockefeller Foundation: the Russell Years," in *International Health Organizations and Movements, 1918–1939*, ed. P. Weindling (Cambridge: Cambridge University Press, 1995), 203–21.

20. Farley, *To Cast Out Disease.*

21. Lion Murard and Patrick Zylberman, "French Social Medicine on the International Public Health Map in the 1930s," in *The Politics of the Healthy Life: An International Perspective*, ed. E. Rodriguez-Ocaña (Sheffield, UK: European Association for the History of Medicine and Health Publications, 2002), 197–218.

22. M. Grmek, "Life and Achievements of Andrija Stampar, Fighter for the Promotion of Public Health," *Serving the Cause of Public Health: Selected Papers of Andrija Stampar*, ed. M. Grmek (Zagreb: Andrija Stampar School of Public Health, 1966), 13–51; Patrick Zylberman, "Fewer Parallels than Antitheses: Rene Sand and Andrija Stampar on Social Medicine, 1919–1955," *Social History of Medicine* 17, no. 1 (2004): 77–93.

23. Murard and Zylberman, "French Social Medicine"; Zylberman, "Fewer Antitheses than Parallels."

24. A. Stampar, "Health and Social Conditions in China," *Quarterly Bulletin of the Health Organization of the League of Nations* 5 (1936): 1090–1126.

25. Stampar, "Health and Social Conditions in China," 1123.

26. Stampar, "Health and Social Conditions in China," 1124.

27. Socrates Litsios, "Selskar Gunn and China: The Rockefeller Foundation's 'Other' Approach to Public Health," *Bulletin of the History of Medicine* 79 (2005): 295–318; Marta Aleksandra Balinska, *Une vie pour l'humanitaire. Ludwik Rajchman, 1881–1965* (Paris: La Découverte, 1995).

28. Subir Sinha, "Lineages of the Developmentalist State: Transnationality and Village India, 1900–1965," *Comparative Studies in Society and History* 50, no. 1 (2008): 57–90.

29. E. Blunt, ed., *Social Service in India: An Introduction to Some Social and Economic Problems of the Indian People,* (London: HMSO, 1939), 382–83; Central Co-operative Anti-Malaria Society, *Annual Reports* (Calcutta: Central Co-operative Anti-Malaria Society, 1927–43); Mridula Ramanna, "Local Initiatives in Health Care: Bombay Presidency, 1900–1920," *Economic and Political Weekly*, October 9, 2004, 4560–67.

30. Victor G. Heiser, *An American Doctor's Odyssey: Adventure in Forty Five Countries* (New York: W. W. Norton, 1936).

31. Stefanie S. Bator, "Women Are the Way Forward: The Rockefeller Foundation in the Philippines, 1923–1932," Rockefeller Archive Center Research Report, 2011, Rockefeller Archive Center website, www.rockarch.org/publications/resrep/bator.pdf.

32. Sunil S. Amrith, *Decolonizing International Health: India and Southeast Asia, c. 1930–1965* (Basingstoke, UK: Palgrave MacMillan, 2006), 30.

33. Amrith, *Decolonizing International Health*, 30.

34. J. L. Hydrick, *Intensive Rural Hygiene Work and Public Health Education of the Public Health Service of Netherlands India* (Batavia-Centrum, Java: n.p., 1937), 45–47; the discussion of Hydrick in the preceding paragraphs draws on Sunil S. Amrith, *Decolonizing International Health*, chap. 1.

35. Eric A. Stein, "Colonial Theatres of Proof: Representation and Laughter in 1930s Rockefeller Foundation Hygiene Cinema in Java," *Health and History* 8, no. 2 (2006): 14–44.

36. Ludwik Anigstein, "Malaria and Anopheles in Siam," *Quarterly Bulletin of the Health Organisation* 1, no. 2 (June, 1932): 233–308.

37. Hell, *Siam and the League of Nations.*

38. Lion Murard, "Designs within Disorder: International Conferences on Rural Health Care and the Art of the Local, 1931–39," in *Shifting Boundaries of Public Health: Europe in the*

Twentieth Century, ed. Susan Gross Solomon, Lion Murard, and Patrick Zylberman (Rochester, NY: University of Rochester Press, 2008), 141–74, quotation on 142.

39. The following discussion draws on Amrith, *Decolonizing International Health,* chapter 1.

40. League of Nations, *Intergovernmental Conference of Far-Eastern Countries on Rural Hygiene: Report by the Preparatory Committee* (Geneva: League of Nations, 1937), [III. Health. 1937.III.3].

41. LNA, Box 6093, 8A, 25509, 8855, Haynes to Private Secretary, Viceroy of India, 22 August 1936.

42. Lenore Manderson, "Wireless Wars in the Eastern Arena: Surveillance, Disease Prevention and the Work of the Eastern Bureau of the League of Nations Health Organization, 1925–1942," in *International Health Organizations and Movements, 1918–1939,* ed. P. Weindling (Cambridge: Cambridge University Press, 1995), 109–33.

43. W. R. Aykroyd, "International Health—A Retrospective Memoir," *Perspectives in Biology and Medicine* 11 (1968): 273–85.

44. League of Nations, *Intergovernmental Conference,* 16–20.

45. League of Nations, *Intergovernmental Conference,* 68.

46. See, for example, League of Nations, *Malaria Commission: Report on Its Tour of Investigation in Certain European Countries in 1924* (Geneva: League of Nations, 1925), C.H. 273.

47. League of Nations, *Intergovernmental Conference,* 93.

48. League of Nations, *Intergovernmental Conference,* 78.

49. League of Nations, *Intergovernmental Conference,* 79.

50. Cf. League of Nations Archives, Organization d'Hygiene, vol. 358, C.H./Conf.Hyg.Rural.Orient/4, Note received by the Secretariat of the Conference from Dr. Leonard Shishlien Hsu, "Rural Reconstruction and Social Planning."

51. Murard, "Designs within Disorder," 164.

52. See League of Nations, *Intergovernmental Conference of Far-Eastern Countries on Rural Hygiene, Preparatory Papers: National Reports: Report of the Netherlands Indies* (Geneva: League of Nations, 1937), [III.Health.1937.III.15]; and A.P. den Hartog, "Towards Improving Public Nutrition: Nutritional Policy in Indonesia before Independence," in *Dutch Medicine in the Malay Archipelago, 1816–1942,* ed. G. M. van Heteren, A. de Knecht-van Eekelen, and M. J. D. Poulissen (Amsterdam: Rodopi, 1989), 105–18.

53. M. Jones, "Infant and Maternal Health Services in Ceylon, 1900–1948: Imperialism or Welfare?" *Social History of Medicine,*15, no. 2 (2002): 263–89.

54. Cited in John Farley, *Bilharzia: A History of Imperial Tropical Medicine* (Cambridge: Cambridge University Press, 1991), 176.

55. David Arnold, *Science, Technology and Medicine, New Cambridge History of India,* vol. 3, pt. 5 (Cambridge: Cambridge University Press, 2000), 203.

56. Economic Advisory Council, Committee on Scientific Research, 5th Report: "Consumption and Supply of Cinchona Alkaloids in the Empire," January 1938, EAC (SC) 31 (Confidential): British Library, Asian and African Studies Collection: India Office Records [hereafter IOR], M/3/180: "Quinine: Question of Production within the Empire."

57. IOR, M/3/180: "Quinine."

58. IOR, M/3/180: "Quinine."

59. IOR, M/3/180: "Quinine."

60. Michael Feher notes that this is a central characteristic of what he calls "nongovernmental politics": the participation in political life, broadly defined, without the aspiration to govern (Michael Feher, ed. *Nongovernmental Politics* [New York: Zone Books, 2007]); see also Charles Rosenberg, "'Anticipated Consequences: Historians, History and Health Policy," in

Putting the Past Back In: History and Health Policy in the United States, ed. R. Stevens, C. Rosenberg, and L. Burns (New Brunswick, NJ: Rutgers University Press, 2005).

61. Amrith, *Decolonizing International Health.*

62. Partha Chatterjee, *The Black Hole of Empire: History of a Global Practice of Power* (Princeton: Princeton University Press, 2012), 273; see also Mrinalini Sinha, *Specters of Mother India: The Global Restructuring of an Empire* (Durham, NC: Duke University Press, 2006).

63. Stein, "Colonial Theatres of Proof."

64. Amrith, *Decolonizing International Health.*

10 Modernizing Yet Marginal

Hospitals and Asylums in Southeast Asia in the Twentieth Century

Loh Kah Seng

In my interview with Kuang Wee Kee, a former leprosy patient, he spoke of the "three brothers" of illnesses that not only drastically affected his life but also caused great anxiety among the public in Singapore since the colonial era. The "little brother," he said, was mental illness, which was "quite light" in its impact; followed by the "second brother," tuberculosis; and finally leprosy, the "big brother." Kuang had suffered from isolation and painful treatment while confined for a long time in a leprosarium under the law of compulsory segregation. Even after his cure and discharge, he and his wife, Ow Ah Mui, also a leprosy sufferer, found that society refused to accept them. Kuang's comments on the three "big brothers" underline the role of institutional treatment and confinement in Southeast Asia, namely, the tuberculosis clinic, the leprosarium, and the mental asylum.[1]

The experiences of Kuang and Ow provide an entry point for investigating the place of hospitals and mental and leprosy asylums in the transnational history of public health in twentieth-century Southeast Asia. Scholars such as Warwick Anderson have argued convincingly for a more nuanced approach to the history of imperial medicine in Southeast Asia. To Anderson, the interaction between Western and Southeast Asian medicine was a two-way, multi-actor process. Developments in the Philippines, for instance, also shaped health care in the United States.[2] This approach differs from the established scholarship, in which colonial medicine was seen as a tool of empire that scientifically extended Western political and cultural domination over inferior Asian "races."[3] In my view, Anderson's approach is useful for mapping new areas of research, rather than to detach completely from older work. Transnationalism has not been always a harmonious exchange between equals: it includes instances in which the relationship was fraught and contested. In colonial Southeast Asia, medical transnationalism involved a largely unequal relationship between metropole and colony as the Western powers colonized most of the region in the late nineteenth century, even if cases of mutual influence occurred. At the same time, the "tool of empire" framework should accommodate not only the complex exchanges between metropole and colony, but also the interfaces between the international, national, and local. In the interactions between the global, national, and local, a therapeutic system may serve to legitimize power but may also provoke resistance against it.[4]

This chapter investigates how hospital- and asylum-based health care originating in the West facilitated the making of modern Southeast Asia. These ideas had an obvious impact during the colonial period, but continued to affect postcolonial Southeast Asia. This chapter traces the complex interactions between the global and local and is mindful of the ways in which Southeast Asian states, societies, and patients have alternately contested and appropriated foreign ideas. Southeast Asia's hospitals have not achieved the degree of state power that Foucault imagined in Europe, and asylums were often not the "total institutions" that Goffman envisaged, which were enclosed places sustained by regimes of formal control.[5] Like other leprosy patients in Singapore and elsewhere in Southeast Asia, Kuang and Ow were able to exercise their agency in coping with life within the leprosarium, meeting their own needs and interests, and—in the long run— transforming the texture of institutional life.

Neither imperial nor postcolonial medicine were hegemonic, and subalterns have an important place in the writing of transnational histories of public health. I use the term "subaltern" broadly to include Southeast Asian groups who exercised their agency not merely through resistance but also by accommodating, appropriating, contesting, or redefining biomedicine—the Western form of medicine based on the scientific method of testing and verification. In doing so, patients and inmates produced new cultures of healing and patient cultures that expressed their worldviews and differed from elite forms of modernity. This maps a social history of hospitals and asylums that acknowledges the multiple agents, processes, and outcomes involved in the making of modern Southeast Asia. The processes involved three groups of actors—namely colonial regimes, postcolonial states, and the peoples of Southeast Asia.

Colonial Neglect and Failings

It was, of course, Foucault who—in several of his books, most notably *Madness and Civilization* and *The Birth of the Clinic*—explored the links between health institutions and the making of the modern state. Foucault examined the overlap between therapeutic and political spaces that allowed states to discipline and transform human bodies. Hospitals and asylums were important sites in the medicalization of Southeast Asian states. By medicalization, I refer to the historical process by which people seek out or are integrated into the Western biomedical system, which becomes the "proper" way to treat illness and is ostensibly superior to indigenous or traditional medicine.

In pairing hospitals and asylums, we acknowledge their similarities and differences. Foucault underplayed the role of asylums in extending the power of the modern state: to him, leprosaria—operating on the principle of segregating the ill—were necessarily inferior to clinics, hospitals, and prisons in reaching into individual and social life. However, there is increasing awareness that leprosaria were social laboratories for engineering modernity and conferring citizenship. In addition to providing sanctuary, they converged toward the functions of a hospital by straddling two roles—healer and jailor.[6] Hospitals can also be prison-like in the way they are platforms from which medical legislation and policy are enforced, where people are mandated to be examined, treated, and even temporarily detained. These persons do not have to be ill—witness the experience of prostitutes in Southeast Asia who had to submit themselves for examination at STD clinics; many of them went underground.[7]

Hospitals and asylums are spatially important in drawing people into the structures and relations of modernity. They mark the divide between health care based on biomedical expertise and informal care provided by members of the community and family, who may only visit the patient in these institutions. Hospitals are places where the sick go for medical treatment and where they are at times warded, whereas asylums extend the thematic separation between the patient and their family and community to a period of often involuntary and possibly indefinite confinement. For patients suffering from mental illness and leprosy, the confinement is justified on the grounds of biomedical expertise as being both for the greater good and in the interest of the patient.[8] The separation from family and community, illustrated so vividly in the social rejection of cured leprosy sufferers such as Kuang and Ow, may persist even after the institutionalization ceases.

In much of the historical literature on colonial Southeast Asia, Foucault does not seem applicable. A common theme in the literature is colonial neglect and failings, which diverge from the "tool of empire" scholarship. However, this obscures the role of public hospitals, as part of the colonial centralized bureaucracy, in transforming local society. The literature also makes distinctions between curative and preventive health care, as well as between the urban and rural, modern, and traditional, and the colonial and postcolonial. Public health programs such as sanitation works are frequently deemed to have been the front line of imperialism, and to have had a greater direct impact on larger numbers of people than did hospitals.[9] In this view, hospitals were marginal nodes in the colonial system, catering mainly to Europeans and upper class Asians. Inadequately staffed, unable to offer effective treatment, too costly, and culturally different, they were shunned by most ordinary Asians, who saw them as places where one simply went to die. Similarly, as the literature maintains, the reach of hospitals in the colonial period was limited to urban areas and plantation estates, and in particular to urban elites, a point that still has some resonance today.[10]

In British Malaya, hospitals were usually located in the Federated Malay States and the Straits Settlements, which were more economically developed and urbanized and had larger migrant populations than the northern and eastern parts of the peninsula.[11] Throughout Malaya, hospitals were so unpopular with smallpox patients that family members were allowed to stay with the patient and even provide food, thus weakening the connection between treatment and separation.[12] During the post–World War I flu epidemic, Malaya's public hospitals were overcrowded, and the government had to use closed-down cinemas as makeshift hospitals. Locals regarded them as places to die, but were more receptive about using services provided by local and ethnic organizations.[13] Similarly, Filipinos avoided hospitals during the cholera epidemic at the beginning of the twentieth century, and temporary tents had to be pitched near hospitals to accommodate relatives and friends of the sick. Many locals, in fact, feared the hospital more than the disease, an ambivalence that was intensified by the recent American conquest of the country.[14] In Cambodia, the Mixed Hospital was established in 1885, offering both French and traditional medicine. But it failed to appeal to locals, who viewed hospitals as intimidating places operated by foreigners. Although they were at times willing to consult Western physicians, Cambodians refused to be admitted to hospitals and were reluctant about undergoing surgery or giving birth there.[15] In colonial Vietnam, too, local doctors had to prescribe traditional remedies or combine them with Western medicine.[16]

In reality, the curative sector in Southeast Asia was and remains more complex. Undoubtedly, public hospitals were few in number, underutilized, and made little effort to accommodate local sensitivities during the colonial period. But we must also not ignore privately funded hospitals in the region's smaller towns, and near mines and plantation estates. These were semi-urban or rural places that were rapidly developed during the period of colonial rule and Western capitalist expansion. Hospitals run by Chinese migrants might also have catered to a larger proportion of non-Western patients than colonial institutions.[17] For example, plantation workers in colonial Malaya and Indonesia preferred local estate hospitals to district or public hospitals, simply because the latter were poorly staffed and traveling there cost workers time and wages.[18] In Indonesia, in addition to urban and estate hospitals, there were a great variety of traveling dispensaries, mobile clinics, and maternal and child health clinics in the rural areas.[19]

The distinction between the curative and preventive is overdrawn because hospitals were places where hygiene and sanitation were practiced while these measures were implemented in the society. They treated contagious diseases that were public health concerns, such as tuberculosis and epidemic diseases.[20] Hospitals, then, were a microcosm of—if not a laboratory for—public health campaigns. In addition, hospitals collect—quite obsessively—statistics on the incidence of illnesses and demographic profiles of patients. This information was useful for organizing public health programs and the medicalization of health care. Public hospitals and asylums were part of the centralized administrations established in the late nineteenth century, which were interested in collecting information and undertaking interventions into local life. In Thailand, hospital staff collected data from patients in order to identify "high-risk" health groups. This labeling, which in effect assigned blame to various groups, showed how personal information collected in a hospital became useful for classifying and mobilizing society at large.[21] As nodes of modernity, hospitals and asylums of the late nineteenth and twentieth centuries were qualitatively different from the institutions established earlier in Southeast Asia, and were funded by humanitarian, religious, and voluntary associations—both Western and non-Western. Over and above how far they were utilized or how they were received by locals, hospitals were important points in a system of social control that, to draw upon Mary Douglas, distinguished between what was clean and unclean.[22]

The view of hospitals as colonial failings has much merit, but has tended to overemphasize the dichotomy between the colonizer and colonized. The claim that Southeast Asians were reluctant to go to hospitals or only went there at an advanced stage of illness is still based on a modernist premise on the superiority of Western medicine. In some cases, the "delay" was not the making of the sick themselves. Driven by profit, European managers in Malaya often did not transfer miners suffering from tuberculosis to a hospital until their disease was at an advanced stage.[23] Although there were real economic and cultural barriers to the wider use of hospitals, ordinary Asians were not altogether antimodern. They responded to biomedicine in various ways, including selective appropriation and accommodation. In addition, hospitals were important tools of political economy in both the colonial and postcolonial periods. As urban-based institutions, hospitals were and remain important to social and economic change in Southeast Asia in the same way cities have been important. The economic factor, relative to race, is particularly salient in the postcolonial period, when governments in the region typically represented the majority ethnic group, although race politics have continued to be important in state policy toward minorities.

Hospitals as Nodes of Modernity

A social history of hospitals in Southeast Asia reveals how the colonial powers, while motivated by profit, were not disinterested in making policy interventions in health care. Health policy in the twentieth century was organized around rationalist-scientific principles of governance. Drawing from James Scott, hospitals were not only intended to cure or prevent illness (to tame nature), but also to transform human nature—in this case people's attitudes toward matters of life and death.[24]

The origins of modern hospitals and asylums lay in developments in germ research in Europe. The new idea of contagion was not uncontested there, but gradually it superseded preexisting notions of disease, particularly miasma theory. Germ theory, bolstered by a series of groundbreaking discoveries of the role played by pathogens, cultivated a view among Western specialists that disease could be understood only through rigorous, empirical research based on the scientific method. In Britain, medical institutions such as the London School of Hygiene and Tropical Medicine, Liverpool School of Tropical Medicine, Pathology Institute, and Institute of Medical Research applied the new method to what were thought to be tropical diseases. Increasingly, colonial governors and "men on the spot" (local European officials and merchants) viewed Southeast Asia as an unsafe tropical world.[25] It is unclear how far developments in germ research affected the imperialist wave of the second half of the nineteenth century, sometimes called the New Imperialism, which precipitated crises and conflicts in north Burma, Aceh, Bali, Luzon, the Malay states, and Vietnam—although Siam survived the Paknam Crisis of 1893. Local developments in politics and commerce probably were more important. But the new ideas were significant after the colonization of the region, when the imperial powers viewed Asian peoples as carriers of disease who had unsanitary ways of life and cultural habits.

Prior to the New Imperialism, European physicians in Southeast Asia had shown a keen interest in local traditions of health care, which had over time been influenced by Chinese, Ayurvedic, and Indian medicine. Although biomedicine gained ascendancy beginning in the late nineteenth century, the process was neither linear nor uncontested. In Indonesia, European physicians remained somewhat less confident about biomedicine and retained an interest in indigenous medicine until the 1930s, although the influence of biomedicine undoubtedly grew over time. The physicians continued to obtain their knowledge of local herbs through patients, local physicians, vendors in the marketplace, and women of Indo-European descent. The women were fluent speakers of Javanese and Malay who were in frequent contact with vendors, merchants, and Chinese pharmacists. They used their knowledge to produce homemade prescriptions—which were a hybrid of Western and local medicine—for the Indonesian middle class. This was an example of a more equal form of medical interaction between the metropole and colony occurring at the local level. The accumulated knowledge of local medicine also had a long-term impact in Indonesia: it became relevant after the country's independence in 1949 when, pressed by economic necessity, the Sukarno government promoted the use of *jamu*, or traditional medicine.[26]

In the early decades of the twentieth century, the modernizing imperative of colonial medicine was expressed in discourses of hygiene and personal responsibility. According to Michael Worboys, the focus prior to World War I was on European health, but subsequently it included the health of locals, with whom Europeans worked in proximity. The war made the Europeans realize that their troops needed to adapt to the local environment in order to operate effectively. The change in emphasis was also due to the establishment of Western-financed mines and plantations in Southeast Asia, where European managers and Asian migrant workers lived close together; as well as to the growth of cities as centers of administration, trade, and immigration.[27] In the 1920s, ideas of trusteeship and dual mandate also emerged in Britain, giving colonial powers the responsibility to preserve local culture while helping the natives develop economically and culturally.[28] Broadly, the shift in health policy was part of the transition of colonial governance from indirect (although usually binding) influence to direct rule. In addition to the state factor, transnational organizations such as the League of Nations and the Rockefeller Foundation also promoted public health measures in the 1930s. Their guiding belief, like that of Western policy makers, was that native bodies could be purified.[29]

These developments created an official interest in knowing and intervening in local society. Hospitals and asylums encouraged individuals to be responsible for their hygiene and well-being. Curative institutions thus practiced public health programs. Patients and inmates were urged to keep their bodies and their immediate living environments clean, and to participate in constructive economic, cultural, and recreational activities. In Malaya, the 1920s witnessed the development of public health programs against tuberculosis, venereal disease, yaws, beriberi, and hookworm.[30] Different circumstances existed in Thailand, which was unique in Southeast Asia in that it remained free from formal colonial rule. Nevertheless, the country still received Western economic and cultural influences, and the Thai state also embraced the intervention-reform imperative of the Western powers. For the state, pursuing the modernization program was a diplomatic move to maintain the country's independence. Like colonies in the region, Thailand embraced Western ideas of health care and accepted a recipient position in the transnational health system, mirroring the unequal relationship between metropole and colony that prevailed elsewhere. The state attempted to establish a nationwide system of health services, including hospitals. These efforts were part of a broader effort to project the country's progressive image, but were also ways of reforming Thai society.[31]

The period after World War II saw an enlargement of the role played by hospitals and asylums. The appearance of ambitious medical development plans—which included the building, rebuilding, and expansion of institutions—was a means to rejuvenate Western colonial confidence and legitimacy following the defeat by Japan during the war. The Colonial Welfare and Development Act funded medical and other welfare programs in the British colonies with a yearly endowment of £120 million, which was often inadequate.[32] In Malaya, these programs, as Tim Harper surmises, nevertheless constituted a form of welfare state imperialism, intended to restore credibility to the colonial regime.[33]

The colonial factor was reinforced by a new belief, prevalent in the postwar period, in the possibility of attaining social progress through the application of technology and expertise. This belief was grounded in modernization theory, whose premises were universality, rationality, and urgency. Crucially, the postwar medical plans, particularly in the British colonies, were framed within discourses of crisis, which emphasized how health conditions had deteriorated to dangerous levels due to the growth of slums and unauthorized settlements. These discourses are traceable to the view of the pathogenic city that emerged in industrializing and urbanizing Europe in the nineteenth century, which postulated undesirable links between health and the urban environment. Belatedly transferred to postwar Southeast Asia, the idea of urban pathology formulated similarly dire connections between housing, water, and sanitation. The purpose, however, was to meet the perceived challenges of the postwar period.[34] Colonial regimes utilized and propagated these discourses, but the original advocates were Anglo-American planners with transnational experiences and expertise. They proposed that a framework of master planning and zoned urban development would not only remove health hazards to the city, attributed to cholera, tuberculosis, and other epidemic diseases, but also fashion responsible citizens.[35] The 1951 United Nations Mission of Experts to South and Southeast Asia, led by American planner Jacob Crane, warned about the "ravages of tuberculosis" caused by living in congested slums and urban kampongs. In underlining the health benefits of proper planning, the mission ignored differing cultural attitudes in the region towards modern concrete housing. It urged that public housing development, although expensive, would be "a sound investment for good citizenship."[36] Although slums and squatter settlements were indeed expanding after the war, they had been a feature of the development and urbanization of prewar Southeast Asia. The discourses of crisis were not so much a response to health problems, but a way to articulate and achieve new social aims.[37]

Another feature of health policy in the postwar period was, as Sunil Amrith demonstrates, the renewal of transnational campaigns to make the world safe from disease. This effort, spearheaded by the World Health Organization (WHO), targeted the "Big Four" diseases: malaria, venereal disease, leprosy, and tuberculosis. Public hospitals, clinics, and asylums were crucial nodes of the WHO's disease prevention and eradication programs; they were gathering points for Western professional expertise, which then penetrated local communities and rural areas. As in urban planning, these efforts were framed within outwardly neutral discourses about scientific expertise and universal applicability—that health issues could be resolved through the use of technology and technical expertise, such as the use of DDT. As Anglo-American housing discourses lauded the merits of master planning and zoning, the WHO's appeal to universalism also ignored cultural differences and was based on an overly optimistic faith in the role of technology.[38] The Orientalist discourses of the late nineteenth century had stressed backward natives with insanitary habits to legitimize the New Imperialism. Likewise, the language of health and housing in the postwar years prepared for colonial retreat by highlighting the universality of Western values and institutions.

The programming of hospitals and asylums as part of ambitious development plans were not merely a colonial process. The postcolonial states of Southeast Asia retained the focus on hospitals and curative medicine that was a hallmark of Western colonial practice.[39] As transnational nodes of modernity, hospitals and asylums bridged the colonial-independence divide that typically marks the political history of modern Southeast Asia. Historians of medicine have more commonly studied the colonial era, with a focus on race, whereas the post-independence period has been less understood, partly due to a lack of primary sources. However, if, as Peter Boomgaard suggests, the medicalization of states in the region is a continuing process, we may see it as a meandering process that extends into the postcolonial period.[40] At some point when the Western regimes abandoned the attempt to reimpose colonial rule, they viewed health programs as projects of orderly decolonization through social policy means. To Western planners, the reform of health services and institutions in the colonies would create viable postcolonial states and safeguard Western interests in the region.[41]

Even in the colonial period, local doctors had shared some similarities with their Western counterparts. Indonesian doctors were as insensitive to cultural difference as European doctors in treating their patients.[42] Filipino physicians embraced the values and methods of their American counterparts, with one notable exception: they were less concerned with racial difference than with class divides.[43] Plausibly, race became a less important factor in health policy in the post-independence years. The transition to independence produced loud noises about the travails of colonial domination, but postcolonial elites retained in large part the centralized administration they inherited. As David Arnold points out, all medicine colonizes, not only colonial medicine.[44] As part of the bureaucracy, public hospitals and asylums were useful for spearheading new projects of national integration and social mobilization. To some extent, the postcolonial states of Southeast Asia resembled the welfare states that were being established in Europe at the time. Policy makers in both regions targeted, as stated in Britain's Beveridge report, the five "Giant Evils": idleness, squalor, want, ignorance, and disease. In arousing people from allegedly idle or squalid states, postcolonial health programs intervened into daily life, as colonial policy had hitherto sought to do. There was also a similar economic motive: postcolonial planners, like their colonial predecessors, viewed public health expenditure not as a burden on the budget but as a form of investment in the nation's development.[45] In Singapore, which appealed to foreign capital investment, public hospitals functioned as part of a national system of health care designed to produce and maintain establish a healthy workforce for foreign industries.[46] In different ways, the postcolonial states of Southeast Asia embraced and adapted modernization theory.

The nature of this postcolonial relationship with biomedicine—partly through so-called colonial inheritance and partly through contemporary Western experts—remains a matter of debate. Some authors have pointed to the continuing influence of neocolonialism. Higginbotham and Marsella argue that local practitioners on mental health care in Southeast Asia occupy a subordinate position in unequal professional networks that are dominated by Western experts. The result has been to privilege biomedicine and institutionalization over traditional treatment and community and family care for the mentally ill.[47] By contrast, Anderson has emphasized the need not to depict the colonial/postcolonial world as a passive receptacle for Western medicine in national history accounts.[48]

Notwithstanding continuing and frequently strong Western influences, Southeast Asian policy makers and planners have adapted the colonial legacy. In the 1970s, hospitals in Thailand and the Philippines facilitated the penetration of health care into local areas, as younger doctors practiced community-based methods of reaching less accessible populations.[49] From the 1980s, the role of the state in Southeast Asia began to diminish as ideas about the corporatization and privatization of health care gained popularity, first in Singapore and subsequently in other countries that followed the city-state's example in reforming its health system. Malaysia, for instance, followed Singapore's approach in corporatizing its public hospitals.[50] The shift to corporatization and privatization could be traced to several factors, some of which were internal, such as demands for better quality care among the rising middle class. The state also sought to tap private capital and expertise, to retain doctors in the public sector, and to free up the budget for other uses.[51] Conflict, as in Indochina between the 1950s and 1970s, hampered the development of national systems of medical care in some parts of mainland Southeast Asia.[52] In Vietnam, Laos, and Cambodia, communist states also embraced privatization and corporatization as part of the transition toward a market-centered economy in the 1980s and 1990s.[53] However, these developments also had a transnational dimension: they mirrored, if not closely followed, trends in the West that saw the expansion of neoliberal ideas of economic development, the dismantling of the welfare state, and the transformation of health care into an industry in the United States and Britain from the beginning of the 1980s.

Leprosaria as Sanctuary, Hospital, Prison, and Laboratory

The leprosaria of Southeast Asia shared many aspects of the history of hospitals. In addition, as places of segregation, they assumed the roles of sanctuary, hospital, prison, and social laboratory. In Malaya, segregation quickly became the basis of a new policy toward leprosy, following the discovery of the bacillus *Mycobacterium leprae* by G. A. Hansen in 1873. By the 1890s, international anxiety over contagion had precipitated local fears over the so-called leprosy problem, although there had been no discernible increase in the number of admissions into the asylums. Nonetheless, the Straits Settlements government decided in 1898 to confine all sufferers in an asylum until they were cured, to bar them from occupations that made them more likely to spread the disease, and to punish those who sheltered or employed them. This draconian approach departed from the earlier British policy of removing vagrants and the destitute from public places. The policy of segregation was implemented—albeit later, in 1923—in the Federated Malay States. In the early decades of the twentieth century, the number of inmates in the asylums in Singapore, Penang, and the Federated Malay States grew, and a large asylum cum hospital was established at Sungai Buloh, at the outskirts of Kuala Lumpur, in 1930. Built on the concept of an open settlement, it was euphemistically termed "The Valley of Hope." Most of the patients interred in the leprosaria were Chinese, male, and of working-class background, but their numbers grew rapidly enough to cause severe overcrowding by the 1930s.[54]

By contrast, the French colonial regime's approach toward leprosy in Cambodia was far less comprehensive and invasive. On the one hand, as in Malaya, sufferers were also mandatorily separated from society by law. In 1903, the first leprosarium in the country was opened at Culao Rong; a decree was passed six years later for the detention of sufferers and the building of asylums to accommodate them. On the other hand, the implementation of the policy was less rigorous than in Malaya. Patients who could guarantee their livelihood without work were allowed to remain at home. This created a bias in the policy against the lower-income group. Women, as in Malaya, were underrepresented in Culao Rong and also in the village-style settlement at Troeung, established in 1916. As Sokhieng Au suggests, French doctors did not know how to gain medical access to the female body.[55] The difference between Malaya and Cambodia may be due to context. British policy was influenced by the political economy of the Straits Settlements and west Malaya: separating healthy and unhealthy bodies was deemed crucial for fast-developing export economies based in the cities, mines, and plantations, where large numbers of workers lived together. The formation of the Federated Malay States in 1895, replacing indirect influence with a more centralized system, showed a colonial appetite for social control and intervention. By contrast, the main pillar of development in Cambodia—tenant-based rice cultivation—did not provoke such anxieties about the connection between economic and medical health.

From the 1920s, received wisdom on healthy and hygienic bodies was implemented in leprosaria in Southeast Asia. The aim was not only to keep society safe from disease, but to purify the bodies and minds of the sufferers in the absence of a medical cure. The new approach was part of an international shift in attitudes toward the control of leprosy. In some countries, a more humane and realistic policy had emerged, based on the argument that leprosy was not really contagious. At the start of the twentieth century, laws of mandatory segregation were repealed in the Philippines, Indochina, and India. In Malaya, the idea was discussed, although ultimately the legislation was retained. The British Empire Leprosy Relief Association attempted to soften attitudes toward segregation throughout the colonies. It urged that leprosy was not very contagious and that a hygienic, non-prisonlike living environment be created in the asylum. Such a view grew partly out of the perception that like tuberculosis, leprosy was a disease of the environment. However, the association also supported draconian measures that characterized this phase of leprosy control, particularly the removal of children from parents with leprosy and the use of chaulmoogra therapy. In Trafalgar, Singapore, Kuang Wee Kee and his co-inmates endured such painful yet ineffective hypodermic treatment.[56] In any case, the association's positive efforts did not last, partly because softening the policy of segregation revived anxieties about the resurgence of the disease. Hampered, too, by financial crises in the 1920s and 1930s, official policy returned largely to segregation by the time war broke out in Europe. What the efforts of the 1920s clearly sought to accomplish was to transform the leprosarium from an almshouse, where inmates were safe but otherwise left to themselves, to a micro-agricultural or industrial settlement where they were organized, and more generally to a social laboratory and model for the outside world.[57]

This was the case in the Philippines, where a leprosarium was established on the remote island of Culion in 1904. Even when segregation was no longer mandated, as Anderson surmises, the institution functioned as a laboratory of citizenship under the umbrella of American colonial tutelage. Here, as elsewhere in the region, confinement was intended to be a liberating experience for Filipinos. Institutional life was closely ordered, with a focus on engineering people from different parts of a socially diverse country into modern Filipinos. The highlight of the American experiment was having the residents govern themselves—in effect, having them institutionalize their own confinement. Culion had its own elected mayor and patients' council, and from 1908 onward women could vote. The leprosarium became an experiment in Philippines self-government, as the United States sought to absolve itself of charges of colonialism. The American regime was so concerned with leprosy that more than a third of the public health budget was allocated to Culion—while the fight against tuberculosis, which killed far more people, received much less official support.[58] Other leprosaria in Southeast Asia also organized elected, self-governing councils, in addition to inmates doubling up as (poorly paid) guards, teachers, medical attendants, and gardeners, but none of these citizenship experiments took place as early and comprehensively as in the Philippines. In the transnational flow of ideas and practices, Anderson points out that Culion's experience also influenced the management of American leprosaria in Molokai and Carville.[59]

In Malaya, the authorities also dreamed of how "[t]he transition from an unkempt, filthy, hunted looking leper . . . to a clean, skin-whole, self-respecting member of an organized community is in most cases a matter of some weeks only."[60] In the absence of a cure for leprosy until after World War II, the poetics of hygiene and individual responsibility were expedient in rationalizing the indefinite segregation of patients. They were exhorted to properly organize their lives—to bathe regularly, rear livestock or engage in some form of paid work, and participate in sports and other meaningful sociocultural activities—within the walls of the asylums, of course. Sungai Buloh even issued its own currency to prevent money passing outside the institution. In effect, such practices urged the sufferers to imagine their independence and integrity while locked up within the asylum.

The other innovation of the early decades of the twentieth century was to keep newborns safe from their parents, although there was little compelling evidence that the babies were at risk. At Culion, they were not separated from their parents at birth, but when they had grown into young children.[61] In Malaya, they were passed along to healthy relatives, or—if this was not possible—given to voluntary associations and subsequently put up for adoption. This has created a splinter of history that is transnational—in my research on leprosy in Malaya and Singapore, I discovered that some of these children were adopted by expatriates and brought up outside their birth countries. The search for their biological parents and personal identity has brought some of these children, now adults, back to Malaysia.[62] But there are still many aging former patients who are living in asylums in Malaysia and Singapore, who have never been contacted by their children.

New Cultures of Healing

The international ideas of health care that passed through hospitals and asylums had a significant impact on local health traditions. Indigenous medicine in Southeast Asia was not an unchanging entity: over time, it had been influenced by various foreign traditions.[63] Nevertheless, the dominance of biomedicine in the twentieth century had qualitatively changed the nature of the encounters between the ill and their healers. In precolonial Indonesia and Cambodia, for instance, recovery from illness involved more than receiving diagnosis and pre-scription from an expert: it was also a ritualistic process in which the sick person had to participate to obtain his or her own recovery.[64] In colonial Cambodia, many people viewed doctors as mere dispensers of drugs and regarded the theory of contagion as mystical and unconvincing.[65]

Boomgaard has rightly observed that precolonial and contemporary indig-enous traditions are not the same.[66] However, when used with caution, anthro-pological studies of current local practices may throw useful light on precolonial traditions, about which there is insufficient written record. These studies suggest that Western medicine did change local attitudes. In precolonial Southeast Asia, it seems that sufferers of mental illness and leprosy did not confront the degree of social stigma that was heightened by the theory of contagion and the act of segregating sufferers in the colonial and postcolonial periods. In Laos and other countries in Southeast Asia, although mental illness was associated with spirit causes and magical cures, the sufferer was not blamed for his or her condition and continued to receive the care and protection of family and community.[67] Stigma against leprosy was not a Western creation either: it has existed in preco-lonial Southeast Asia, China, and India, although its intensity varied according to context.[68] In colonial Cambodia, leprosy sufferers at Troeung worshipped the old legend of the Leper King, despite the Buddhist injunction in favor of perfect bodies.[69] Cambodians and Malays who suffered from leprosy were frequently still accepted as part of the community and were not cast out from the village or confined in an institution.[70] Part of the reason Malays were underrepresented in mental and leprosy asylums was the availability of community and family care. It was also because as foreign imports, the institutions for a long time did not address their cultural needs, such as that for halal food.[71] Many Malays were also suspicious of hospitals: in response to cholera outbreaks, the British govern-ment had to build isolation houses for Malay sufferers; the alternative would have been to force them to be admitted into hospitals.[72] Hospitals and asylums were distinctly Western creations that demonstrated the logic, failure, and stigma of biomedicine.

Nonetheless, the response of local people to biomedicine has been nuanced and pragmatic. They variously retained, adapted, or transformed their cultures of healing, which differed from Western forms since they were defined by local circumstances and constraints. Still, Southeast Asian practices remained entan-gled with biomedicine in terms of optimism about coping with illness and get-ting well. Part of the reason for the underutilization of modern medical services in the developing areas of the region, such as urban slums or rural areas, was practical and economic: high costs, physical inaccessibility, inadequate staffing, and ineffective treatment still deter many locals from using hospitals.[73] In rural Sabah, access to district hospitals, dispensaries, outpatient clinics, and maternal and child clinics in the 1980s varied according to the quality of roads, availability of transport, and physical distance.[74] In other cases, however, Southeast Asians based their choice of medical treatment on their own experiences and the experiences of people they knew.[75] To some extent, the conflict between traditional medicine and biomedicine has been overstated and ignores the ways Southeast Asians move fluidly between them.

Practical problems have at times been surmounted. In rural Indonesia, nurses have appropriated doctors' expertise to treat people, thus operating beyond their formal role as carers. In response, many villagers came to trust both the nurses' ability and the efficacy of biomedicine.[76] In one study, villagers in Sasak, Indonesia, viewed traditional medicine and biomedicine as complementary. Many of them possessed a faith in biomedicine as an authoritative form of health care. They typically obtained their prescriptions from a pharmacy, rather than the hospital, where the experience was culturally alienating and bureaucratic. Other villagers were found to be more skeptical because Western medicine was less affordable: they chose to retain customary methods that revolved around practices of sorcery and rituals.[77] In another study in Singapore, a very different urban context, a similar form of medical pluralism existed. Singaporeans typically use Chinese, Ayurvedic, Malay, and Sidda Vaidya forms of traditional medicine and biomedicine, or tried one when the other had been ineffective. Many Singaporeans viewed Western and Chinese medicine as opposed yet complementary: the former was regarded as useful for diagnosis, the latter for treatment. Others were critical of young Western-trained doctors' detachment in dealing with patients. For some Singaporeans, visiting general practitioners or hospitals was not necessarily driven by a belief in Western medicine, but by the need to obtain an acceptable medical certificate for employers and schools.[78]

Differences within social groups and communities underline how medical traditions and modern medicine interact to create historical change. The process is nonlinear and is determined by local circumstances and individual and community factors. A number of developments have taken place in Vietnam since the 1980s as a result of the *doi moi* program of economic decentralization, where the state's role has shaped Vietnamese responses. The move to privatized health care has meant that medical services were being more frequently utilized by higher-income groups, and people increasingly preferred private clinics and practitioners to the commune health centers that were established under socialist rule. Formal, urban services were also being sought after by medical insurance enrollees, who were likely to be civil servants, urban residents, and salaried employees—and generally middle class. Higher-income Vietnamese have sought better health care, and the average length of hospital stays increased in the 1990s.[79]

An anthropological study of contemporary attitudes in Indonesia underlines Southeast Asians' sophistication in their responses towards biomedicine. In a nutrition clinic based in a hospital in Yogyakarta, a meeting between a Western-trained local doctor and patients from the nearby urban kampong produced contested transcripts on the relative roles of biomedicine and traditional medicine at the community level. On the one hand, the doctor attempted, à la Foucault, to emplot the patient's descriptions of their condition and lifestyle within the biomedical tradition. He prescribed not only medical remedies but also regimes of self-control or discipline: that is, what the patient must do or avoid in order to get well. On the other hand, the patients countered with subversive interpretations and objections, in effect undermining and transforming the professional discourse. Their responses were ways of negotiating between medical expertise, personal belief, and the daily challenges faced by an urban community. They reconciled between biomedicine and their cultural belief that illness was variously due to natural causes, other humans, spirits, and themselves. They maintained that illness is inevitable and were skeptical about the possibility of prevention and cure that the doctor suggested. For Javanese, recovering from illness was not merely about taking drugs, but making non-medicinal efforts to get well, in which one succeeds with the grace of God. According to the study, "[t]he clinical encounter is usually unfinished business," leaving the physician's attempts at emplotment and hegemony frustrated. Among older patients, who had experienced the lack of Western health care in the colonial and early postcolonial periods, biomedicine was simply an addition to existing medical traditions.[80] Such views did not constitute fatalism or ignorance, but were logical in accepting one's constraints and existing circumstances.

In the asylums of Southeast Asia, patient cultures emerged over time that thwarted the discipline of the gatekeepers and improved the actual lived experiences of the residents. Similar developments have occurred in mental and leprosy asylums outside of Southeast Asia.[81] As Anderson discovers, Culion was a classic total institution, expressed in its similarity to an army camp and an American small town. This veneer of progressive modernity belied the experience of many inmates, for whom it was the "Island of Pain." But even here, American-prescribed modernity suffered occasional rupture. In the 1930s, the residents contested the authority of the management by drawing up a petition and organizing a public hearing to demand the rights to movement and marriage.[82]

Patient cultures were, however, more commonly expressed in acts of agency and passive resistance in everyday life over the long haul. "Weapons of the weak" helped transform the experience and meaning of living indefinitely within an institution. They included privately circulating oral transcripts such as gossip, rumors, and complaints, but also actual resistance to work, occupational therapy and treatment, escaping from the asylum, and participating in social activities that verged on the morally reprehensible and even illegal.[83] In Malaysia and Singapore, long-term residents viewed Sungai Buloh and Trafalgar as constituting their own country, built and run by their own efforts. In the colonial period, inmates organized secret societies (which at times fought among themselves), smoked opium, and sang communist songs. In the post-independence years, social gambling, hawking, and moonshining constituted the underside of life in the asylum. Yet social and cultural life was not always counter-hegemonic, for the residents also organized and joined cultural dance, song, and music groups. Over time, many of them accepted roles as patient-workers in the institution.[84] For long-term residents and married couples, the leprosy shelter lost its roles as hospitals, prisons, and even safe havens, but had become their homes.

In Cambodia, segregation was complicated by the country's traumatic passage from colony to nationhood. In the late colonial period, Troeung, unlike Culion, was not a total institution but a forgotten place as the policy of segregation was withdrawn and inmates were left to their own devices. As Au notes, the institution was "a failure in the exercise in modernity." Nevertheless, leprosy became a state concern again after World War II, and the postcolonial regime revived the French policy of segregation into the 1960s.[85] With the country's entanglement in the Vietnam conflict, the inmates endured a decrease in medical and food supply under the Khmer Republic, and lived in constant fear of American bombings. In the Pol Pot era, the regime forced patients into unsafe and hazardous medical experiments, as the asylum was converted into a concentration camp. Many of them were killed in a massacre of the camp's inmates in 1976, but some survived. The hospital at Troeung continued to operate during the Khmer Rouge period, and also treated cancer patients, and Troeung itself reopened in 1979. Many of the survivors of that period continued to do quarry work, although at risk of damaging their limbs. Yet despite the grim history of both country and asylum, some residents still asserted their agency in their desire to return home and in teaching fellow residents.[86]

Conclusion

The patient cultures and cultures of healing in the leprosaria have negative sides: cured sufferers decided to remain within the asylum because of the rejection they encountered outside, yet their self-institutionalization and identification as a closed group have made their return to society even more difficult. In some cases, family members had been ready to accept them, but the residents have preferred to be with people with whom they shared binding experiences.[87] Their ability to establish a viable community within the asylum has come at a price of their continued isolation outside of it. Local responses are ultimately constrained by long-term transnational and national developments in the policy of segregation. It is in subjective meaning and interpersonal relations that individual and community experiences are at times qualitatively independent and liberating.

The function of leprosaria as a node of modernity in Southeast Asia is quickly disappearing. Leprosy is still a medical issue in some countries, but it is conceivable that the disease will no longer be a major health problem in the near future, as inexpensive drugs become more widely available to sufferers. As in other parts of the world, asylums are or will be summarily forgotten, demolished, or converted to new uses, both medical and non-medical. This has already happened in Singapore and Malaysia. The needs and rights, too, of dwindling numbers of active and cured patients risk being ignored as budgets shrink and patients face relocation to new housing and settlements.

In contrast, hospitals in the region will continue to evolve and expand their roles. The trend toward privatization and corporatization underlines how Southeast Asians are being socialized as world citizens to adapt to the imperatives of the global capitalist economy. The retreat of the welfare state is uneven and fraught with difficulties in implementation and securing popular support in countries like Indonesia, Malaysia, the Philippines, and even Singapore.[88] But it shows how Southeast Asian lives are being integrated into the transnational flows of capital even when they are ill. National boundaries have become more porous than before, as states themselves pursue neoliberal programs of development. This new phase of transnationalism extends from the social history of hospitals and asylums in Southeast Asia in the twentieth century. These institutions had assisted the transformation of natives and Asian sojourners into the subjects and labor force of new states and primary export economies dominated by Western capital during the colonial era, and into worker-citizens of nation-states and industrial economies in the postcolonial period. As health care decisions are increasingly overlaid by questions of how and how much Southeast Asians should organize their adult lives—to work, save, and pay for illness—the nexus between the international and local will be of even greater importance within the framework of the global economy of the twenty-first century.

Notes

1. Loh Kah Seng, *Making and Unmaking the Asylum: Leprosy and Modernity in Singapore and Malaysia* (Petaling Jaya, Malaysia: SIRD, 2009).

2. Warwick Anderson, "Where Is the Postcolonial History of Medicine?" *Bulletin of the History of Medicine* 72, no. 3 (1998): 522–30; also "Going through the Motions: American Public Health and Colonial 'Mimicry,'" *American Literary History* 14, no. 4 (2002): 686–719.

3. See, for instance, Lenore Manderson, *Sickness and the State: Health and Illness in Colonial Malaya, 1870–1940* (New York: Cambridge University Press, 1996); Michael Worboys, "The Colonial World as Mission and Mandate: Leprosy and Empire, 1900–1940," *Osiris* 2nd ser., 15 (2000): 207–18.

4. Vinh-Kim Nyugen and Karine Peschard, "Anthropology, Inequality, and Disease: A Review," *Annual Review of Anthropology* 32 (2003): 447–74.

5. Erving Goffman, *Asylums: Essays on the Social Situation of Mental Patients and Other Inmates* (New York: Doubleday, 1961).

6. Richard Keller, "Madness and Colonization: Psychiatry in the British and French Empires, 1800–1962," *Journal of Social History* 35, no. 2 (2001): 295–326.

7. Milton Lewis, Scott Bamber, and Michael Waugh, eds., *Sex, Disease and Society: A Comparative History of Sexually Transmitted Diseases and HIV/AIDS in Asia and the Pacific* (Westport, CT: Greenwood Press, 1997).

8. Mary Douglas, "Witchcraft and Leprosy: Two Strategies of Exclusion," *Man*, n.s. 26 (1991): 723–36.

9. Manderson, *Sickness and the State*.

10. Peter Boomgaard, "Writing Medical Histories of Southeast Asia: Comparative Approaches to Health, Disease, and Healing," in *Colonial Medicine in Spanish Philippines*, ed. Raquel A. G. Reyes (Manila: Ateneo de Manila University Press, forthcoming); Manderson, *Sickness and the State*; Liew Kai Khiun, "Terribly Severe Though Mercifully Short: The Episode of the 1918 Influenza in British Malaya," *Modern Asian Studies* 41, no. 2 (2007): 221–52; David G. Marr, "Vietnamese Attitudes Regarding Illness and Healing," in *Death and Disease in Southeast Asia: Explorations in Social, Medical and Demographic History*, ed. Norman G. Owen (Singapore: Oxford University Press, 1987), 162–86.

11. Manderson, *Sickness and the State*.

12. Manderson, *Sickness and the State*.

13. Liew, "Terribly Severe Though Mercifully Short," 221–52; Manderson, *Sickness and the State*.

14. Reynaldo C. Ileto, "Cholera and the Origins of the American Sanitary Order in the Philippines," in *Discrepant Histories: Translocal Essays on Filipino Cultures*, ed. Vicente L. Rafael (Manila: Anvil, 1995).

15. Sokhieng Au, *Mixed Medicines: Health and Culture in French Colonial Cambodia* (Chicago and London: University of Chicago Press, 2011).

16. Marr, "Vietnamese Attitudes Regarding Illness and Healing."

17. Manderson, *Sickness and the State*.

18. Manderson, *Sickness and the State*; Kathryn M. Robinson, "Village Health Services and the Indonesian Family Planning Program," in *The Political Economy of Primary Health Care in Southeast Asia*, ed. Paul Cohen and John Purcal (Canberra: Australian Development Studies Network, Australian National University, 1989), 149–58; Amarjit Kaur, "Indian Labour, Labour Standards, and Workers' Health in Burma and Malaya, 1900–1940," *Modern Asian Studies* 40, no. 2 (2006): 425–75; J. Norman Parmer, "Estate Workers' Health in the Federated Malay States in the 1920s," in *The Underside of Malaysian History: Pullers, Prostitutes, Plantation Workers*, ed. Peter J. Rimmer and Lisa M. Allen (Singapore: Singapore University Press, 1990), 179–92.

19. Rosalia Sciortino, "Rural Nurses and Doctors: The Discrepancy between Western Concepts and Javanese Practices," in Boomgaard et al., *Health Care in Java: Past and Present*, 111–29.

20. Boomgaard, "Writing Medical Histories of Southeast Asia."

21. Nyugen and Peschard, "Anthropology, Inequality, and Disease"

22. Mary Douglas, *Purity and Danger: An Analysis of the Concepts of Pollution and Taboo* (London: Routledge Classics, 2002).

23. Manderson, *Sickness and the State*.

24. James C. Scott, *Seeing Like a State: How Certain Schemes to Improve the Human Condition Have Failed* (New Haven, CT: Yale University Press, 1998).

25. Manderson, *Sickness and the State*.

26. Hans Pols, "European Physicians and Botanists, Indigenous Herbal Medicine in the Dutch East Indies, and Colonial Networks of Mediation," *East Asia Science, Technology and Society: An International Journal* 3 (2009): 173–208.

27. Manderson, *Sickness and the State*.

28. Worboys, "The Colonial World as Mission and Mandate."

29. Sunil S. Amrith, *Decolonizing International Health: India and Southeast Asia, c. 1930–1965* (Basingstoke, UK: Palgrave MacMillan, 2006).

30. Manderson, *Sickness and the State.*

31. Davisakd Puaksom, "Of Germs, Public Hygiene, and the Healthy Body: The Making of the Medicalizing State in Thailand," *The Journal of Asian Studies* 66, no. 2 (2007): 311–44.

32. Michael Ashley Havinden and David Meredith, *Colonialism and Development: Britain and Its Tropical Colonies, 1850–1960* (London and New York: Routledge, 1993).

33. T. N. Harper, "The Politics of Disease and Disorder in Post-War Malaya," *Journal of Southeast Asian Studies* 21, no. 1 (1990): 88–113.

34. Manderson, *Sickness and the State.*

35. Loh Kah Seng, *Squatters into Citizens: The 1961 Bukit Ho Swee Fire and the Making of Modern Singapore* (Singapore: NUS Press and ASAA Southeast Asia Publications Series, 2013).

36. United Nations Mission of Experts, *Low Cost Housing in South and Southeast Asia*, ST/SOA/3/Rev.1 (New York: United Nations, 1951), 10–11, 20, 142, 163.

37. Loh, *Making and Unmaking the Asylum.*

38. Amrith, *Decolonizing International Health.*

39. World Health Organization, *Collaboration in Health Development in South-East Asia 1948–88, Fortieth Anniversary Volume* (New Delhi: World Health Organization, 1988).

40. Boomgaard, "Writing Medical Histories of Southeast Asia."

41. Nicholas Tarling, *The Fall of Imperial Britain in South-East Asia* (Singapore: Oxford University Press, 1993).

42. Terence H. Hull, "Plague in Java," in *Death and Disease in Southeast Asia: Explorations in Social, Medical and Demographic History*, ed. Norman G. Owen (Singapore: Oxford University Press, 1987): 210–30.

43. Anderson, "Going through the Motions."

44. David Arnold, *Colonizing the Body: State Medicine and Epidemic Disease in Nineteenth-Century India* (Berkeley: University of California Press, 1993).

45. Paul Cohen and John Purcal, eds., *The Political Economy of Primary Health Care in Southeast Asia* (Canberra: Australian Development Studies Network, Australian National University, 1989).

46. John T. Purcal, "Some Aspects of the Political Economy of Health and Development in Singapore," in *The Political Economy of Primary Health Care in Southeast Asia*, ed. Paul Cohen and John Purcal (Canberra: Australian Development Studies Network, Australian National University, 1989), 124–39.

47. Nick Higginbotham and Anthony J. Marsella, "International Consultation and the Homogenization of Psychiatry in Southeast Asia," *Social Science and Medicine* 27, no. 5 (1998): 553–61.

48. Anderson, "Where Is the Postcolonial History of Medicine?" "Going through the Motions."

49. Paul Cohen and John Purcal, eds., *Health and Development in South East Asia* (Canberra: Australian Development Studies Network, 1995).

50. Simon Barraclough, "Constraints on the Retreat from a Welfare-Orientated Approach to Public Health Care in Malaysia," *Health Policy* 47 (1999): 53–67; Kai Hong Phua, "Attacking Hospital Performance on Two Fronts: Network Corporatization and Financing Reforms in Singapore," in *Innovations in Health Service Delivery: The Corporatization of Public Hospitals*, ed. Alexander S. Preker and April Harding (Washington, DC: World Bank, 2003), 451–84.

51. Virasakdi Chongsuvivatwong, Kai Hong Phua, Mui Teng Yap, et al., "Health and Health-Care Systems in Southeast Asia: Diversity and Transitions," *Lancet* 377 (January 29, 2011): 429–37; Rozita Halina Tun Hussein, Syed Al-Junid, Soe Nyunt-U, Yahaya Baba, and Wil-

ly De Geyndt, "Corporatization of a Single Facility: Reforming the Malaysian National Heart Institute," *Innovations in Health Service Delivery: The Corporatization of Public Hospitals,* ed. Alexander S. Preker and April Harding (Washington, DC: World Bank, 2003), 425–50; Phua, "Attacking Hospital Performance on Two Fronts."

52. Jan Ovesen and Ing-Britt Trankell, *Cambodians and Their Doctors: A Medical Anthropology of Colonial and Postcolonial Cambodia* (Copenhagen: NIAS, 2010).

53. Anil B. Deolalikar, "Access to Health Services by the Poor and the Non-Poor: The Case of Vietnam," *Journal of Asian and African Studies* 37 (2002): 244–61.

54. Loh, *Making and Unmaking the Asylum;* A. Joshua-Raghavar, *Leprosy in Malaysia: Past, Present, Future* (Selangor, Malaysia: A. J. Raghavar, 1983).

55. Au, *Mixed Medicines;* Ovesen and Trankell, *Cambodians and Their Doctors.*

56. Loh, *Making and Unmaking the Asylum.*

57. Worboys, "The Colonial World as Mission and Mandate."

58. Warwick Anderson, *Colonial Pathologies: American Tropical Medicine, Race, and Hygiene in the Philippines* (Durham, NC: Duke University Press, 2006).

59. Anderson, *Colonial Pathologies.*

60. Loh, *Making and Unmaking the Asylum,* 7.

61. Au, *Mixed Medicines;* Anderson, *Colonial Pathologies;* Loh, *Making and Unmaking the Asylum;* Ovesen and Trankell, *Cambodians and Their Doctors.*

62. Loh, *Making and Unmaking the Asylum.*

63. Boomgaard, "Writing Medical Histories of Southeast Asia"; Ina E. Slamet-Velsink, "Some Reflections on the Sense and Nonsense of Traditional Health Care," in *Health Care in Java: Past and Present,* ed. Peter Boomgaard, Rosalia Sciortino, and Ines Smyth (Leiden: KITLV Press, 1996), 65–80.

64. Steve Ferzacca, *Healing the Modern in a Central Javanese City* (Durham, NC: Carolina Academic Press, 2001); Ovesen and Trankell, *Cambodians and Their Doctors.*

65. Au, *Mixed Medicines.*

66. Boomgaard, "Writing Medical Histories of Southeast Asia."

67. Joseph Westermeyer, "Folk Concepts of Mental Disorder among the Lao: Continuities with Similar Concepts in Other Cultures and in Psychiatry," *Culture, Medicine and Psychiatry* 3 (1979): 301–17.

68. Loh, *Making and Unmaking the Asylum;* Jane Buckingham, *Leprosy in Colonial South India: Medicine and Confinement* (New York: Palgrave, 2002); Barbara Lovric, "Bali: Myth, Magic and Morbidity," in Owen, *Death and Disease in Southeast Asia: Explorations in Social, Medical and Demographic History,* ed. Norman G. Owen (Singapore: Oxford University Press, 1987), 117–41.

69. Ovesen and Trankell, *Cambodians and Their Doctors.*

70. Loh, *Making and Unmaking the Asylum;* Au, *Mixed Medicines.*

71. Ng Beng Yeong, *Till the Break of Day: A History of the Mental Health Services in Singapore, 1841–1993* (Singapore: Singapore University Press, 2001).

72. Manderson, *Sickness and the State.*

73. Santhat Sermsri, "Health and the Urban Poor in Bangkok," in Cohen and Purcal, *Health and Development in South East Asia,* 49–58.

74. Glen Chandler, "Access to Health Care in the Interior of Sabah," in Cohen and Purcal, *The Political Economy of Primary Health Care in Southeast Asia,* 101–23.

75. Au, *Mixed Medicines.*

76. Sciortino, "Rural Nurses and Doctors."

77. Cynthia L. Hunter, "Sorcery and Science as Competing Models of Explanation in a Sasak Village," in *Healing Powers and Modernity: Traditional Medicine, Shamanism, and Science*

in Asian Societies, ed. Linda H. Connor and Geoffrey Samuel (Westport, CT: Bergin & Garvey, 2000), 152–70.

78. Vineeta Sinha, "Theorizing the Complex Singapore Health Scene: Reconceptualizing 'Medical Pluralism'" (PhD diss., Johns Hopkins University, 1995).

79. Deolalikar, "Access to Health Services by the Poor and the Non-Poor."

80. Ferzacca, *Healing the Modern in a Central Javanese City,* 86.

81. See Zachary Gussow, *Leprosy, Racism, and Public Health: Social Policy in Chronic Disease Control* (Boulder, CO: Westview Press, 1989); Buckingham, *Leprosy in Colonial South India;* Eric Silla, *People Are Not the Same: Leprosy and Identity in Twentieth-Century Mali* (Portsmouth, NH: Heinemann, 1998).

82. Anderson, *Colonial Pathologies.*

83. James C. Scott, *Weapons of the Weak: Everyday Forms of Peasant Resistance* (New Haven, CT: Yale University Press, 1985).

84. Loh, *Making and Unmaking the Asylum.*

85. Au, *Mixed Medicines,* 178.

86. Ovesen and Trankell, *Cambodians and Their Doctors.*

87. Loh, *Making and Unmaking the Asylum.*

88. Samuel S. Lieberman and Ali Alkatiri, "Autonomization in Indonesia: The Wrong Path to Reduce Hospital Expenditures," in *Innovations in Health Service Delivery,* ed. Alexander S. Preker and April Harding (Washington, DC: World Bank, 2003), 511–32; Barraclough, "Constraints on the Retreat from a Welfare-Orientated Approach to Public Health Care in Malaysia"; Phua, "Attacking Hospital Performance on Two Fronts."

11 Healing the Nation

Politics, Medicine, and Analogies of Health in Southeast Asia

Rachel Leow

IN COLONIAL SITUATIONS around the world, the relationship among modernity, health, and political power has frequently been invoked by both colonizer and colonized. In India, for example, David Arnold has argued that introduction and spread of Western medical discourses was intended in part to demonstrate the superiority of Western science over "Eastern prejudice" and scientific inertia, to persuade through concrete practices the legitimacy of colonial rule.[1] Yet when invoked by nationalist resistance, leaders often did not dispute the scientific superiority of Western health, merely the colonial state's monopoly over it. In Vietnam, medical self-reliance was one of the most widely available forms of resistance, and in the rallying cry "hygiene is the love of one's nation" (*ve sinh la yeu nuoc*) is embedded a view of health inherited from colonial science.[2] Ruth Rogaski has traced the shifts in Chinese perceptions of what health (*weisheng*) has meant over the course of the nineteenth and twentieth centuries in engaging with Western imperial domination, and shown that in this period, notions of Chinese health were dislocated from their deep association with Chinese cosmology, and reoriented towards what she calls "hygienic modernity," comprising such concerns as bodily cleanliness, racial fitness, and national sovereignty. These new concerns, she argues, were articulated in the idiom of modern Western science, and were in fact precisely qualities that foreign observers criticized China for lacking.[3]

The fetishization of modern science in the name of the nation may be in part due to the disproportionate presence of Western-trained medical students and doctors among the ranks of pioneering Asian nationalists of the twentieth century. There are some qualities of medicine as a profession that dispose its practitioners to social work, particularly in places where levels of education and social development, and the availability of local intellectual capital, have been historically low. In colonial societies, the practice of medicine was often de facto political, because the role of healing was so entwined with public policy. Agitation against opium, for example, has historically attracted doctors to its ranks of activists, because the issue is positioned at a critical juncture between medical expertise, social health, morality, and policy reform.[4] In many societies in Southeast Asia, contra Weber, professionalization has thus not necessarily entailed a withdrawal from state and power; on the contrary, vocational professionals are more frequently socially oriented. Doctors who move to dabble in politics often find the transition from one to the other is never really complete; their politics and medical practice are rarely mutually exclusive.[5] The nature of their training no doubt played a role, too. Early generations of indigenous doctors, like lawyers, were highly educated, and occupied an important social stratum as a professional nationalist intelligentsia. They were mobile subjects, often educated abroad and exposed to many different forms of government, social systems, and ideological influences; yet the medical training they received disposed them to view their sociopolitical environment as a subjective plurality through which ran the rational, objective truth of modern science.[6]

Disproportionately in Southeast Asia, medical training was frequently one of the earliest exposures of colonized, educated elites to science. The first generation of nationalist doctors began to emerge and play an important role in society from the late nineteenth century. José Rizal, Philippine nationalist and polymath, studied medicine and ophthalmology in the Philippines, Spain, France, and Germany in the 1880s. In 1892, Sun Yat-sen earned his degree in medicine at the Hong Kong College of Medicine. In the same year, Lim Boon Keng, prominent Straits Chinese intellectual, reformer, and philanthropist, earned his medical degree at Edinburgh University. In 1908 in Indonesia, one of the earliest indigenous political societies, Budi Utomo, was founded at the School for Training of Native Doctors in Batavia. Subsequent generations of Southeast Asian doctors continued to move easily between politics and medicine. Benjamin Sheares, the second president of Singapore (1971–81), undertook his medical training in the 1920s; Mahathir Mohammad, the longest-serving prime minister of Malaysia (1981–2003), undertook his in the 1950s. Both were largely unwilling to relinquish their medical practices and teaching during their political tenures in the independent nations they rose to govern. M. K. Rajakumar, also trained in the 1950s, sustained a philanthropic medical practice in Singapore while forging a parallel career as a veteran socialist politician.

Analogies of National Health: Mixing Politics and Medicine

For these groups of physicians and medical students, the close relationship between political and medical practice frequently lent itself, as Warwick Anderson and Hans Pols have suggested, to the promulgation of "organic analogies and evolutionary models" of politics.[7] The analogy of health and hygiene to a nation's well-being is not just fanciful, especially if political actors themselves invoke such analogies to invest their actions with ideological force. Rizal, for example, wrote powerfully of Spanish colonialism as the "social cancer" of the Philippine nation, and spoke metaphorically of its extirpation.[8] In the 1950s and 1960s, as nations decolonized, the combination of medical scientism and what James Scott has called "high modernism" drove a formidable engine of progress and development, stimulating programs of vaccination, public sanitation, hygiene education, and maternal and child health that were built into burgeoning capital cities and spread with somewhat neoimperial enthusiasm in the countryside.[9] The cleansing of unwanted elements in culture in the name of the nation's well-being has also taken many forms throughout the twentieth century—some more sinister than others. Campaigns to "whiten" or clean (*membersihkan*) states during the Malayan Emergency, for example, were often vested with the language of hygiene, a war on behalf of the ideological health of the nation. BERSIH,[10] the grassroots movement for free and fair elections some forty years later, too, drew on the same analogy to speak publicly of "cleansing" Malaysia's corrupt election practices.

It is also easy to entertain another analogy: that doctors, in politics, have a diagnostic relationship to country and society, claiming through their expertise an ability to heal, fix, experiment, save, and—above all—prescribe. Rudolf Virchow, German father of social medicine and one of José Rizal's inspirations, famously wrote that "medicine is a social science, and politics is nothing but medicine on a larger scale."[11] This is a view shared, perhaps unsurprisingly, by Mahathir, himself a graduate of the King Edward VI College of Medicine in Singapore. Invited to give the Neo-centennial Lecture at the University of Santo Tomas on June 11, 2012, Mahathir remarked that "doctors sometimes make better leaders than lawyers because doctors are trained to objectively analyze diseases, including those of nations."[12] As he has written elsewhere,

> Politics is a good profession for people with medical training. Doctors go through the process of observing a patient, recording his or her medical history, then you make a physical examination, do lab tests, and finally arrive at a diagnosis. The process is basically the same in politics.[13]

One may, without undue exaggeration, read Mahathir's controversial text, *The Malay Dilemma*, as Mahathir's diagnosis of the causes of the May 13 riots and a prescription for political action.[14]

Known as "Pak Doktor," Burhanuddin Al-Helmy is an interesting foil to Mahathir, who is also frequently referred to by his full vocational title (Dr. Mahathir). I say foil, because Burhanuddin is often characterized as a "path not taken"' for Malaysian history, a "failed political enterprise"; he is even sometimes referred to as a "could-have-been" Prime Minister of Malaya.[15] Unlike Mahathir, Burhanuddin was trained not at the King Edward VII College of Medicine, but at the Ismaeliah Medical College in New Delhi, India. Burhanuddin was the first Malay doctor to graduate in the field of homeopathy, and established a Malay homeopathic center, the Gedung Homeopati, in Singapore in 1937.

Burhanuddin is better known as a political theorist of Malay nationalism. His *Asas Falsafah Kebangsaan Melayu* (The philosophy of Melayu nationalism), a collection of essays written for *Mingguan Melayu*, was published in 1954, and is fairly well known.[16] It is less well known, however, that while in detention during the Maria Hertogh riots in 1950, Burhanuddin used the long solitary hours in prison to write a collection of essays on *Falsafah perubatan homeopathy* (The philosophy of homeopathic medicine), which has only recently been rescued from oblivion.[17] His forays into Islamist politics, through his membership of the Pan-Malaysian Islamic Party (PAS), and into homeopathic practice, through his personal medical entrepreneurship, proceeded hand in hand. In 1953 he founded a homeopathic research institute in his house in Kampung Pachitan, Singapore; in 1955 he attended the Afro-Asian Conference at Bandung and joined PAS as its president the following year. While serving in the *Dewan Rakyat* (House of Commons) for PAS between 1959 and 1964, he also founded the Homeopathic Association of Malaysia in 1961 and presided over it until his arrest in 1965.

The curious intermingling of his politics and medicine has gone virtually unremarked, and there is no space to do any justice to it here, apart from speculatively. What is arresting about Burhanuddin, however, is the counterpoint he provides to the "scientistic" modernism often perceived to characterize late colonial nationalist movements, as well as the postcolonial projects of the development-obsessed 1960s and 1970s. What does a politics that emerges from a radically different sort of medical training look like?

Alternative Medicines, Alternative Nations

Certainly many of Burhanuddin's ideas about political behavior derive their spiritual weight from Sufism. He believed that both glory and decline of the nation were predicated on the character of its people, the bodies of whom were places of *amrad al-qab*—diseases of the heart: arrogance and conceit, ostentation, jealousy, suspicion, and love of *jah* (money, fame). Sufism could foster nobility of character and cure the disease; the decline of the Malay character was due to Western imperialism, and the struggle (*jihad*) against it an Islamic obligation. The principles of homeopathy, as Burhanuddin understood and practiced them, fell along related lines. Modern or Western medicine, he said, assumed the sources of disease to be "pests and small organisms," "as though humans are nothing but machinery [*jentera*], and treating or preventing disease were a matter of fixing a broken machine [*seperti membela jentera yang rosak*]." Homeopathy, on the other hand, returned humanity to the "first cause, the basis of human life: reason and soul (mind) are the source of all illness."[18]

This view of illness, scientifically unorthodox and running counter to modern conceptions of medicine, may strike us as so much quackery.[19] Certainly I am no homeopath. But can we understand anything of worth in the mixing of politics and medicine in these two Malay leaders? Both Burhanuddin and Mahathir were profoundly concerned about the future of the Malay race, and more broadly about the future of Malaya; both devoted an enormous portion of their lives towards nation-building politics. Race and ideologies about race have always been and continue to be central to the Malaysian nation-building project; in Malaysia, race *is* politics. What do Burhanuddin's and Mahathir's different conceptions of race and politics look like in light of their respective medical backgrounds?

Here, Mahathir is the scientific modernist extraordinaire. *The Malay Dilemma* is clear on his eugenicist convictions. The Malays, he said, are unable to compete with the Chinese because of genetic, evolutionary reasons: the latter are hardened by centuries of warfare, struggle, harsh climates, and diaspora, and the former fat on the easy richness of Malaysian soil. Referring to the Malays, and as justification for his infamous affirmative action policies, he said, in a nod to social Darwinism: "We do not have 4000 years to play around with."[20] The solution—one which Lee Kuan Yew would also arrive at by different channels of rationalization—was a sustained effort to improve racial communities by tinkering with their culture. (Lee, incidentally, remarked approvingly of Mahathir that the latter believed in the essential backwardness of the Malays "as a medical man"; and indeed, that Lee himself was "in agreement with three-quarters of his analysis").[21] For both Lee and Mahathir, eugenicist, social Darwinian conceptions of race went hand in hand with a lab-based approach to high modernist nation-building. Like Lee, Mahathir is content to view people as "machines" (to use Burhanuddin's word) to be manipulated, rearranged, and even rebred for their own good. Illnesses of the nation, just like illnesses of the body, were fundamentally physiological afflictions.

Burhanuddin, on the other hand, wanted to cure people's bodies through their minds. Spiritual and rational health was the same as, or would lead to, physical health. Scholars frequently mention Burhanuddin in conjunction with the left-wing PUTERA-AMCJA discussions in 1947,[22] over which he chaired and from which eventually issued a controversial set of counterproposals to the Anglo-Malay Federation Proposals, called the People's Constitution. Idealistic and running radically counter to powerful conservative currents of the time, this document, as well as the left-wing movement surrounding it, died the following year when the Malayan Emergency was declared.[23] One of the more controversial proposals put forward by the People's Constitution, attributed principally to Burhanuddin, was that *Melayu*, a word frequently denoting a racial or ethnic category, should be the title of any proposed citizenship and nationality in Malaya. Burhanuddin wanted, in other words, to divorce nationality (*kebangsaan*) from the issue of racial descent (*bangsa*). In his *Asas falsafah,* Burhanuddin laid out two important principles which distinguished between *bangsa* and *kebangsaan.* The first was that *Melayu*-ness was not something which one simply *was*—genetically, you might say—but something which one *lived* and *fulfilled:*

> Malay nationality [*kebangsaan*] is not just based on the grounds that the person is *bangsa* Malay, or his father is Malay, or his grandfather or grandmother is Malay, or that he is of Malay descent or ancestry, if that person has not *fulfilled* the meaning and the objectives of Malay nationality.[24]

He also believed that *kebangsaan* or *Melayu* nationality ought not to be defined by race, but conferred by law and politics:

> Every person, no matter from what group or *bangsa,* whose ties and relationships with this original nationality [*kebangsaan*] have been severed, or who severs such ties, and proceeds to unreservedly and totally commit allegiance to, as well as fulfill the conditions and demands of, Malay nationality [*kebangsaan Melayu*]; such a person becomes of Malay nationality, *in the political sense.*[25]

The emphasis on the force of will, rationality, and mind—that all those who lived and thought themselves to be *Melayu* could *actually be Melayu*—characterized Burhanuddin's faith and politics as well as his medicine. One was not restricted or condemned to one's biology; what mattered was the daily fulfillment and performance—and by inference the absolute malleability—of the national self. In this, Burhanuddin himself perceived his homeopathic work as another kind of national service: "I believe that homeopathy as a medical science is a national asset [*milik bangsa*], one which I proffer as an eternal legacy for our nation's independent future."[26]

Burhanuddin's medical training and its impact on his conceptions of the nation seems to run counter, then, to the "scientific patriotism" which Anderson and Pols correctly identify across large parts of Southeast Asia. At the very least, Burhanuddin stands in the history of Asian modernity as a gentle reminder that religion, spirituality, and so-called unscientific resources are frequently an unremarked idiom of social organization, national regeneration, and critical thought.[27] Homeopathy may not count as scientific, progressive modern medicine; but embedded into Burhanuddin's politics, it was certainly no "atavistic vision of the new nation," and no less a motive force for nationalist mobilization.[28] One may even suggest that, in the case of the cancer of race politics in Malaysia, it briefly offered a more congenial metaphor for national self-fashioning than evolutionary genetics.

Notes

1. David Arnold, *Colonizing the Body: State Medicine and Epidemic Disease in Nineteenth-Century India* (Berkeley: University of California Press, 1993), 158.

2. David Craig, *Familiar Medicine: Everyday Health Knowledge and Practice in Today's Vietnam* (Honolulu: University of Hawai'i Press, 2002), 56.

3. Ruth Rogaski, *Hygienic Modernity: Meanings of Health and Disease in Treaty-Port China* (Berkeley: University of California Press, 2004).

4. One example of such an activist is Wu Lien-Teh, Malayan-born Chinese doctor who founded an Anti-Opium Association in Penang in the early 1900s. See Hean Teik Ong, *To Heal the Sick: The Story of Healthcare and Doctors in Penang, 1786–2004* (Penang: Penang Medical Practitioners' Society, 2004), 26–29.

5. Warwick Anderson and Hans Pols, "Scientific Patriotism: Medical Science and National Self-Fashioning in Southeast Asia," *Comparative Studies in Society and History* 54 (2012): 113.

6. See, for example, Miriam Ming-Cheng Lo, *Doctors within Borders: Profession, Ethnicity, and Modernity in Colonial Taiwan* (Berkeley: University of California Press, 2002).

7. Anderson and Pols, "Scientific Patriotism," 96.

8. José Rizal, *Noli Me Tangere*, published in one English translation as José Rizal, *The Social Cancer: A Complete English Version of* Noli Me Tangere *from the Spanish of José Rizal*, trans. Charles Derbyshire (Manila: Philippine Education, 1950).

9. James Scott, *Seeing Like a State: How Certain Schemes to Improve the Human Condition Have Failed* (New Haven, CT: Yale University Press, 1998).

10. Gabungan Pilihanraya Bersih dan Adil (Coalition for clean and fair elections).

11. See J. P. Mackenbach, "Politics Is Nothing but Medicine at a Larger Scale: Reflections on Public Health's Biggest Idea," *Journal of Epidemiology and Community Health* 63 (2009): 181–84.

12. See Manual Almario, "Doctors Rizal and Mahathir," *The Inquirer*, June 19, 2012, opinion.inquirer.net/30979/doctors-rizal-and-mahathir.

13. Mahathir bin Mohammad, "An Asian View of the World," in Mahathir bin Mohammad, *A New Deal for Asia* (Subang Jaya: Pelanduk, 1999), 11–24.

14. Mahathir bin Mohamad, *The Malay Dilemma* (Singapore: Asia Pacific Press, 1970).

15. See, for example, Cheah Boon Kheng, "Ethnicity in the Making of Malaya," in *Nation-Building: Five Southeast Asian Histories*, ed. Wang Gungwu (Singapore: Institute for Southeast Asian Studies, 2005), 92; Hussin Mutalib, *Islam in Malaysia: From Revivalism to Islamic State* (Singapore: NUS Press, 1993), 24.

16. The full text of Burhanuddin's *Asas falsafah kebangsaan Melayu* is contained in, and henceforth cited as, Kamaruddin Jaffar, ed., *Dr. Burhanuddin Al-Helmy: Politik Melayu dan Islam* (Kuala Lumpur: Yayasan Anda, 1980).

17. This collection has recently (2011) been compiled and published by the HBI Homeopathy Center in Kota Bharu, Terengganu, from photocopies made by Dr. Dali Muin, who was a homeopathy disciple and friend of Dr. Burhanuddin's. I have not, however, had the opportunity to view the volume personally.

18. Burhanuddin qualifies in parentheses his use of the Malay word for "soul" or "spirit" (*roh*) with the English word "mind." Burhanuddin Al-Helmy, "Sepintas lalu perkembangan ilmu perubatan: Homeopati: Teori dan praktik," *Majalah Perubatan Homeopathy* 1, no. 1 (1985): 26–31. This essay is republished in full at the HBI Health and Homeopathy Center website, www.homeolibrary.com/NewHomeo_2011/ESEI/PerkembanganPerubatan2.htm.

19. The scientific literature criticizing the principles, efficacy, and the mechanisms of homeopathic remedies is vast. See, for example, E. Ernst, "A Systematic Review of Systematic

Reviews of Homeopathy," *British Journal of Clinical Psychology* 54, no. 6 (December 2002): 577–82; Aijing Shang, Karin Huwiler-Müntener, Linda Nartey, et al., "Are the Clinical Effects of Homoeopathy Placebo Effects? Comparative Study of Placebo-Controlled Trials of Homoeopathy and Allopathy," *Lancet* 366, no. 9487 (August 2005): 726–32; Ayo Wahlberg, "A Quackery with a Difference: New Medical Pluralism and the Problem of 'Dangerous Practitioners' in the United Kingdom," *Social Science and Medicine* 65, no. 11 (December 2007): 2307–16.

20. Mahathir bin Mohammad, *The Malay Dilemma* (Kuala Lumpur: Federal Publications, 1981), 31.

21. Interview with Lee Kuan Yew, *New Straits Times,* October 14, 1989; see Michael Barr, "Lee Kuan Yew: Race, Culture and Genes," *Journal of Contemporary Asia* 29, no. 2 (1999): 145–66.

22. PUTERA-AMCJA was a postwar united front formed in opposition to the Federation Constitutional proposals, from an alliance between the All-Malaya Council of Joint Action (AMCJA), a coalition of civil society and political organizations, and the Pusat Tenaga Rakyat (PUTERA), a coalition of Malay left-wing parties. For a thorough survey of events surrounding the PUTERA-AMCJA and the People's Constitutional proposals mentioned below, see Yeo Kim Wah, *Political Development of Singapore, 1945–1955* (Singapore: NUS Press, 1973).

23. For a reappraisal of Burhanuddin along these lines, see Farish A. Noor, "The Red-Green Alliance: The 'Left-Leaning Years' of the Pan-Malaysian Islamic Party (PAS)," in *What Your Teacher Didn't Tell You: The Annexe Lectures,* ed. Farish A. Noor (Petaling Jaya, Malaysia: Matahari Books, 2009), 181–231.

24. Kamaruddin, *Burhanuddin,* 111.

25. Kamaruddin, *Burhanuddin,* 113.

26. Burhanuddin al-Helmy in the inaugural speech at the opening of the Homeopathic Association of Malaysia in 1961. Cited in Mohamed Hatta Abu Bakar, *Perubatan Homeopathy* (Terengganu, Malaysia: HBI Homeopathy Center, 1977), the relevant excerpt of which can be found at the Homéopathe International website, www.homeoint.org/articles/malay/malaysia.htm.

27. For this observation, see Christopher Bayly, *The Birth of the Modern World, 1780–1914: Global Connections and Comparisons* (Oxford: Blackwell, 2004), 76–80.

28. Anderson and Pols, "Scientific Patriotism," 97.

12 Health or Tobacco

Competing Perspectives
in Modern Southeast Asia

Loh Wei Leng

In spite of the wide acceptance of tobacco since its introduction from the New World of the Americas to Europe in the mid-sixteenth century, and thereafter disseminated farther afield to other continents by the seventeenth century, there have been those who have been very critical of its use.[1]

As early as 1604, King James I of England, in his now well-known "Counterblaste to Tobacco," a diatribe against "this vile custome of Tobacco taking," which he felt was "a custom loathsome to the eye, hateful to the nose, harmful to the brain, dangerous to the lung"; and even as the smoking habit became popular in the twentieth century, dubbed the "cigarette century," the negative effects of addiction on the consumer have long been recognized.[2] What accounts then for the "deadly persistence" of this product when nicotine, the primary addictive agent in cigarettes, chewing tobacco, cigars and pipe tobacco, has been said to be "the leading preventable cause of disease, disability, and death"?[3]

Indeed, taking a broader and comparable look at drugs in general, of which tobacco is one among many psychoactive substances, an intriguing question raised by David T. Courtwright in his global history on drugs is why some—such as opium, cocaine, and marijuana—have been designated illicit substances in nearly all countries, while what Courtwright deems the "Big Three"—alcohol, tobacco and caffeine—have for the most part been legal.[4]

Notwithstanding the seemingly similar stance of most governments in their selection of which drugs are acceptable, it is quite unlikely that one answer suffices for all countries in terms of the nature and range of policies adopted over time. For instance, reviews of books in a recent issue of the journal *Social History of Alcohol and Drugs* convey distinctively different drug experiences in Iran,

Table 12.1. Tobacco in Southeast Asia: Area planted and production (1960–2000)

	Area planted (hectares)					Production (metric tons)				
Year	1960	1970	1980	1990	2000	1960	1970	1980	1990	2000
Indonesia	173,836	208,822	141,225	241,170	210,000	63,030	92,649	72,700	333,211	157,052
Philippines	95,913	105,250	81,165	49,830	40,296	59,896	93,760	70,719	63,718	62,550
Thailand	60,793	85,111	92,561	63,095	43,300	26,022	41,153	70,950	69,469	40,705
Myanmar	40,470	55,443	58,000	55,000	36,000	33,682	31,153	64,600	28,170	16,560
Cambodia	12,140	25,091	9,000	9,000	9,669	6,035	14,670	4,500	4,500	7,282
Malaysia	2,744	3,237	13,243	10,659	16,595	1,488	2,231	9,447	9,967	7,390
Laos	2,024	6,070	4,000	4,000	6,700	850	3,230	1,700	2,700	33,400
Vietnam			32,000	26,478	24,400			25,000	19,644	27,200

Source: U.S. Department of Agriculture, cited at indexmundi website, www.indexmundi.com /agriculture, accessed August 26, 2012.

China, and the United States.[5] Hence, this chapter will look into the specificities that can be discerned for a number of locations in Southeast Asia, to ascertain the developments that have shaped the approaches of different countries.

An epidemic of tobacco use is a crucial driver of the rise of non-communicable chronic disease in Southeast Asia. As both a major producer and a major consumer of tobacco, Southeast Asia occupies a prominent place in the global effort to control the health effects of tobacco; and it is in Southeast Asia that some of the firmest obstacles to that effort lie. This chapter provides a long-term perspective on the development of the tobacco industry in the region, thus providing a context for understanding one of the most pressing health challenges facing the region today.

In 1990, Asia contributed 4,235,000 metric tons (60 percent) of the world tobacco crop, with China as the largest Asian producer, its output 2,692,000 metric tons (38 percent).[6] Southeast Asia's share was 531,379 metric tons (12.5 percent) from 459,232 hectares in area planted (see table 12.1).

In terms of crops and production, in the second half of the twentieth century, Indonesia, Philippines, and Thailand are the top three for the 1960s and 1970s, followed by Myanmar and Cambodia with Malaysia and Laos trailing behind. In the 1980s and 1990s, Thailand and Philippines switch places, followed by Myanmar and Vietnam, with Malaysia's production picking up. In 2001, Indonesia was one of the leading producers of tobacco leaves, ranked seventh behind the first five (China, India, Brazil, United States, and Turkey), which produce two-thirds of the world's tobacco, and Zimbabwe in sixth place.[7] As comparable data is not available for the first half of the twentieth century, the order of magnitude of tobacco cultivation in particular, and the industry in general, in the specific

Table 12.2. Tobacco in Southeast Asia: Area planted and production (1910–1945)

Year	Area planted (hectares)					Production (metric tons)				
	1910	1920	1930	1940	1945	1910	1920	1930	1940	1945
Indonesia						109,000	72,000	124,000	100,000	
Siam	11,360	8,640	9,920	8,960	13,120					
Burma	38	49.8	47.3	55.8						
Malaysia			1,429*	2370	524**					

Sources: W. M. F. Mansvelt and P. Creutzberg, *Changing Economy in Indonesia: A Selection of Statistical Source Material from the Early 19th Century up to 1940* (The Hague: M. Nijhoff, 1975), 55; J. C. Ingram, *Economic Change in Thailand, 1850–1970* (Kuala Lumpur: Oxford University Press, 1971), 51; Teruko Saito and Lee Kin Kiong, *Statistics on the Burmese Economy: The 19th and 20th Centuries* (Singapore: ISEAS, 1999), 43–44; Tan Wan Hin, "The Development of the Tobacco Growing Industry in Peninsular Malaysia," *Journal Geographica* (Geographical Society, University of Malaya) 13 (1978): 3. The years for Siam (Thailand) are 1911 (1910 column), 1918–9 (1920 column), 1928–9 (1930 column), 1938–9 (1940 column), 1944 (1945 column). The years for Malaysia are 1932 (1930 column), 1948 (1945 column).

Southeast Asian countries would very likely be along the same lines—namely, that Indonesia, Philippines, and Thailand (then Siam) were significant producers, with Myanmar (then Burma), Cambodia, Malaysia, Laos, and Vietnam trailing behind.

The high profitability to the state in the form of revenue from primary commodity production has long been associated with colonial export economies of the nineteenth century. In spite of the vastly different administrative structures and historical precedents from earlier centuries, the various Western powers faced a similar imperative, namely to be self-financing and maintain themselves with sufficient funds, which they sought from the development of one or more export staples. This can be borne out in the case of Malaysia under the British, Indonesia under the Dutch, and in the Philippines—where the Spanish colonial authorities ran its own Tobacco Monopoly from 1781.[8,9] The private sector was also able to reap profits, where monopoly can make the fortunes of the one company that had secured it as exemplified by the most prominent private firm after the end of the Tobacco Monopoly in 1880, Compania General de Tabacos de Filipinas (also known as Tabacalera), which survived even after American rule between 1899 and 1946, having expanded into many other allied businesses such as trade and shipping.[10]

To recall what was just mentioned, certain data may not be available for specific periods, such as employment figures, for which crop data has to serve as the proxy as to the size of the industry. So, too, when data on crops are unavailable, for an indication of the economic importance of the tobacco industry in a given locality, production and export figures may have to be used.[11] A reminder here may be in order, that figures presented in table 12.2 are not necessarily comparable and merely serve to indicate ongoing tobacco cultivation. Nonetheless, as non-quantitative accounts are available, sketches of state objectives and their strategies are drawn from them.

Indonesia and the Philippines never fail to feature in the sixteenth-century picture of global diffusion of tobacco, a part of broader worldwide historical processes, the mercantilist expansion of the early modern era and later the rise of colonial empires. In the nineteenth century, both the Dutch and the Spanish built on experiences (from the Dutch East Indies Company [VOC in Dutch] and from Mexico) in their quest to control their Southeast Asian territories, to partake in the trade of Asian commodities and cultivate cash crops for the requisite finances to maintain their settlements.

The Cultivation System (1830–70) drew on the VOC model of "the forced production of agricultural products . . . for export . . . to collect a certain amount of rent from those who farmed the land . . . in the form of agricultural products suitable for export."[12] Land was opened up after 1870—long leases—to private enterprise with European plantation companies developing vast tobacco states in Sumatra, yielding the well-known Deli tobacco.[13] Jacobus Nienhuys, a Dutch planter, played a major role in making the region into a leading tobacco production area, and Deli tobacco achieved a monopolistic position in the world market within five decades.[14] The shift to large-scale agricultural enterprises for export crops from the last quarter of the nineteenth century is in part due to the Industrial Revolution and its inventions—such as the new shipping technology, from sail to steam, which enabled goods to be economically transported in bulk.[15] Rapid growth from this period until the 1930s Depression years—with no drastic reversal for tobacco, whose output had more than doubled between 1880 and 1914, having been so firmly established—can also be attributed to the phenomenal growth of the world economy, and the concomitant European overseas expansion and rise in demand for primary commodities.[16,17]

The pattern set from the nineteenth century—the state extracting its share of the profits from cash crops with export potential—provided a strategy worth pursuing into the twentieth century. The caveat is that the general upward trend in exports hides changes in the commodity composition of trade and spatial variations, even as new mantras were crafted—the Liberal Policy giving way to the Ethical Policy in the Dutch East Indies. Similarly, as Spanish rule changed to American control in the Philippines at the turn of the twentieth century, responding to world market forces, commercial agriculture could continue to be counted on: "By the early 1840s the principal exports in order of value were, in the first group sugar, tobacco leaf and cigars, abaca cordage and fiber; in the second group, indigo, coffee, cotton. The first group contributed 86% of the value of the leading exports.... In 1929, sugar, coconut products, abaca and tobacco made up 86.7 per cent of total exports, and in 1932, 91.6 per cent."[18]

We now turn to Thailand (Siam until 1949), the Southeast Asian nation not colonized by any Western power. What was Siam's economic structure and the role of the state? If there was no imperial objective of sending surplus revenue to the metropolitan center in Europe, what was owed to the absolute monarch (until the change to a constitutional monarchy in 1932)? Thai kings owned all the land, custom gave the free man the right to as much land as he could cultivate and his obligation was a portion of produce and services which he owed his patron (officials or nobles), who collected on behalf of the king.[19] As for trade, Siam had minimal contact with Europeans from 1688 to 1850s, when it was opened to the West. The lists of exports reported by different foreign observers in the nineteenth century were quite similar and included "everything of importance which Siam exports *even today*, except for rubber."[20] Tobacco was on the list of exports; however, W. A. Graham noted that the Siamese preferred foreign brands after 1850.[21] This is reflected in "quite large" imports of cigarettes until a new and increased tariff in 1926, aimed at encouraging domestic production of cigarettes using imported leaf, as reflected in a rise in unmanufactured tobacco imports.[22] This development has to be viewed in the context of the emergence of the standardized, mass-produced cigarette, an American invention, which had just come on the scene at the turn of the century, and in no time developed into a global industry.[23] British American Tobacco Company (BAT) seized the opportunity to set up a factory in Bangkok in 1936, started the cultivation of Virginia tobacco in the North and Northeast, which had long grown tobacco, and developed local brands.[24] In 1941, the Thai government formed a Tobacco Monopoly and bought up BAT's operation—a measure of the success of BAT's global expansion. Since the Tobacco Monopoly was able to realize profits from the factory output as well as tax revenue, tobacco in Siam had definitely been a boon to the state since the mid-nineteenth century, when the returns from trade tariffs would very likely have overshadowed produce payments from peasant subjects.[25]

When we consider another player, the consumer, it becomes clear that in recent decades the topic of the social and health impacts of tobacco continues to be highly contentious; thus, casting the discussion in binary terms is unavoidable given diametrically opposing interests. As we have seen, there are those with much to gain from tobacco use—business (the industry directly plus the other parties indirectly involved) and state (with reference to collection of revenue and employment generated). The latter, however, can also be aligned with the other side, the voices raised on behalf of the consumer—a range of anti-smoking bodies, both governmental and non-governmental (NGOs). In addition, it should also be noted that the consumer can wear two hats, as a user as well as a cultivator with a stake in the industry. As tobacco is a labor-intensive crop, long in existence before the Spanish sought to establish a monopoly in the Philippines, it had been cultivated in small garden plots.[26] Among the tasks any monopoly encounters is the problem of control of supply, the concomitant being contraband trade, regarding which the tobacco revenue police in 1783 were given "secret orders to ignore the small plots . . . illegally cultivated near their houses for their own consumption."[27] In other words, we cannot assume that all consumers are positively inclined toward regulation and control of usage; many resist such measures that curb their freedom of choice—a sentiment applicable from the past into the present!

The leading Southeast Asian organization is the Southeast Asia Tobacco Control Alliance (SEATCA), established in 2001, which receives funding from the Rockefeller Foundation and the Thai Health Promotion Foundation. In turn, SEATCA lends its support to the Tobacco Industry Surveillance Network (TISN) which has teams in Cambodia, Laos, Malaysia, Philippines, Thailand, and Vietnam. Each Southeast Asian country has its own set of NGOs: examples include the Thai Health Promotion Foundation; the Indonesian Smoking Control Foundation; Framework Convention on Tobacco Control Alliance, Philippines (FCAP); Vietnam Committee on Smoking and Health; the Malaysian Council for Tobacco Control; and the Malaysian Women's Action for Tobacco Control and Health.[28]

Although tobacco has long had its detractors, advocates for tobacco control (TC) maintain that it has been an uphill struggle against the tobacco industry, that "[i]n contrast to the size of the challenge, global tobacco control has, until recently, lacked sustained global leadership, been severely underfunded and wanted for strategic direction."[29] It was only in 2003 that the World Health Organization (WHO) managed to get the Framework Convention on Tobacco Control (FCTC) open for signature and to be ratified later by national legislatures, the process having started in 1994 at the Ninth World Conference on Health or Tobacco in Paris. From Southeast Asia, among the first forty to sign were Myanmar, Singapore, Brunei, and Thailand. Nonetheless, despite the imbalance vis-à-vis the powerful Transnational Tobacco Companies (TTCs), TC advocates have amassed evidence of the human costs of tobacco with documentation of a litany of detrimental consequences backed by medical research, "the large-scale epidemiological studies of the mid-twentieth century."[30] From the 1950s, the deleterious cost effects of dependence on tobacco took on more prominence in the public eye with a shift to heightened awareness of tobacco's toxic nature. In 1962, a report of the Royal College of Physicians of London on smoking and health stated that cigarette smoking was a cause of lung cancer. This was followed by the first of many reports of the U.S. Surgeon General's Advisory Committee on Smoking and Health, which confirmed a similar finding. These seminal works laid the basis for steps toward reducing tobacco use. Prior to this, in the initial decades of the twentieth century, in much of Asia attention was given to efforts to ban the consumption of opium, an intoxicant which has been shown to produce a condition of diminished mental and physical ability; tobacco is at the other end of the spectrum, considerably milder than the drugs widely legislated as illicit. After all, one explanation, facetious but apt, on "why some drugs have remained legal . . . [is that] cigarettes rarely start brawls and their carcinogens take years to kick in, which allowed tobacco conglomerates to maintain a smokescreen of harmlessness until recently."[31]

World Bank and WHO studies on various Southeast Asian countries have found that among the negative effects of income diverted from necessities such as food, shelter, and education due to tobacco use are malnutrition, death from tobacco-related illnesses—"cancers of the oesophagus, stomach, lungs and larynx . . . [and] tuberculosis," the latter being a list of illnesses identified in Myanmar in 2001.[32] A recent study of lung cancer conducted from 1984–89 in Malaysia, where "[s]eventy five percent of patients (84% of men and 26% of women) were smokers." concluded that "[c]arcinoma of the lung is the commonest type of cancer, accounting for about 12 to 24 percent of all cancer mortality in Malaysia."[33] Fifteen years later, the problem had not been solved; it was "the commonest tumour to afflict males and the most common cause of cancer deaths accounting for 19.8% of all medically certified cancer related mortality in this country."[34] At any rate, advocates at international, regional, and national levels have been active in circulating irrefutable scientific evidence but, as reports on the prevalence of smoking in Southeast Asia show, much remains to be done to reverse the habit.

Although space does not permit a lengthy discussion of why tobacco has so successfully found markets and users wherever it was introduced, in Asia, since the commercially minded Portuguese traders brought it from port to port along Asian trade routes in the sixteenth century, one powerful force has been identified as a major contributory factor towards its acceptance—namely, the promotion efforts of Western merchants in previous centuries, which morphed into the tobacco lobby by the twentieth century.[35] This, however, does not touch on the recipients of the product and messages transmitted in a variety of forms, resulting in the creation of "cultures of dependence," with their temporal and spatial variation.[36] Essays in *Consuming Habits: Drugs in History and Anthropology* seek to assess the role of psychoactive substances in the construction of culture, since

> the categories of licit or illicit are neither static nor rigid. . . . In some times and places, both tobacco and coffee have been classed as illicit with heavy penalties for use. . . . Some substances, moreover, are classed as licit in one culture and illicit in another: alcohol, for instance is forbidden in Islamic societies but in most of the rest of the world it has usually been legally available, at least to adult males.[37]

Indeed, two groups of potential users, the young and women, are promising targets. The industry has been found to employ "six vehicles and themes to construct a tobacco culture in Asia: music, entertainment (including nightclubs, discos, and movies), adventure, sport (including motorsports, soccer, and tennis), glamour (beauty and fashion), and independence . . . to make smoking desirable, even normal," and "that smoking was an apposite and integral part of these milieu."[38] Evidence of lobbying (besides the other methods just itemized) in Southeast Asia's top two producer nations may have propelled them to meet rising domestic demand, and in the process retain their ranking. The Philippines tobacco industry is reputed to have "the strongest tobacco lobby in Asia"; while in Indonesia, "influencers" on social media—Facebook, Twitter, and the like—were to be "offered incentives to plug its ['tobacco giant'] brands."[39,40] Additionally, recent increases in female smoking have been reported in Cambodia and Malaysia.[41] WHO smoking statistics confirm that Indonesia and the Philippines top all categories, with female smokers as the next frontier (See table 12.3). It would appear that in the intersection between consumer culture and medicine—the role of science versus fashion in the evolving attitudes to drugs for recreational use—health concerns and the tobacco user are at the mercy of extremely inventive sponsorship and promotional strategies of the industry. In short, culture provides the context for consumption patterns.

A closing note on the chief concerns of Modern Southeast Asia governments and the resultant social and health impact on their peoples. Fiscal exploitation of primary commodities in colonial economies is a well-trodden theme in economic and business history. Consideration of this subject in conjunction with aspects of sociocultural, medical, and health history has served to underscore the significance of the state-business nexus in determining policies since the pre-independent, colonial era and continuing into the present. The current scenario seems to indicate that the imperative of rewards from commercial cash crop cultivation and the manufacture of cigarettes remains paramount, a powerful motivation which has resulted in state ambivalence toward broader societal concerns. A survey of the role of ASEAN states in their tobacco control measures speaks volumes, as it reports that

> all but Indonesia have embraced the Framework Convention on Tobacco Control and all endorse some form of tobacco control policy. Nevertheless, except for Brunei, all these states are, to varying degrees, *complicit in investing in or promoting* the tobacco industry.[42]

The study documented the role of the state: from promotion to regulation and control, oftentimes with contrastingly divergent policies concurrently in place, and provided a description of contemporary policies in Southeast Asia that are clearly contradictory.[43] The argument of poverty alleviation explored by Barraclough and Morrow has been offered as the main rationale for continued state support of the industry, to counter the emerging recognition of the health and economic costs of the adverse effects of addiction.

What one historian has depicted as "cultures of dependence" appears to be extremely difficult to dislodge, up against TTCs' advertising, promotion, and sponsorship onslaught, which captures new consumers (the young and wom-

Table 12.3. WHO age-standardized estimated prevalence of smoking those aged fifteen years or older (2009)

	Any smoked tobacco						Cigarettes					
	Current			Daily			Current			Daily		
	Male	Female	Total	Male	Female	Total	Male	Female	Total	Male	Female	Total
Indonesia	61	5	33	54	4	29	57	4	30	49	3	26
Thailand	45	3	24	39	2	20	45	3	24	38	2	20
Philippines	47	10	29	38	8	23	47	10	28	38	8	23
Myanmar	40	8	24	31	6	18	35	5	20	26	4	15
Cambodia	42	3	23	40	3	22	41	3	22	39	3	21
Malaysia	50	2	26	41	2	21	46	2	24	36	1	19
Laos	51	4	28	43	3	23	47	3	25	38	2	20
Vietnam	48	2	25	40	1	20	40	1	21	31	1	16
Singapore	35	6	21	25	4	15	33	5	19	23	4	13

Source: "WHO Report on the Global Tobacco Epidemic, 2011: Warning about the Dangers of Tobacco," World Health Organization website, www.who.int/tobacco/global_report/2011/en.

en), seducing them with "images such as glamour, fashion and independence as well as affluence, sophistication, modernity and success . . . well documented [strategies]."[44] Coupled with the fact that since its global diffusion from the mid-sixteenth century, tobacco "as an instrument for purely personal gratification" appears to have been able to override the warnings labels incorporated into cigarette packaging![45] Once induced into tobacco use, aping the new fashion—then and now—addiction takes over.

With the change in recent years in global consumption of tobacco and the shift of smoking patterns—in which the percentage of people who smoke in higher-income countries are decreasing, versus increasing percentages in low- and middle-income countries—a 2002 WHO study informs us, "Around 4.9 million deaths were attributable to tobacco use worldwide in 2000, an increase of 45 percent since 1990, with the most rapid increase seen in developing countries which now account for 50 percent of these deaths."[46] However, countries with more comprehensive TC legislation, such as Thailand and Singapore, are more likely to reduce consumption resulting in lower rates of tobacco-attributed diseases and deaths.[47] "In Thailand, per capita cigarette consumption decreased by over 30% from 1996 to 2000, due to national policies that ban cigarette marketing and discourage smoking"—surely a remarkable achievement in a four-year period.[48] Singapore had the lowest smoking prevalence in 2009, except among females (table 12.3). The implication to draw from this is that the only hope for the developing countries at risk today from the tobacco epidemic is tobacco control advocates' persistent efforts counter the industry's aggressive and ever-creative strategies. Advocacy is the way forward for Southeast Asian countries seeking to reverse current trends and to ensure that tobacco-related morbidity and mortality consequences for its peoples are consigned to the rubbish heap, relegating the legacy of tobacco to the past.

Since its emergence on the global stage as one of a number of psychoactive substances, such as coffee and cocoa, that have become integral components of world trade, tobacco has been cultivated for domestic consumption, developed for foreign markets, and transformed into the global cigarette in the twentieth century; it is currently under siege on all fronts—international, regional, and national. Through the lens of tobacco, Southeast Asian countries have borne witness to all these phases in the evolution of the world economy, and continues to be an active participant in the making of global history, in the contest toward a tobacco-free future.

Notes

1. J. Crawford, "On the History and Consumption of Tobacco," *Journal of the Statistical Society of London* 16, no. 1 (1853): 45–52; A. Steinmetz, *Tobacco: Its History, Cultivation, Manufacture, and Adulterations: Its Use Considered with Reference to Its Influence on the Human Constitution* (London: Richard Bentley, 1857); A. Charlton, "Tobacco or Health 1602: An Elizabethan Doctor Speaks," *Health Education Research* 20, no. 1 (2005): 110–11.

2. King James I of England, "A Counterblaste to Tobacco," www.laits.utexas.edu/poltheory/james/blaste/blaste.html, accessed February 22, 2014; Allan M. Brandt, *The Cigarette Century: The Rise, Fall, and Deadly Persistence of the Product That Defined America* (New York: Basic, 2007).

3. National Institute on Drug Abuse, *NIDA Research Report—Nicotine Addiction*, NIH Pub. No. 01-4342, printed July 1998, revised June 2009, National Institute on Drug Abuse website, www.drugabuse.gov/researchreports/nicotine/nicotine.html.

4. David E. Courtwright, *Forces of Habit: Drugs and the Making of the Modern World* (Cambridge, MA: Harvard University Press, 2001).

5. *Social History of Alcohol and Drugs*, 21, no. 2 (2007).

6. Jordan Goodman, *Tobacco in History: The Cultures of Dependence* (London: Routledge, 1993), 6.

7. J. Mackay and M. Erikson, *The Tobacco Atlas* (Geneva: WHO, 2002), 46, World Health Organization website, libdoc.who.int/publications/2002/The%20tobacco%20Atlas.pdf.

8. Lim Teck Ghee, *Origins of a Colonial Economy, Land and Agriculture in Perak 1874–1897* (Penang: Penerbit Universiti Sains Malaysia, 1976); Tan Wan Hin, "The Development of the Tobacco Growing Industry in Peninsular Malaysia," *Journal Geographica* (Geographical Society, University of Malaya) 13 (1978): 1–10.

9. W. M. F. Mansvelt and P. Creutzberg, *Changing Economy in Indonesia: A Selection of Statistical Source Material from the Early 19th Century up to 1940* (The Hague: M. Nijhoff, 1975).

10. Ed. C. de Jesus, *The Tobacco Monopoly in the Philippines, Bureaucratic Enterprise and Social Change, 1766–1880* (Manila: Ateneo de Manila University Press, 1980), xiv.

11. Mansvelt and Creutzberg, *Changing Economy in Indonesia*, 13.

12. Wim van den Doel, "The Dutch Empire. An Essential Part of World History," *BMGN— Low Countries Historical Review* 125, no. 2–3 (2010): 187.

13. Mansvelt and Creutzberg, *Changing Economy in Indonesia*, 24.

14. Thee Kian Wee, *Plantation Agriculture and Export Growth: An Economic History of East Sumatra, 1863–1942* (Madison: University of Wisconsin Press, 1977), 6, 85.

15. Mansvelt and Creutzberg, *Changing Economy in Indonesia*, 15.

16. Mansvelt and Creutzberg, *Changing Economy in Indonesia*, 113, 21.

17. J. Thomas Lindblad, "Economic Aspects of the Dutch Expansion in Indonesia, 1870–1914," *Modern Asian Studies* 23, no. 1 (1989): 16–17.

18. Onofre D. Corpuz, *An Economic History of the Philippines* (Manila: University of the Philippines Press, 1997), 109, 252.

19. J. C. Ingram, *Economic Change in Thailand, 1850–1970* (Kuala Lumpur: Oxford University Press, 1971), 12–16.

20. Ingram, *Economic Change in Thailand*, 21, 25.

21. W. A. Graham, *Siam*, 3rd ed. (London: A. Moring, 1924), 2:24–25.

22. Ingram, *Economic Change in Thailand*, 136–37.

23. H. Cox, *The Global Cigarette: Origins and Evolution of British American Tobacco 1880–1945* (Oxford: Oxford University Press, 2000), 3.

24. Cox, *The Global Cigarette*, 282–83.

25. Ingram, *Economic Change in Thailand*, 140–43.

26. Jesus, *The Tobacco Monopoly in the Philippines*, 43, 36.

27. Jesus, *The Tobacco Monopoly in the Philippines*, 48.

28. T. Djutaharta, "Research on Tobacco in Indonesia: An Annotated Bibliography," World Bank HNP Discussion Paper, Economics of Tobacco Control Paper No. 10. (2003), World Bank website, siteresources.worldbank.org/HEALTHNUTRITIONANDPOPULATION/Resources/281627-1095698140167/Djutaharta-ResearchOn-whole.pdf; Mackay and Erikson, *The Tobacco Atlas;* The Bloomberg Initiative to Reduce Tobacco Use Grants Program (2009), www.tobacco controlgrants.org.

29. Derek Yach and Douglas Bettcher, "Globalization of Tobacco Industry Influence and New Global Responses," *Tobacco Control* 9, no. 2 (2000): 211, tobaccocontrol.bmj.com/content/9/2/206.full.

30. Rosemary Elliot, "Body," in *Tobacco in History and Culture: An Encyclopedia*, ed. Jordan Goodman (Farmington Hills, MI: Charles Scribner's Sons, 2005), 84.

31. Robert Perkinson, review of *Forces of Habit: Drugs and the Making of the Modern World*, by David E. Courtwright, *Journal of World History* 15, no. 2 (June 2004): 255–58, quotation on 256.

32. N. N. Kyaing, "Tobacco Economics in Myanmar," HNP Discussion Paper, Economics of Tobacco Control Paper No. 14 (Washington, DC: World Bank, 2003), xviii–xix.

33. Ismail Yaacob, Zulkifli Ahmad, and Zainol Harun, "Lung Cancer in Kelantan," *Medical Journal of Malaysia* 45, no. 3 (1990): 220.

34. A. Sachithanandan and B. Badmanaban, "Screening for Lung Cancer in Malaysia: Are We There Yet?" *Medical Journal of Malaysia* 67, no. 1 (2012): 3.

35. V. G. Kiernan, review of *Tobacco in History: The Cultures of Dependence*, by Jordan Goodman, *Social History of Medicine* 7, no. 2 (1994): 329.

36. Goodman, *Tobacco in History.*

37. Jordan Goodman, Paul E. Lovejoy, and Andrew Sherratt, *Consuming Habits: Drugs in History and Anthropology*, 2nd ed. (London: Routledge, 2007), xiii.

38. J. Knight and S. Chapman, "'Asian Yuppies . . . Are Always Looking for Something New and Different': Creating a Tobacco Culture among Young Asians," *Tobacco Control* 13, Suppl.

2 (2004): ii22–ii29, quotations on ii22 and ii26, tobaccocontrol.bmj.com/content/13/suppl_2/ii22.full.pdf+html.

39. K. Alechnowicz and S. Chapman, "The Philippine Tobacco Industry: 'The Strongest Tobacco Lobby in Asia,'" *Tobacco Control* 13 (2004): ii71–ii78, tobaccocontrol.bmj.com/content/13/suppl_2/ii71.

40. "The Tobacco Industry: The Last Gasp," *Economist,* March 31, 2011, www.economist.com/node/18486173.

41. O. Shafey, S. Dolwick, and G. E. Guindon, eds. *Tobacco Control Country Profiles 2003,* (Atlanta, GA: American Cancer Society, 2003), 10, World Health Organization website, www.who.int/tobacco/ global_data/country_profiles/en.

42. S. Barraclough and M. Morrow, "The Political Economy of Tobacco and Poverty Alleviation in Southeast Asia: Contradictions in the Role of the State," *Global Health Promotion* Suppl. 40, 17, no. 1 (2010): 40. (Italics added.)

43. "Smoking In Asia: Can't Kick the Habit," *Economist,* September 20, 2007, www.economist.com/node/9833717.

44. Knight and Chapman, "Asian Yuppies," 127.

45. Jesus, *The Tobacco Monopoly in the Philippines,* 1.

46. Cited in Jeff Collin and Anna B. Gilmore, "Developing Countries," in *Tobacco in History and Culture: An Encyclopedia,* ed. Jordan Goodman (Farmington Hills, MI: Charles Scribner's Sons, 2005), 193.

47. Mackay and Erikson, *The Tobacco Atlas,* 76.

48. Shafey, Dolwick, and Guindon, *Tobacco Control Country Profiles 2003,* 8.

13 The Role of Non-governmental Organizations in the Field of Health in Modern Southeast Asia

The Philippine Experience

Teresa S. Encarnacion Tadem

Introduction

The role of non-governmental organizations (NGOs) in the field of health in the Philippine experience could be best understood in the context of the emergence of individuals and NGOs advocating for "health for the poor." For these NGOs one way of attaining this is through community-based health programs (CBHPs), with emphasis on primary health care (PHC) in the rural areas. These individuals and NGOs also view their health advocacy as part of the struggle to address the massive poverty and socioeconomic inequalities in the country. Although such efforts emerged during the pre–martial law period, it was during the martial law period (1972–86) that this health movement grew. Given their long-term objectives and the nature of their work, rooted as they were at the community level, it was inevitable that during the martial law period, these health advocates and NGOs would ally themselves or even be part of the mainstream left movement in the country—that is, the Communist Party of the Philippines (CPP), its military arm, the New People's Army (NPA), and its illegal united front, the National Democratic Front (NDF) or the CPP-NPA-NDF. During its incipience, individual community-based health (CBH) advocates and NGOs were given much impetus by church-based movements, whose mission was to serve the poor, particularly in the countryside. The church's foremost concern of was the health of the church's constituencies, thus making CBHP advocates natural allies. Aside from being strongly linked with the mainstream left movement and the church movement in the country, CBH individuals and NGOs also drew financial and logistical support externally—either from international church-based movements or funding from foreign governments, mainly through their respective NGOs. With the downfall of the dictatorship in 1986, the post–martial law period ushered in new aspects of CBHP advocacies. One was attaining CBHP goals by joining, or engaging, or confronting government. Another was the emergence of reproductive health rights for women as an important dimension of the CBHP program. Such advocacy would gain support from the mainstream left movement, and following external developments such as the emergence of women's rights as a priority in United Nations agencies. The split in the CPP-NPA-NDF in 1992, however, would prove fatal to CBHP advocacy. Aggravating this is the opposition of the Catholic Church's hierarchy to the reproductive health rights of women.

This chapter will, therefore, highlight these important factors affecting the role of NGOs in establishing CBHPs in the Philippines. It will draw mainly from interviews conducted with three major proponents of CBHP and women's reproductive rights in the country: Jaime "Jimmy" Galvez-Tan, a medical doctor and professor of medicine in the University of the Philippines, Manila; Sylvia Estrada Claudio, who has a PhD in psychology, is a medical doctor and professor of community development and social work at the University of the Philippines (UP) Diliman, and is currently director of the UP Diliman Center for Women's Studies; and Ana Maria "Princess" Nemenzo, executive director of WomanHealth. All three NGO activists advocate CBHP programs in general and in the case of Estrada Claudio and Nemenzo, link CBHP with reproductive health rights.

The Emergence of Community-Based Health NGOs in the Philippines during the Pre–Martial Law Period

During the pre–martial law period, what generally existed in the health sector were NGOs that were medical or professional societies. NGOs, as defined by the Philippine National Economic Development Authority (NEDA), are "private, non-profit volunteer organizations that are committed to the task of what is broadly termed as 'development.'" This is to differentiate it from its generic meaning—that is, that NGOs refer to all organized formations outside the government. Medical students at the College of Medicine, University of the Philippines (UPCM) in the 1970s, such as Jaime Galvez-Tan, generally had student organizations that were part of the national ferment of that period, which was fueled by issues of anti-imperialism and nationalism and the demand for the removal of the U.S. military bases and the end of parity rights. The latter two issues were viewed as continuing symbols of American colonialism in the country. Such issues were shared by other developing countries demanding their national liberation from their Western colonizers. This was further fueled by the American involvement in the Vietnam War.[1,2] These activist organizations in which the medical community was involved were not specific to health and were closely identified with the mainstream left movement, the CPP-NPA-NDF. The CPP-NPA-NDF, also referred to as the new Communist Party of the Philippines, was established in 1968 and drew its inspiration from Marxist-Leninist-Maoist thought.

This period, therefore, provided fertile ground for recruiting students into the communist movement; this gave form to the Kabataang Makabayan (KM), which was looked upon as the student arm of the CPP. From KM branched out progressive health organizations such as the Makabayang Samahan ng mga Nurses (MASA; the Association of nationalist nurses). This was followed by the emergence of the Progresibong Kilusang Medikal (Progressive medical movement). These health movements differentiated themselves from non-activist health NGOs during this period, which were mainstream and apolitical voluntary professional and non-profit organizations.[3] This was the kind of political environment which Galvez-Tan was immersed in as a medical student. Upon graduating from the UPCM in 1975 and becoming a medical doctor, Galvez-Tan felt that the only way to pursue his goal of "health for the poor" was through the establishment of CBHPs in the countryside. "Although CBHPs have been implemented in the early 1960s by independent practitioners affiliated with hospitals and clinics, . . . these efforts were limited in scope and did not reach national scale until the introduction of CBHP in many parts of the country by the Rural Missionaries of the Philippines (RMP)."[4] As early as 1969, the RMP Community Based Health Development Program was established in various parts of the country, with farmers and agricultural workers, cultural minorities, and fishing communities as its major clientele-partners.[5] The RMP, which is under the Catholic Church's Catholic Bishops Conference of the Philippines (CBCP), would provide Galvez-Tan the network to pursue his advocacy. The RMP considered themselves the progressive wing of their religious order, and with the declaration of martial law, they continued to pursue their activities under the auspices of their respective dioceses. A number of them were nurses who were nuns.[6] Galvez-Tan said it was by chance that he was brought into RMP's network. This came when he was working as a medical intern in Tondo, home of one of the major slum areas in Manila. Galvez-Tan was training paramedics and community health volunteers. He was introduced to an Italian priest with the RMP who was also assisting the urban slum dwellers in Manila, particularly in a factory strike. He found out that the Italian priest was part of a religious congregation that had health programs that trained paramedics and community health volunteers all over the Philippines. These included the provinces of Isabela in northern Philippines, Samar in the Visayas, and Lanao in Mindanao.[7]

In the course of his vocation, Galvez-Tan got to know and work with Dr. Jesus "Jess" de la Paz, who he considers was very vital in reinforcing his commitment to health care NGOs. They started the Katiwala (overseer) program. He said that this program was very much inspired by China's barefoot doctors; they came to have paramedics and the development of *barangay* health workers.[8] Galvez-Tan's health-based community work would link him with other CBHP advocates in the country. He came to know the medical doctor George Viterbo, who owned a hospital in the province of Iloilo, where he was a pioneer in community-based health medicine. In the Cordillera region in Northern Luzon, Galvez-Tan linked up with Andres Bognocell, a foreigner and a member of the Protestant National Christian Churches of the Philippines (NCCP), which was at the forefront of the progressive movement in the Philippines. According to Galvez-Tan, these people were the forerunners of community health NGOs. Although they were clinicians or specialists, they decided to go for primary health care in the communities they were working in. What motivated them was the discontent with the state of health services in the late 1960s and early 1970s.[9]

The Pursuit of Community-Based Health Care during the Martial Law Period

When martial law was declared on September 21, 1972, all these health progressive movements, which consisted mainly of the UPCM academic community, disappeared.[10] But the advocates for CBHP were able to continue their advocacy; and a reason given for this was that it was difficult to repress health NGOs during the martial law period, as no one would oppose people fighting for their health needs.[11] The martial law period also witnessed the emergence of medical students who became members of the CPP and whose medical careers would be determined by the party. This was the case for Sylvia Estrada Claudio and her husband, Rafael, who were party members while they were UPCM medical students. The Claudios linked up with Galvez-Tan in his CBHP efforts. An organization they established toward this end was the Pangkalusugan Lingkod Bayan (Health for the Nation), which consisted mainly of the UPCM community. On their free days, these medical students gained exposure to CBHPs among the squatter areas such as in Magdalena, Tondo. Tondo is known for having one of the biggest squatter areas in Metro Manila. For the Claudios, this was one way whereby, as medical students, they were able to supplement their medical education.[12]

It was in the late 1970s that the innovative strategy of CBHP, renamed primary health care (PHC), attained official significance. According to Maria Ela L. Atienza, "The Philippine government adopted PHC as its overall health management strategy in consonance with the country's commitment when it joined the World Health Assembly in Alma Ata in Russia in 1978."[13,14] The real essence of

PHC, however, was not achieved during the martial law years, when there was emphasis on a participatory approach among community residents and intersectoral collaboration among various institutions in health.[15,16]

The Church as a Network for CBHP Advocacy

For CBHP advocates such as Galvez-Tan, what continued to provide a vital umbrella for their activities during the martial law period was the church network in the Philippines. For Galvez-Tan, the RMP continued to be at the forefront of this advocacy. The lead would soon be taken by the Catholic Church's National Secretariat for Social Action (NASSA) and their respective regional organizations. Like the RMP, the NASSA was under the CBCP and among its major advocacies was the fight against the dictatorship's violation of human rights. Its inspiration would come from Latin America's Paulo Freire's liberation theology, which for Galvez-Tan was unavoidable given the activist ferment of the martial law era.[17] The importance of the church as a cover for their CBH activities was also experienced by the Claudios, when the party instructed them to go to Cebu province in the Visayas. While there, the Claudios embarked on a CBHP project proposal and they launched it in the Diocese of the Church of Cebu, which was at the forefront of the anti-dictatorship movement during this period. They felt that it was quite safe to do this because church organizations were "tolerated" by the martial law regime.[18]

External Assistance for CBH NGOs

Aside from support from the church networks, advocates of the CBHP also received external financial assistance. NASSA, for example, was supported by the German Catholic development foundation, MISEREOR, as well as those from the Dutch Catholic Church as represented by CEBEMO in the Philippines. They helped fund Alternatibong Kalamboan Katilingbanong Panglawas (AKKAP; Alternative community health development program) which was established mainly through NASSA. AKKAP consisted of social activists from the medical community. CEBEMO also assisted in establishing health NGOs, one of which was Galvez-Tan's health NGO in Mindoro Province.[19] Funding from foreign agencies and NGOs was not unusual during the martial law period; NGOs during this period were perceived as safer conduits of development assistance coming from donor countries. Several studies have shown that almost 90 percent of donor countries' development assistance during the martial law period did not reach its intended beneficiaries as these ended up with President Ferdinand E. Marcos's relatives and cronies.[20] The other foreign NGOs that supported CBHP in the country were the German Protestant NGO Bread for the World and Dutch NGOs such as the Inter-Church Organization for Development Cooperation(ICCO) and the Netherlands Organization for International Development (NOVIB).

These foreign NGOs are generally supported by funding from their respective governments.[21]

EXPANSION OF THE CBHP

For Galvez-Tan, the landmark year for CBHPs was 1975, when the RMP decided to go out to the communities; this was followed in 1978 by another important landmark, when AKKAP became a nationwide program. By this time, AKKAP had a critical mass of doctors and nurses who established the Council for Primary Health Care wing of the AKKAP.[22] From 1977 to 1979, Protestant churches, mainly through the NCCP, joined the ferment of the martial law years. The NCCP went on to create the National Ecumenical Health Concerns (NEHC). The NEHC was the Protestant counterpart of the Catholic Church's rural missionaries.[23] What gave further impetus to the expansion of the CBHP was its link to the Basic Christian Communities (BCC) in the Philippines, which emerged during the late 1960s and early 1970s. The establishment of BCCs was a response by activist church individuals and groups to the political as well as economic oppression experienced by Philippine society's poor sectors during the martial law period. They supported in particular the struggle of the peasants whose lands were illegally expropriated by multinational corporations and whose villages were plundered by the military.[24] Because of its liberationist thrust, it was inevitable that these organizations were subject to military harassment and even the killing of BCC priests and members.[25] BCCs have also been viewed as communist fronts and have also been tagged as conduits for financial assistance, whether internationally or locally for the underground movement.[26] By 1979–80, Galvez-Tan observed that there emerged a lot of lay nurses, lay midwives, and community health workers in general, with an increase in the number of *barangays*. This could be attributed to the government's adoption of PHC, which was able to shift from a doctor-centered type to a community-oriented type with the harnessing of the involvement of voluntary workers, who came to be known as *barangay* health workers (BHWs).[27] CBHPs were greatly helped by foreign funding such as by CEBEMO and MISEREOR, which funded national meetings and assemblies during the martial law period.[28] The global movement for CBHPs exhibited its members' discontent with the manner in which health care was being carried out in various countries. The movement, these CBHP advocates believed, should expand to include not only the physical—that is, the absence of diseases—but also the mental and social well-being of a person.[29]

ENGAGEMENT AND CONFRONTATION WITH THE GOVERNMENT

An impact of this global advocacy during the martial law period was the emergence of government *barangay* health workers, which was led by the Department of Health (DOH). Secretary Jesus Azurin, who—like other health activists such as Galvez-Tan—was also a UPCM graduate. Azurin called the members of the health NGOs for consultations.[30] Galvez-Tan felt that Azurin had no qualms about talking to activist health NGOs because of his "old orientation"; that is, he believed in acupuncture, since he was trained in China. His experience in China also made him open to herbal medicine. Unlike his predecessors, who were specialists (one was a cardiologist), Azurin was also into public health and his thrust was health for the poor. Thus, his orientation was in line with the interests of CBHP health activists. At this time, the mainstream left movement was also at the forefront of establishing the Council for Health Development, which was a national health NGO.[31]

It was during this period, when health NGO activists were talking to Health Secretary Azurin, that Bobby de la Paz, an activist medical doctor who was doing community health care in Samar Province, was assassinated by the military in 1981. This gave rise to the Medical Action Group (MAG), which linked the issue of health with human rights headed by Sylvia de la Paz, his widow. Their motto was "Justice for Bobby de la Paz." The face of de la Paz, together with those of other high-profile victims of martial law repression, was used by the anti-dictatorship movement to rally people to oust the dictator. De la Paz represented the health sector; other prominent victims of military repression included Macliing Dulag of the indigenous peoples of the Cordillera Region in Northern Philippines, Ed Jopson of the student movement, and—the most well known—ex-senator Benigno "Ninoy" Aquino, Marcos's chief political foe.[32] The advocacy for health issues in general and CBHPs in particular were thus very much part of the left movement, which was subsumed under the anti-dictatorship movement. Galvez-Tan pointed out that their health pursuits were guided by the CPP and that everyone tacitly knew they were part of the NDF. What was, thus, very clear was the intertwining of medical and political issues. This also made medical activists like Galvez-Tan vulnerable to military attack, and it was for this reason that in 1985 he accepted a post in UNICEF, where he stayed for seven years.[33]

Community-Based Health NGOs during the Post–Martial Law Period

Under the Corazon C. Aquino administration (1986–92), the military threat against health NGO workers identified with the left movement continued. Estrada Claudio, who worked for MAG, pointed out it was very difficult even to go to her NGO's office for fear of getting assassinated by the military. Aside from giving assistance to human rights victims, MAG has also taken up the cudgels for the urban poor facing eviction, workers on strike, and political detainees and their families.[34] She was a young mother at that time, and the threat to her life as well as to that of her bodyguard (who was provided by the CPP), led her to resign from MAG. She, however, continued her work with Bagong Alyansang Makabayan (BAYAN; New patriotic alliance), a political movement associated with the CPP, as its health sector representative.[35] Despite this continuing repressive atmosphere, the democratic openings that were ushered in by the end of martial law also witnessed the emergence of all sorts of health NGO coalitions; the major forces behind this were the Council for Primary Health Care, AKKAP, RMP, and NEHC, among others. Their advocacy was given further impetus with the Declaration of Primary Health Care.[36] UNICEF was one of the international agencies that supported primary health care (PHC) and with Galvez-Tan's work, it came to have an NGO expression which was the Bukluran ng Kalusugan ng Sambayanan (BUKAS; Unite the nation for health), which was established during the new government's first three months, after holding several weekly meetings and assemblies.[37] BUKAS, which came out with its own health declaration, was also a product of the new political dispensation under President Aquino. The strategy for health NGOs was partnership or critical collaboration with the government. It was in this context that BUKAS served as the umbrella organization for all the different health activist NGOs—such as MAG and those run by Catholics, Protestants, and laypersons, as well as the Manggagawang Kalusugan (Workers for health) and the Community Medicine Foundation, which was led by medical students. The particular issue Galvez-Tan pursued in BUKAS was primary health care.[38]

The Split in the Mainstream Left Movement

According to Galvez-Tan, what brought all these activities to an abrupt halt was the 1992 split of the CPP-NPA-NDF into two camps: the "Reaffirmists," or "RAs," and the "Rejectionists," or "RJs." He pointed out that this would not only prove detrimental to health NGOs but also spelled instant death for BUKAS. The split was triggered by differences in the analysis of the current political dispensation and the consequent strategies to pursue. The RAs in general believe that the overthrow of the dictatorship did not bring about any political and socio-economic changes to society, and they believe that their strategy should still involve the armed struggle emanating from the countryside. Furthermore, hardliners in the party look at socioeconomic work, which includes health activities, as generating "reformism" and "economism" among the people.[39] As for the RJs, they believe that the downfall of the dictator created democratic openings that gave impetus to the legal struggle above the armed struggle.[40] They have also argued that socioeconomic activities should no longer be subordinated to the armed struggle.[41] In the health sector, even when the RAs and the RJs were concerned with the same issues, their respective members simply could not work together. Furthermore, there were also differences in strategies. For example, unlike the RJs, the RAs refuse to collaborate with or have any ties to the government.[42]

HEALTH ADVOCACY AND GOVERNMENT SERVICE

The split in the party did not stop left allies like Galvez-Tan from pursuing his CBHP advocacy, but this time he did so as a government official. As undersecretary of health under the Ramos Administration (1992–98), Galvez-Tan helped to provide funds to health NGOs, and together with Juan Flavier—a rural physician who was then secretary of health—he advocated for primary health care. A particular policy they wanted to implement was to have community workers in *barangays*. What emerged was a federation of *barangay* health workers organized under the DOH. During their term in government, Flavier and Galvez-Tan also institutionalized NGO participation in policy making in the health sector.[43] According to Gerald Clarke, "Under the Partnership for Community Health Development, for instance, the DOH in alliance with local government units, has sub-contracted the provision of services such as training to NGOs."[44] This development was a change in government organization (GO)–health NGO relations, where the GO had initially found difficulty in establishing effective working relations with the NGO sector. There were issues of different approaches to health, fear of co-optation of NGOs by the government, and absence of resources for NGO participation. But these concerns were addressed, leading to GO-NGO collaboration in various community-based health programs.[45]

The Emergence of Reproductive Health Rights Advocacy

Estrada Claudio realized that one limitation of the CBHP approach was that it had no gender component. She partly blamed the left movement for this, as it focused mainly on class issues; other concerns, such as gender and ethnicity, were given lower priority. A window of opportunity came when the head of the Commission on Women's Health (CWH) of the General Assembly Binding Women for Reform, Integrity, Equality, Leadership, and Action (GABRIELA), a women's political movement identified with the CPP, broached to Estrada Claudio the idea of starting a women's health and reproductive rights program. This would be part of the GABRIELA CWH's general activities, which include health services, education, campaigns for women, as well as the setting up of health centers and homes.[46] Estrada Claudio felt that this was one of the more successful commissions in GABRIELA, as it had its own funding and international relations and engaged in community work. Disagreements, however, arose as to whether to accept funds from the United Nations Fund for Population Activities (UNFPA).[47] Because of this, Estrada Claudio left GABRIELA and pursued her CBHP advocacy through Likhaan, an NGO she helped to establish in 1995.

Following basic CBHP techniques, Likhaan's core programs involves community-based clinic or health programs where the reproductive health agenda is rooted and where the leaders come from the communities. Because it is community based, it is able to work through the social ties of health workers from the community, and Estrada Claudio believes that this results in better quality services and organized villages.[48] Organizationally, Likhaan encourages the CBHPs in their respective *barangays* to hold annual elections to attain a functioning democratic organization.[49] Likhaan also placed the different CBHP organizations under a federation called Pinagsamang Lakas ng Kababaihan at Kabataan (PILAK; Federation representing the strong unity of women and the youth). According to Estrada Claudio, PILAK's claim to fame is that it is the first urban poor organization that is outwardly socialist and feminist. In particular, its constitution emphasizes the freedom of sexual orientation and sexual rights.[50]

REPRODUCTIVE HEALTH RIGHTS AND THE WOMEN'S MOVEMENT

For Ana Marie "Princess" Nemenzo, the campaign for reproductive health rights is very much part of the emergence of the women's movement in the country. Like Estrada Claudio, Nemenzo was active in GABRIELA through her women's NGO, Kalayaan. Nemenzo said that their advocacy was very much inspired by the Equal Rights Amendment (ERA) in the United States, particularly the issues of women's rights to divorce and abortion. Among the particular concerns they campaigned against was the church's attempt to include in the 1987 constitution the "right to life of the unborn." The campaign led to the realization that there was a need for an organization that would focus mainly on the reproductive rights of women, and this became the mandate of Nemenzo's NGO, WomanHealth, which was founded in 1987.[51] Both Likhaan and WomanHealth rely on external funding. The two NGOs have as donors Hewlett-Packard, the Ford Foundation, UNFPA, and the Canadian NGO Interpares, among others.[52] The reproductive rights advocacy of WomanHealth received an additional boost in 1987 when it was chosen to be the lead secretariat in organizing the 1987 International Conference on Women, which was held in Manila. WomanHealth made sure that the issue of reproductive rights would be part of the program. According to Nemenzo, other international conferences that gave a boost to the promotion of women's reproductive rights were the 1994 International Conference on Population and Development in Cairo (ICPD), the 1995 World Social Summit in Copenhagen, and the 1995 Beijing Conference on Women.[53] The adoption of the Program of Action in the 1994 ICPD conference and the 1995 Beijing World Conference on Women marked the turning point in health and development concepts and policies that emphasized that the well-being of a person includes matters related to the reproductive system; and emphasis began to be placed on the right to family planning.[54,55]

WORKING WITH GOVERNMENT

Nemenzo narrated how the new political dispensation in 1986 opened the doors for the advocacies of health NGOs. The NGOs were, for example, called by the health officials of the Aquino administration (1986–92) to a dialogue on how they could work together. A result of this was the convening of the First and Second National Conferences on Health in 1987 and 1988, respectively; the conferences were sponsored by the DOH. WomanHealth is also part of a network called Women's Alliance, which engages in dialogue with the DOH. Estrada Claudio also does not oppose working with the government, but at the same time, Likhaan is always cautious to maintain their autonomy. Health NGOs like Likhaan and WomanHealth also have informants in the DOH who are sympathetic to their advocacies. Nemenzo and Estrada Claudio, for example, both narrated how the DOH planned to put up a Woman's Health Center in the National Kidney Hospital to service medical tourism. There were DOH insiders who opposed this and sought the help of health NGOs. Likhaan has also been in the forefront in insisting that PhilHealth, which is the health insurer of government employees, keep abreast of changes in reproductive health; they do this by keeping the dialogue open.[56]

Pushing for the Reproductive Health (RH) Bill

Likhaan and WomanHealth, together with other women's groups, are also active in the Reproductive Health Advocacy Network (RHAN) which is currently in the forefront in the push for the passage of the Reproductive Health (RH) Bill, which the Catholic Church is vigorously campaigning against. They emphasize that they are not for population control but for women's control, as this is the very essence of reproductive rights. Their main concern was how women could be educated on health issues and family planning and the safe and effective choice of artificial contraception.[57] Both Nemenzo and Estrada Claudio feel that DOH officials, in general, have been very supportive of their reproductive health rights advocacy.[58] The campaign for the RH Bill also highlights the contentious nature of the relationship of NGOs with government officials. Health NGOs, for example, have found themselves allied with a number of congressmen who support the bill. But a problem emerges when these NGOs have differences with these political partners over other issues, such as the impeachment of former president Gloria Macapagal Arroyo, which the NGOs did not agree with.[59]

Conclusion

This chapter has detailed the internal as well as external factors that have led to the emergence and pursuit of the community-based health programs (CBHP) in the Philippines. Internally, CBHPs have their roots in the activism of the late 1960s, which saw their advocates very much linked with the mainstream left movement in the country. Among its major allies were church organizations, which were doing social work in communities in which health care was one of the more vital needs. Externally, it was funded by foreign NGOs. During the martial law period, a major hindrance to CBHP efforts was military repression, as these CBHP advocates were viewed as members of the CPP-NPA-NDF. The post–martial law period opened new avenues of strategies for CBHPs; a particularly important one was the opportunity to work in and with government. A fresh dimension that emerged was the linkage of reproductive health rights with CBHPs. This has been greatly supported by international agencies and NGOs advocating for women's rights in general. The split in the left movement in 1992 and opposition from the Catholic Church hierarchy, however, has stymied the growth of CBHPs and the reproductive health rights campaign, respectively.

Notes

1. Teresa S. Encarnacion Tadem, "Philippine Social Movements before Martial Law," in *Philippine Politics and Governance: Challenges to Democratization and Development,* ed. Teresa S. Encarnacion Tadem, and Noel M. Morada (Diliman, Quezon City: Department of Political Science, College of Social Sciences and Philosophy, University of the Philippines, 2006), 1–22.

2. Petronila Bn Daroy, "On the Eve of Dictatorship and Revolution," in *Dictatorship and Revolution: Roots of People's Power,* ed. Aurora Javate-de Dios, Petronilo Bn. Daroy, and Lorna Kalaw-Tirol (Manila: Conspectus Foundation Incorporated, 1988), 1–25.

3. Jaime Galvez-Tan, interview by Teresa S. Encarnacion Tadem, October 26, 2011, Living Life Well Health Hub, SM MegaMall, Manila, Philippines.

4. Maria Ela L. Atienza, "The Politics of Health Devolution in the Philippines with Emphasis on Experiences of Municipalities in a Devolved Set-up" (PhD diss., Kobe University, 2003), 32.

5. The First National Convention of NGOs for Health, *Philippine Directory of NGOs for Health* (Manila: The First National Convention of NGOs for Health, 1990).

6. Jaime Galvez-Tan, interview by Teresa S. Encarnacion Tadem.

7. Jaime Galvez-Tan, interview by Teresa S. Encarnacion Tadem.

8. *Barangay,* which was established during the martial law period, is the smallest political unit in the Philippines.

9. Jaime Galvez-Tan, interview by Teresa S. Encarnacion Tadem.

10. Jaime Galvez-Tan, interview by Teresa S. Encarnacion Tadem.

11. Jaime Galvez-Tan, interview by Teresa S. Encarnacion Tadem,

12. Sylvia Estrada Claudio, interview by Teresa S. Encarnacion Tadem, November 28, 2011, Center for Women's Studies, University of the Philippines, Diliman, Quezon City, Philippines.

13. Atienza, "The Politics of Health Devolution in the Philippines" (PhD diss.), 125.

14. Maria Ela L. Atienza, "The Politics of Health Devolution in the Philippines: Experiences of Municipalities in a Devolved Set-up," *Philippine Political Science Journal* 25, no. 48 (2004): 25–54, quotation on 32.

15. Atienza, "The Politics of Health Devolution in the Philippines" (PhD diss.), 32.

16. Atienza, "The Politics of Health Devolution in the Philippines" (article), 25–54.

17. Jaime Galvez-Tan, interview by Teresa S. Encarnacion Tadem.

18. Sylvia Estrada Claudio, interview by Teresa S. Encarnacion Tadem.

19. Sylvia Estrada Claudio, interview by Teresa S. Encarnacion Tadem.

20. *Diliman Review* staff, "Interview with Horacio B. Morales and Isagani R. Serrano," *Diliman Review* 36, no. 5 (1988): 31–36.

21. Liaison Committee of Development NGOs, "National Specificities and Realities," *Partners for Development: The NGOs, the EEC and the People of the Third World Working Together for New Solidarity* (Brussels: Liaison Committee of Development NGOs, 1986).

22. Jaime Galvez-Tan, interview by Teresa S. Encarnacion Tadem.

23. Jaime Galvez-Tan, interview by Teresa S. Encarnacion Tadem.

24. Tadem, "Philippine Social Movements before Martial Law," 1–22.

25. James Goodno, *The Philippines: Land of Broken Promises* (London and Atlantic Highlands, NJ: Zed Books, 1991).

26. Goodno, *The Philippines.*

27. Atienza, *The Politics of Health Devolution in the Philippines.*

28. Jaime Galvez-Tan, interview by Teresa S. Encarnacion Tadem.

29. Jaime Galvez-Tan, interview by Teresa S. Encarnacion Tadem.

30. Jaime Galvez-Tan, interview by Teresa S. Encarnacion Tadem.

31. Sylvia Estrada Claudio, interview by Teresa S. Encarnacion Tadem.

32. Jaime Galvez-Tan, interview by Teresa S. Encarnacion Tadem.

33. Jaime Galvez-Tan, interview by Teresa S. Encarnacion Tadem.

34. The First National Convention of NGOs for Health, *Philippine Directory of NGOs for Health* (Manila: The First National Convention of NGOs for Health, 1990).

35. Sylvia Estrada Claudio, interview by Teresa S. Encarnacion Tadem.

36. Jaime Galvez-Tan, interview by Teresa S. Encarnacion Tadem.

37. *Bukas* in Filipino also literally means "open."

38. Jaime Galvez-Tan, interview by Teresa S. Encarnacion Tadem.

39. Joel E. Rocamora, "The New Political Terrain of NGO Development Work," *DEBATE: Philippine Left Review* 10 (1994): 47–65.

40. FOPA Crisis of Socialism Cluster Group, "The Dual Crisis of the Philippine Progressive Movement," in *Re-examining and Renewing the Philippine Progressive Vision: Papers and Proceedings of the 1993 Conference on the Forum for Philippine Alternatives (FOPA), San Francisco Bay Area, California, 2–4 April 1993,* ed. John Gersham and Walden Bello (Quezon City: Forum for Philippine Alternatives, 1993), 11–23.

41. Rocamora, "The New Political Terrain of NGO Development Work," 47–65.

42. Jaime Galvez-Tan, interview by Teresa S. Encarnacion Tadem.

43. Sylvia Estrada Claudio, interview by Teresa S. Encarnacion Tadem.

44. Gerard Clarke, *The Politics of NGOs in South-East Asia: Participation and Protest in the Philippines* (London and New York: Routledge, 1998), 93.

45. Victor E. Tan, and Rose Marie Nierras, *Philippine Sociological Review,* 1–4 (1993): 37–58.

46. The First National Convention of NGOs for Health, *Philippine Directory of NGOs for Health.*

47. Sylvia Estrada Claudio, interview by Teresa S. Encarnacion Tadem.

48. Sylvia Estrada Claudio, interview by Teresa S. Encarnacion Tadem.

49. Sylvia Estrada Claudio, interview by Teresa S. Encarnacion Tadem.

50. Sylvia Estrada Claudio, interview by Teresa S. Encarnacion Tadem.

51. Ana Marie Nemenzo, interview with Teresa S. Encarnacion Tadem, November 3, 2011, Via Mare Restaurant, University of the Philippines, Diliman, Quezon City, Philippines.

52. Sylvia Estrada Claudio, interview by Teresa S. Encarnacion Tadem.

53. Ana Marie Nemenzo, interview with Teresa S. Encarnacion Tadem.

54. Diwata A. Reyes, "Population and Reproductive Health Policies: Lessons from Thailand's Experience" (paper presented in the Fourth Asia Scholarship Foundation Conference, n.d.).

55. Jeanne Frances I. Illo, Carolyn I. Sobritchea, Cecilia G. Conaco, Diwata A. Reyes, and Aurora E. Perez, *Assessing the UNFPA Ted Turner Projects in the Philippines (PHI/98/PO7): An Assessment Report Submitted to the United Nations Population Fund, Makati City* (Diliman, Quezon City: University of the Philippines, Center for Integrative and Development Studies, December 1999).

56. Sylvia Estrada Claudio, interview by Teresa S. Encarnacion Tadem.

57. Ana Marie Nemenzo, interview with Teresa S. Encarnacion Tadem.

58. Ana Marie Nemenzo, interview with Teresa S. Encarnacion Tadem.

59. Sylvia Estrada Claudio, interview by Teresa S. Encarnacion Tadem.

Contributors

SUNIL S. AMRITH is reader in modern Asian history at Birkbeck College, University of London. He is author of *Crossing the Bay of Bengal: The Furies of Nature and the Fortunes of Migrants, Migration and Diaspora in Modern Asia,* and *Decolonizing International Health: India and Southeast Asia, 1930–65.*

TIM HARPER is associate director of the Centre for History and Economics, reader in Southeast Asian and imperial history, University of Cambridge, and a fellow of Magdalene College, Cambridge.

NOPPHANAT ANUPHONGPHAT received his MA in History from Chulalongkorn University, Thailand, in 2003. He is currently a senior researcher and managing director of the National Health Archive and Museum (NHAM), Thailand. His research looks at the history of Buddhism in Thai society and the social history of health. He also works as a volunteer for Buddhika, the Buddhist network for Buddhism and society.

SOKHIENG AU is an independent scholar specializing in the history of medicine and Southeast Asian studies. She has published both historical and public health operational research studies. She recently published a book entitled *Mixed Medicines: Health and Culture in French Colonial Cambodia.* Her interdisciplinary research focuses on a range of topics including colonial medicine, gender and health, medicine and technology, and—most recently—international public health. She currently lives in Paris, France.

GREG BANKOFF works on environmentally related topics. In particular, he writes on environmental-society interactions with respect to natural hazards, resources, human-animal relations, and issues of social equity and labor. He is currently completing projects on the urban fire regime, flooding, and social forestry. His most recent work is *Flammable Cities: Urban Fire and the Making of the Modern World* (co-edited with Uwe Luebken and Jordan Sand). He is professor of modern history at the University of Hull.

PETER BOOMGAARD is senior researcher at KITLV, Leiden; professor (emeritus) of history, University of Amsterdam; 2012/13 fellow at the Rachel Carson Center, Munich; and 2013/14 Fernand Braudel Senior Fellow at the European University Institute, Florence. Among his publications are *Frontiers of Fear:*

Tigers and People in the Malay World, 1600–1950, and *Southeast Asia: An Environmental History.* He has (co-)edited many volumes, including *Globalization, Environmental Change, and Social History,* and *Empire and Science in the Making—Dutch Colonial Scholarship in Comparative Global Perspective, 1760–1830.*

KOMATRA CHUENGSATIANSUP is the director of Society and Health Institute (SHI) at the Bureau of Health Policy and Strategy, Ministry of Public Health, Thailand. He is interested in the intersections among the fields of health, social sciences, and humanities. His current work includes research programs on history of medicine and public health, philosophy of science and medicine, anthropology and community health, civil society and health systems reform, and indigenous healing systems in Thailand. He has written extensively on social and cultural aspects of health and human development, and his principal publications include *Community Approach: A Field Book on Anthropological Tools for Community Work in Primary Care; Power and Corruption: A Cultural Analysis of Health Bureaucracy; Medicine and Ethnicity; Drug in Community: A Socio-Cultural Aspect; Deliberative Action: Civil Society and Health Systems Reform in Thailand;* and *Village Health Volunteers in the Contexts of Changes* (2007).

THERESA W. DEVASAHAYAM holds a PhD in anthropology from Syracuse University, New York. She was a fellow and Gender Studies Programme Coordinator at the Institute of Southeast Asian Studies (ISEAS), Singapore, from 2008 to 2014. Theresa has authored and edited several books on women's labor force participation, low-skilled migrant women, gender and aging, and women and politics, including *Gender, Emotions and Labour Markets: Asian and Western Perspectives* (2011) (co-authored with Ann Brooks). Additionally, she has published in numerous international and regional journals. Theresa enjoys working at the intersections between academia, research, and international development. She has been a consultant to various United Nations agencies and is currently an independent consultant for gender issues.

ALBERTO G. GOMES is the director of the Centre for Dialogue and professor of anthropology at La Trobe University in Melbourne, Australia. His anthropological research on the Orang Asli (Malaysian aborigines), spanning more than thirty years, has produced numerous articles and three books. Among his recent publications is the highly acclaimed *Multi-ethnic Malaysia: Perspectives on Past, Present and Future* (co-edited with Lim Teck Ghee and Azly Rahman); "AlterNative Development: Indigenous Forms of Social Ecology," in *Third World Quarterly;* and "Anthropology and the Politics of Indigeneity," in *Anthropological Forum.* He is currently working on the anthropology of civility and on the nexus between equality, sustainability, and peace.

LOH KAH SENG is assistant professor at the Institute for East Asian Studies, Sogang University. His research investigates the transnational and social history of the making of Southeast Asia after World War Two. Loh is author and editor of five books, including *Squatters into Citizens: The 1961 Bukit Ho Swee Fire and the Making of Modern Singapore; Oral History in Southeast Asia: Memories and Fragments* (co-edited with Ernest Koh and Stephen Dobbs); *The University Socialist Club and the Contest for Malaya: Tangled Strands of Modernity* (co-authored with Edgar Liao, Lim Cheng Tju, and Seng Guo Quan); and *Making and Unmaking the Asylum: Leprosy and Modernity in Singapore and Malaysia.*

LOH WEI LENG is a retired professor in history at the University of Malaya, Kuala Lumpur. Among her recent publications are two chapters in *Penang and Its Region: The Story of an Asian Entrepot,* and two chapters in the December 2009 special issue of the *Journal of the Malaysian Branch of the Royal Asiatic Society,* "Peranakan Chinese in Penang and the Region." Her research interests include the economic, business, and maritime history of Malaysia.

RACHEL LEOW is lecturer in East Asian History at Cambridge University, and research associate of the Joint Centers for History and Economics at Harvard and Cambridge. Her present research projects all explore ways in which political, social, literary, and scientific ideas circulate and transform during the first half of the twentieth century in China and Southeast Asia.

ATSUKO NAONO is visiting research fellow at the Institute for Advanced Studies on Asia (University of Tokyo) and a research associate with the Centre for South East Asian Studies at SOAS. She is also subject consultant to the "Revealing Hidden Collections: Buddhist Literature in UK and SE Asian Collections" project at the Bodleian Library, University of Oxford. Her book *State of Vaccination* examines how a colonial medical establishment (Burma) coped with the neglect under the Raj. She has a special interest in colonial public health history, various health organizations activities in Southeast Asia, and religious and cultural understandings of the body.

VIVEK NEELAKANTAN recently completed his PhD at the University of Sydney. His dissertation critically explored Indonesia's engagement with the World Health Organization during the 1950s, particularly the specific ways in which Indonesian physicians engaged with biomedical ideas. He was the 2011 recipient of the highly competitive Australia Netherlands Research Collaboration Travel Fellowship that facilitated archival research in Switzerland and the Netherlands. He earned his MA from the University of Iowa in 2008, and was nominated as the University of Iowa Crossing Borders Fellow for the academic year 2006/7.

TERESA S. ENCARNACION TADEM is professor at the Department of Political Science at the University of the Philippines, Diliman. She previously served as its department chair as well as director of the UP Third World Studies Center and editor of its journal *Kasarinlan*. Teresa has published articles on Philippine social movements, the anti-ADB campaigns in Thailand, the Basque and Moro separatist movements, and the Philippine technocracy. Her latest publications include the edited volume *Localizing and Transnationalizing Contentious Politics: Global Civil Society Movements in the Philippines;* and the co-edited volume *Marxism in the Philippines: Continuing Engagements* (co-edited with Laura L. Samson).

ERIC TAGLIACOZZO is professor of history at Cornell University, where he teaches mainly on Southeast Asia. He is author of *The Longest Journey: Southeast Asians and the Pilgrimage to Mecca;* and *Secret Trades, Porous Borders: Smuggling and States along a Southeast Asian Frontier,* which won the Harry J. Benda Prize from the Association of Asian Studies in 2007. He is also editor or co-editor of four other volumes that explore Sino-Southeast Asian contact; the inter-civilizational dialogue between Southeast Asia and the Middle East; the conversation between history and anthropology as disciplines; and Indonesian culture, politics and society over a two-thousand-year period.

KIRSTY WALKER is a Prize Fellow in Economics, History, and Politics at the Center for History and Economics, Harvard University. Her doctoral research at the University of Cambridge has explored interethnic intimacy and creole family histories in Southeast Asia. In connection with the Centre for History and Economics, University of Cambridge, she has also published a review article on economic crises and health in historical perspective, examining the transnational history of public health in Southeast Asia during the interwar period.

MARY WILSON, MD, is adjunct associate professor, Global Health and Population, Harvard School of Public Health. She serves on the board of trustees of the International Centre for Diarrheal Disease Research, Bangladesh (icddr,b). In Cambridge, Massachusetts, Wilson was site director for the GeoSentinel Network, a global disease surveillance network. She is associate editor for *Journal Watch Infectious Diseases;* author of *A World Guide to Infections: Diseases, Distribution, Diagnosis;* editor of *New and Emerging Infectious Diseases;* and editor (with Richard Levins and Andrew Spielman) of *Disease in Evolution: Global Changes and Emergence of Infectious Diseases.*

Index

Lightning Source UK Ltd.
Milton Keynes UK
UKOW03f0312091014

239737UK00001B/44/P